Foundation Clinical Nursing Skills

Transforming essential principles into practical nursing skills

Clinical nursing skills from Oxford will take you, step-by-step, from student to nurse, giving you the knowledge to perform clinical skills with accuracy and confidence.

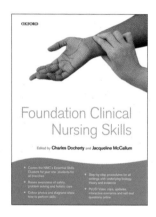

Starting with *Foundation Clinical Nursing Skills* for first years and working your way up through the series you'll find essential background theory explained and supported with evidence-based rationale. Each clinical skill is set out in a step-by-step process, richly illustrated with diagrams and photographs, whilst a range of scenarios help you apply theory to practice.

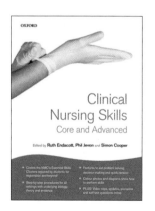

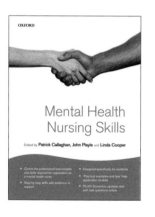

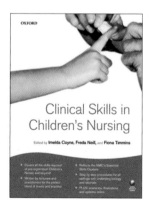

Visit the website to reinforce your learning, with tips, exercises, video examples, to prepare you for placement and exams

www.oxfordtextbooks.co.uk/orc/clinicalnursingskills

Smart nursing from Oxford

Foundation Clinical Nursing Skills

EDITED BY

**Charles Docherty and
Jacqueline McCallum**

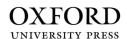

OXFORD
UNIVERSITY PRESS

OXFORD

UNIVERSITY PRESS

Great Clarendon Street, Oxford OX2 6DP

Oxford University Press is a department of the University of Oxford.
It furthers the University's objective of excellence in research, scholarship,
and education by publishing worldwide in

Oxford New York

Auckland Cape Town Dar es Salaam Hong Kong Karachi
Kuala Lumpur Madrid Melbourne Mexico City Nairobi
New Delhi Shanghai Taipei Toronto

With offices in

Argentina Austria Brazil Chile Czech Republic France Greece
Guatemala Hungary Italy Japan Poland Portugal Singapore
South Korea Switzerland Thailand Turkey Ukraine Vietnam

Oxford is a registered trade mark of Oxford University Press
in the UK and in certain other countries

Published in the United States
by Oxford University Press Inc., New York

British Library Cataloguing in Publication Data
Data available

Library of Congress Cataloging in Publication Data
Data available

Typeset by SPI Publisher Services, Pondicherry, India
Printed in Italy
on acidfree paper by
L.E.G.O. S.p.A—Lavis TN

ISBN 978-0-19-953445-6

3 5 7 9 10 8 6 4

Oxford University Press makes no representation, express or implied, that the drug
dosages in this book are correct. Readers must therefore always check the product
information and clinical procedures with the most up-to-date published product
information and data sheets provided by the manufacturers and the most recent codes of
conduct and safety regulations. The authors and the publishers do not accept responsibility
or legal liability for any errors in the text or for the misuse or misapplication of material in
this work. Except where otherwise stated, drug dosages and recommendations are for the
non-pregnant adult who is not breast-feeding.

Preface

This book is the result of many years teaching experience and the realisation that there was a void that needed to be filled as we could never find a single textbook that provided every skill for the first year student. Instead we were using a number of different texts and our students had to do the same. This problem encouraged us to write a core text for learning clinical skills for students of all branches (adult, child, learning disability & mental health) participating in the first year common foundation programme.

The content of this book will provide you the student reader with the necessary skills to facilitate your progression to your chosen branch. These skills are required by everyone studying nursing and with the context of nursing evolving, we have linked each skill to acute, continuing or community settings where appropriate.

There are a number of people that we wish to thank for bringing this book to fruition, but our biggest thanks is to Val Ness. Val made a number of contributions to different chapters, and her enthusiasm, knowledge and motivation are second to none. We also wish to thank the many contributors who provided expertise in their chapters, they are, in alphabetical order; Mary Ballentyne, Jayne Donaldson, Peter Johnstone, Kirsteen Lang, Linda Loftus, Ellen Malcolm, Willie McDonald, Claire McGuinness, John Murray, Bridget Reade, Liz Simpson, Ken Taylor and John Timmons. With a special thank you to Heinrich Heidinger for his expertise in learning disability and making sure these particular scenarios were appropriate.

Particular gratitude is due to the people who have made the skills recordings on the website possible. These are Kenny Munro, Audio Visual technician at Glasgow Caledonian University and Claire Brewer at Oxford University Press (OUP). But these resources would not have been possible without the help of those who took part in the recordings and so special thanks again go to the contributors, not only for their writing, but also their ability to perform professionally for the camera.

You will notice throughout the book there are many figures and pictures. We wanted to help you learn by encouraging you to visualise skills being practised, and our thanks go to the photographer Andy Forman, the artist David Gardner and the art editor at OUP, Erica Martin.

Our thanks to the editorial staff of Oxford University Press, Geraldine Jeffers, Leonie Sloman and Marionne Cronin for their patience with us. We kept them waiting much longer than we care to mention at times, pushing deadlines back, partially because many of us were unrealistic about the magnitude of the task. We would also like to thank the reviewers. Every text owes a great deal to those academics across the country who ensured that the content is correct and factual, providing helpful advice.

Finally we have some personal acknowledgements.

Charles - I would like to thank my wife, Jacqueline, and family, Joanna, Claire, and Liam.

Jacqueline – I would like to thank my husband Colin, and two children, Heather and Niall. Heather hopes to start adult nursing in September 2009 and therefore I hope she finds this text invaluable.

Jacqueline McCallum and Charles Docherty 2009

Acknowledgements

Oxford University Press and the authors are very grateful to the many nurses, lecturers, students, and other healthcare professionals who provided peer review feedback on the draft chapters of this book. To maintain their anonymity, they are not listed here but their thoughtful advice has been invaluable and is highly appreciated.

About the authors

The editors

Charles Docherty PhD, MN, DN, RNT, RN, MBSC. has 20 years of teaching experience and has researched and published in a number of relevant areas. Previously Senior Lecturer in practice based learning, he is new Director of Clinical Simulation, in the Royal College of Surgeons in Ireland—Medical University of Buhrain where he is developing the infrastructure and capacity to teach clinical skills to undergraduate medical and nursing students in a multiprofessional context.

Jacqueline McCallum EdD, MN, PgCert, RNT, BA, RN is Acting Senior Lecturer in Clinical Simulation at Glasgow Caledonian University. She provides strategic direction for clinical simulation in the School of Nursing, Midwifery and Community Health. Having spent eleven years as a cardiac nurse, Jacqueline has written numerous articles on cardiac and critical care nursing, as well as skills acquisition.

The contributors

Mary Ballentyne, BSC, RN, RNT, FHEA, PGCE Senior Clinical Nurse Specialist, Southern General Hospital and Lecturer, Glasgow Caledonian University.

Jayne Donaldson PhD, MN, BN, RN, PGCE, Senior Lecturer, School Director Academic Development (Undergraduate), Napier University, Edinburgh. Areas of interest: development of clinical skills and fitness to practice within nursing and midwifery.

Peter Johnstone RN, RSCN, RCNT, RNT, Nursing Lecturer, Glasgow Caledonian University.

Kirsteen Lang BN, RN, Practice Education Facilitator, NHS Greater Glasgow and Clyde.

Linda Loftus MN(Oncology), BA(Hons), RCT, RNT, RN, Nursing Lecturer, Glasgow Caledonian University.

Ellen Malcolm MSc, PgDip Critical Care, RN, Charge Nurse ITU, NHS Greater Glasgow and Clyde.

John Murray MSc, BSc, DPSN, FHEH, RMN, RN, Lecturer in Nursing, Glasgow Caledonian University. Areas of expertise: adult nursing; movement and handling; critical care.

William McDonald MSc PGCert (LTHE), BSc with SPQ, RMN, Lecturer in Nursing, Glasgow Caledonian University. Areas of expertise: mental health nursing; old age psychiatry.

Claire McGuinness Msc, BSc, LPE, FHEA, RN, Lecturer in Nursing, Glasgow Caledonian University. Areas of Expertise: child nursing; intensive care.

Valerie Ness MN, PGCert (TLHE), RNT, ENP, RN, Lecturer in Nursing, Glasgow Caledonian University. Areas of expertise: adult nursing; accident and emergency; continence; moving and handling.

Bridget Reade RN, Charge Nurse, Glasgow Royal Infirmary Medical Unit.

Elizabeth Simpson MSc, BSc, LPE, FHEA, RN, Lecturer in Nursing, Glasgow Caledonian University. Areas of expertise: adult nursing, resuscitation service.

Ken Taylor MN, BSc, RMN, Cert Ed (nursing), RNT, RN, Nursing Lecturer, Glasgow Caledonian University.

John Timmons MN, Dip NS, PgCert (TLHE), RNT, RN, Wounds-UK, Aberdeen.

How to use this book

Foundation Clinical Nursing Skills explores and demonstrates the clinical skills required of all first year nursing students through the use of specific features and learning tools. This brief tour shows you how to get the most out of this textbook package.

2.5.1 Cardiopulmonary resuscitation for adults

Definition

Cardiopulmonary resuscitation is the act of artificially maintaining respiratory and cardiac function. It involves maintaining a clear airway, artificial breathing, and compressing the chest to circulate blood.

When to perform cardiopulmonary resuscitation

The skill should be performed in any casualty who has suddenly collapsed and is unresponsive with absence of signs of circulation. Basic life support measures, as shown in **Fig. 2.20**, may be commenced in any environment in hospital, where expertise is at hand, these will quickly be supplemented by more advanced, however

Background knowledge

Each skill is introduced, defined, and explained with reference to anatomy and physiology, safety, holistic care, nursing theory and the evidence base before the procedure is given so students understand why and when to undertake a clinical skill.

Step-by-step guidance

Each skill is broken down into clear steps with accompanying rationale so students can see what to do and why. These have been carefully laid out to help learning.

▶ When this icon appears in the Procedure Box a video of the skill is available on our Online Resource Centre (see overleaf for details).

Responding to cardiopulmonary resuscitation in adults

Step	Rationale
Danger	
1 Remove any obvious danger to the rescuer.	To prevent causing harm to the rescuer and prevent harm to the victim and rescuer.
Response	
2 Check response of the casualty by shaking and asking, 'Are you alright?'	Confirm the conscious level of the casualty and assist in diagnosis.
3 If the casualty responds, leave in position in which found and alert help if you need it.	To check the casualty's condition, and allow an opportunity to reassess.
4 If the casualty does not respond, shout, 'HELP!'	To obtain assistance if you should need it.
Airway	
5 Check the airway for obvious signs of obstruction. If a solid obstruction is detected, remove this with a hooked finger and sweeping motion.	To clear airway and optimize the casualty's airway.

Why does everyone know about the 'naughty step', 'chill out chair' or other child control mechanisms? It would seem that behaviour can be modified or ameliorated with appropriate inputs. There is a lot of information available concerning behaviour modification and microscopic detail is not essential at this early stage of nursing. Theoretically, by positive and negative reinforcement; behaviour that is rewarded will be repeated and behaviour that is not rewarded will be extinguished.

Behaviour-modification programmes and cognitive behaviour therapy are two of the many therapies available in the adult sector that fundamentally work on the above principle: further reading may be required when you enter your branch programme.

ⓢ Scenarios

Consider what you should do in the following situations, then turn to the end of the section to check your answers.

Further scenarios are available at 🌐 **www.oxford-textbooks.co.uk/orc/docherty/**

👁 Scenario 1

Eighteen-month-old Cameron is visually impaired and, whilst he is able to mobilize relatively independently, he is hesitant to move or interact without parental presence. How can Cameron be encouraged to mobilize, interact, and play?

💬 Scenario 2

Twelve-year-old Ashleigh has experienced multifactorial abuse leading to low trust with all adults and, as a result, has low self-esteem and is self-abusive. How can therapeutic play contribute to Ashleigh's recovery?

♿ Scenario 3

Angela has a multiple-diagnosis learning disability causing spastic paralysis of her limbs. She is 18 years old with a mental age of 8. She is unable to communicate verbally and as a result of her spasticity is unable to utilize sign language. Her aural and vision senses are intact and she reacts to vocal input. How can play be utilized to contribute to Angela's care plan?

👤 Scenario 4

Mabel, aged 83 years, is active, articulate but unsteady on her feet. How could you help to maintain her activity, in a safe manner?

Website

🌐 **www.oxfordtextbooks.co.uk/orc/docherty/**
You may find it helpful to work through our short online quiz and interactive scenarios intended to help you to develop and apply the skills in this chapter.

References

Brooker C and Waugh A (2007). *Foundations of Nursing Practice: Fundamentals of Holistic Care*. Mosby Elsevier, London.
A useful generic source of information concerning fundamentals of holistic care, potentially applicable to all branches as detailed and broad examples are utilized in text.
Darbyshire P (1994). *Living With a Sick Child in Hospital*, pp. 89–93. Chapman and Hall, Glasgow.
Ginsburg KR, the Committee on Communications, and the Committee on Psychosocial Aspects of Child and Family Health (2007) The importance of play in promoting healthy child development and maintaining strong parent-child bonds. *Pediatrics*, **119**(1), 182–91.
Grandis S, Long G, Glasper EA, and Jackson P, eds (2003). *Foundation Studies for Nursing*. Palgrave MacMillan, London.
Heath H (2001). *Foundations in Nursing Theory and Practice*, 4th edn. Mosby, London.
Hubband S and Trigg E (2000). *Practices in Children's Nursing,Guidelines for Hospital and Community*. Churchill Livingstone, Edinburgh.
Price J and McNeilly J (2006). Developing an educational programme in paediatric care. *International Journal of Palliative Nursing*, **12**(11), 536–41.
Russell-Johnson H (2000). Adolescent survey. *Paediatric Nursing*, **12**(6), 15–19.
Taylor J, Muller DJ, Wattley L, and Harris P (1999). *Nursing Children, Psychology, Research and Practice*, 3rd edn. Stanley Thornes, Cheltenham.

All nursing branches and settings

At the end of each skill scenarios from each branch of nursing explore how skills can be undertaken in light of the unique needs of individual patients. Examples are taken from community and hospital settings ensuring students can deliver skills on every placement. Students are asked what they would do before answers are revealed (they can be found after the references).

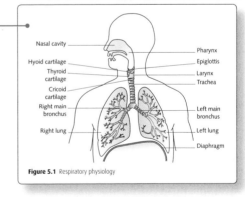

Figure 5.3 Pulse check and feeling respiratory rate at the same time

Visual demonstration

Colour drawings help to relate the underlying anatomy to the clinical skill whilst colour photographs demonstrate to students how to undertake a skill.

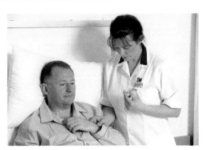

Nasal cavity

Hyoid cartilage

Thyroid cartilage

Cricoid cartilage

Right main bronchus

Right lung

Pharynx

Epiglottis

Larynx

Trachea

Left main bronchus

Left lung

Diaphragm

Figure 5.1 Respiratory physiology

Developing your skills

In acute and community care the nurse's knowledge, skills, and actions in assessing the patient can have a huge influence on the patient's outcome. It is, therefore, important that, as a student nurse, you practice and become competent in these skills. It is also important to keep your knowledge up to date at all times. It is vitally important in assessing the patient's respiratory status, since there is a very close link with respiratory dysfunction and adverse events and **mortality** (Considine 2005).

It is essential that you become accustomed to and practice the skill of assessing a patient's breathing and providing assistance depending on what the assessment shows

Designed for beginners

Clinical terms are helpfully highlighted in blue throughout the text and are explained in a glossary at the end of the book. The authors have used straightforward language throughout to explain concepts and procedures clearly.

How to use the Online Resource Centre

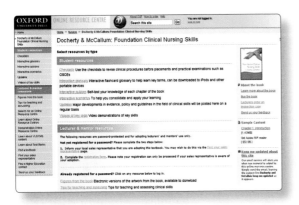

This textbook is accompanied by an Online Resource Centre (ORC) that provides students and lecturers with interactive resources to develop clinical nursing skills. You can access the ORC from any computer with internet access and so you will find it helpful to save the web address in to your 'favourites' at the earliest opportunity: **www.oxfordtextbooks.co.uk/orc/docherty/**

Videos

A selection of key clinical skills videos are available to watch on the ORC. Where you see the video icon in the chapter text, watch the accompanying video at your earliest convenience to consolidate the procedures in the book.

 To access the videos, visit the home page for the ORC and click on the 'videos' link.

Updates

Major developments in evidence, policy and guidelines in the field of clinical skills will be posted to the Online Resource Centre on a regular basis. Sign up to be alerted to the updates by clicking on the link 'Keep me updated about this site' on the home page of the ORC **www. oxfordtextbooks.co.uk/orc/docherty/**

Chapter specific resources

Each chapter is supported by a range of online resources to help readers apply and develop their skills in each chapter.

Scenarios Interactive scenarios give students the opportunity to try out their skills in a safe environment prior to placements.

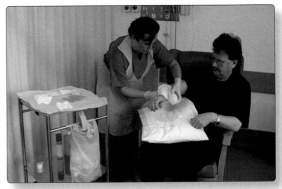

Quizzes To help reinforce students' knowledge and understanding the authors have written short online quizzes.

Checklists Brief checklists allow students to revise the clinical procedures before placements and practical examinations such as OSCEs.

Hyperlinked bibliography These provide direct links to online articles referenced in the chapter (institutional subscriptions are required for access to full papers)

Interactive glossary Technical terms are presented in an interactive 'flashcard' format to help students learn and revise terms and concepts.

For lecturers and mentors

Figures from the book to download and use in teaching and tips for teaching clinical skills

Contents

Detailed Contents

List of procedures

1 Introduction

CHARLES DOCHERTY AND JACQUELINE MCCALLUM

Why do I need to learn clinical skills?

As a nursing student beginning the first year of your course you require theoretical knowledge of health and illness to explain how an individual person functions at a variety of levels, from the biological to the social and psychological. You will also learn some of the fundamental principles of caring and treatment, and through this become aware that nursing is a very practical profession, encompassing a large number of clinical skills that must be mastered. This theory and practice together constitute what you are required to learn and these are the **skills** that are needed for a term that you may have heard: 'fitness for practice' or 'fitness for purpose,' which, basically, means that at the end of your nursing education you have the skills, knowledge, and attitudes required to work as a nurse in your chosen branch.

In the first year of the programme (referred to as the common foundation programme), there are common clinical skills that you are required to master prior to entering the second and subsequent years of your course (usually called the 'branch' years). This book has been specifically designed to enable you to learn and perform these valuable and necessary skills and give you the best start.

Which skills am I learning?

The skills included here are a result of asking a large number of universities that teach first-year nursing which skills they include. Some universities differ very slightly in which skills they include in the first year, however, in general you will find that you will learn almost all, if not all, of the skills in the book. We have also ensured that we address the NMC Essential Skills Clusters for year one to prime you for the rest of your course. We have also asked lecturers, practitioners, and experienced students to design an 'ideal' clinical skills book and this is the result – all the skills you need in exactly the right way to learn them.

Getting started: what you need to know

As a future nurse you need to understand not just *how* to undertake a skill but *why* and *when*, and to think about the *patients* you are working with and their individual circumstances. There are certain essential theoretical elements to learning clinical skills, to which we refer throughout this book. However, you need to do some extra work too. In no particular order these elements are:

Firstly, you must use this book alongside a good quality **anatomy and physiology** book. We endeavour to make as many helpful links and summaries as we can; however, we can't include everything without writing a book twice the size! Only you are responsible for learning the biology that you need to know as a good nurse.

Secondly, you will be introduced to the idea of **evidence-based practice** – put simply this is the idea that no nurse would ever undertake a procedure without checking that she or he knows and understands why it is done that particular way. Just as the way you learn the rules of the road so as not to crash a car, or learn about food safety so as not to give your family food poisoning, so too a nurse learns the 'rules' of clinical skills. You will see references to articles, guidelines and protocols in the text – use them, and also refer to our online resource centre, where we will update you about major developments.

Thirdly, clinical skills are not simply tasks we carry out on anonymous people. Our patients are whole human beings with multidimensional lives. We use important nursing theories, such as the Activities of Living of Roper, Logan, and Tierney (2000), and the concept of **holistic care** to ensure that when we perform a clinical task, we do it in a sensitive manner, caring for the person and treating them with respect.

Roper, Logan, and Tierney's twelve activities of living form the basis of many care plans and nursing assessments. These activities are well known, not just in nursing but also in occupational therapy, and have been chosen as the basic structure for this book. For more information on these, refer to Holland *et al.* (2008). For the purposes of this book, we have identified ten of these activities for particular attention:

- Maintaining a safe environment
- Communication
- Breathing
- Eating and drinking
- Eliminating
- Personal cleansing and dressing
- Controlling body temperature
- Mobilizing
- Working and playing
- Dying

The remaining two activities from Roper, Logan, and Tierney's 12 activities of living – expressing sexuality and sleeping – have an influence on many of the other activities and we have, therefore, incorporated these as appropriate throughout the text.

Last but not least, there are some **legal and professional requirements** that you must meet. For every skill you undertake, you must think of patient safety and ethical considerations, including:

- **Consent** – permission from the patient to have the procedure performed on them
- **Capacity** – the ability to give you consent, which is compromised through mental illness, loss of consciousness, age, and immaturity, and learning disability
- Correct identification of the patient (no one wants to be given the wrong drug!)

- Understanding that you are accountable (responsible) for all of your nursing actions
- Paying attention to health and safety – you must ensure that your actions and use of equipment are safe and correct

You must read the professional code of conduct for nurses (NMC 2008) and local policies and procedures.

On one level, legal and professional practice means having clean hands, using gloves when necessary, asking permission to perform a procedure, but on another it means being motivated to learn anatomy, reading new clinical guidelines and thinking all the time, 'Is my care as good as it could be?'

So how do I learn all this?

In light of the above, as a new nursing student, whether you have undertaken clinical tasks before in a previous job or never at all, you must read about the skill to learn why the skill is necessary, what part of the body you are dealing with, what evidence justifies your action, and what the patient may be thinking and feeling. These topics will be covered in many lectures and may often feature in assignments and in exams. On a more practical note, you also need to work out what equipment is required, the actual performance of the task, and then the 'aftercare', which can include documentation and record keeping. Many of these elements are taught in clinical skills laboratories.

University and placements

It is current practice to learn a range of clinical skills first at university. This will provide you with some confidence and a degree of competence to take to your placement. You will have time to practice and refine the skill usually on a mannequin (and perhaps on your classmates!) before you use the skill for real on a patient.

Some skills can be tricky to master the first time and you will need to practice these over and over again. It is common for students to make mistakes, especially the first time at attempting something new. By practising skills on mannequins in the university, with your lecturer for support in a safe environment, it does not matter if mistakes are made. You will find that you can learn from mistakes and will probably never make the same mistakes again. It is important, therefore, to practice, practice, practice, because you can improve and learn all the time until you feel comfortable performing clinical skills at university. By the time you go on placement, you will be ready to do it for real.

Learning the skills does not end with you using them for the first time on a real patient. This is where you can start to reflect on your performance and identify areas for further improvement. You will learn about reflection in nursing during your three years of education and there is a great deal of literature available on how to do it. Our advice is that after performing clinical skills, this is an ideal time to carry out reflection using a chosen model of reflection. This can be discussed with your mentor and included in your clinical record of achievement. Such reflection and records of evidence can help to show your achievement of some of the first-year clinical 'competencies'. Your university needs to provide proof that you have achieved these as well as the clinical skills clusters, in order to move onto your branch programme.

Using this book

You will have gathered by now that learning clinical skills is not quite as simple as learning how to 'do' something. This book has been specifically designed to help you learn practice and appropriate theory in **one** place. You will have seen in the opening pages just how the features in this book have been designed to help you (see the walk-through preface). Here are some useful short points!

Finding information

Each chapter follows a similar layout so that you can quickly move to the most relevant point for focused reading, whether it's theoretical background information or practical guidance. We hope that you will enjoy browsing when reading the book for the first time or for revision. To help you write assignments we have included hyperlinks to cited articles where possible on our online resource centre – these will easily take you to the original articles for further reading. You will also find it useful to browse the references to get a sense of the sources of information

we used in order to identify suitable literature for your own essays and group work.

Preparing to use a skill

You can use this as an aide-memoire in preparation for the performance of a procedure by reading a chapter and then printing a checklist from our website. You can also use these checklists as tools to help reflect on and evaluate a particular performance. In addition, the website provides access to videos, presentations, photographs, and more real-life scenarios. All of these activities are designed to improve engagement with clinical skills, ultimately leading to their mastery.

Some of the skills involve the use of equipment that you may not have used before. To help you with this, there are a number of pictures included in the book for each skill to help you become familiar with what the equipment looks like. In addition to this, the website that accompanies the book shows photographs and video clips to help follow the steps of certain procedures.

Scenarios

Reality checks are provided in abundance through real-life scenarios – we advise that you read these, consider what you would do, either in your head or on paper, decide on your course of action and only **then** read our suggested answers!

Mentors and lecturers

This book is designed to be useful to students, their mentors, and university lecturers, for different reasons.

For mentors unsure of what constitutes the current curriculum in the first year, this book gives an excellent coverage of the skills expected to be achieved by students, and may help the mentor to guide and direct the student as to what is to be learned as well as how it is to be learned. Using the resources of the website and the step-by-step approach to performance outlined in the book, the mentor and student can mentally and verbally rehearse the performance of a task prior to practising with patients. This will improve the student's confidence, and should impact positively on patient comfort and safety. The checklists and detailed descriptions can help the mentor focus **objectively** on the skill while providing feedback to students on their performance.

For lecturers, clinical demonstrators, and simulation laboratory technicians based in a university, this book has many helpful features.

Recommended reading

We have worked extremely hard to ensure that you can reliably recommend this text to your first-year students to truly support their learning needs both at university and placement. We cover the skills that first-year students must learn, we do not assume prior knowledge, we explain material at the right level, and give lots of practical tips via illustrations, scenarios and a website.

Illustrations

Useful illustrations can be found in the 'teachers' section of our online resource centre for you to download into your virtual learning environment (VLE) and use in lectures.

Scenarios

Each chapter includes useful scenarios for all patients' needs, be they children, adults, or those with mental health issues or learning disabilities (there are a total of 80 scenarios in the book). Our online resource centre has over 40 further interactive scenarios and 50 interactive self-test questions.

Additional tips for teaching on our online resource centre

This has further tips to help you teach, including:

- Planning simulated learning experiences
- Using our online skills checklists to assess performance objectively
- Using video clips to represent an ideal or 'model' demonstration of a skill with which to compare actual student performance

- Guidance for the construction of 'objective structured clinical evaluations' or OSCEs, which are increasingly used in universities to assess clinical performance

Conclusion

In conclusion, this book is a vital tool for the acquisition of clinical skills presented at a time when it is increasingly important that students acquire these to a required standard. This is also a time to be aware that patient safety and comfort are paramount and that preparation for practice and reflection on practice are as important as the actual practice itself. Acquiring clinical skills is, therefore, an important component of any clinical placement. This coincides with an emerging paradox: clinical placements demand more skilful performances from practitioners while at the same time they are becoming so busy and pressurized that the time allowed for acquiring these skills is greatly reduced. This book, therefore, is an invaluable support for first-year students and will provide guidance and facilitate improved performance through the tools of reflection, and will be welcomed by the profession.

References

Holland K, Jenkins J, Solomon J, and Whittam S (2008). *Applying the Roper-Logan-Tierney Model in Practice*, 2nd edn. Churchill Livingstone, Edinburgh.

NMC (2008). *The Code: Standards of Conduct, Performance and Ethics for Nurses and Midwives*. Nursing and Midwifery Council, London.

Roper N, Logan WW, and Tierney AJ (2000). *The Roper-Logan-Tierney Model of Nursing: Based on Activities of Living*. Churchill Livingstone, Edinburgh.

Useful further reading and websites

Check 🌐 **www.oxfordtextbooks.co.uk/orc/docherty/** for changes and new developments. Updated research, guidelines, or equipment will be added every three months.

2 Mandatory skills

WILLIAM MCDONALD, VALERIE NESS, KEN TAYLOR, CLAIRE MCGUINNESS, AND ELIZABETH SIMPSON

Skills

Introduction

We have created this chapter because these **mandatory** skills underpin good nursing practice and are required for the safety of people in care and those who care for them. Hence, these skills tend to be the compulsory skills that placement providers expect **first-year students** to be familiar with **prior to their first placement**. It is, therefore, *essential* that you read this chapter before you do anything else.

This chapter aims to give you a brief outline of each skill, explaining its importance before providing separate introductory sections on each skill, for example, Section 2.1 on communication. You will also see that these skills are further developed in separate chapters, for example, Chapter 4 on communication, where more detailed information allows you to become more fully familiar with and competent in that skill. *Note, it should be recognized that these short pieces only give guidance on all of these skills; full practical training in these skills is also required, particularly resuscitation, drug administration, and dealing with violence and aggression.*

Mandatory skills

- Communication
- Moving and handling
- Violence and aggression
- Infection control
- Resuscitation
- Administration of medicines

Why these skills underpin nursing practice

Nurses are expected to keep the people in their care, and themselves, safe by practising in a way that has been made safe by the consideration of evidence gained from research and experience. These skills are currently regarded as the best way to carry out each task, but they might change over the years, as new evidence becomes available; it is, therefore, important that your practice is kept up to date.

Legal and ethical frameworks for nursing

Nurses are in a very privileged position in that they are trusted with the health and lives of other human beings; they are more intimately involved in the physical, psychological and **emotional world** of individuals than most other professions. When a patient offers this trust, nurses have a responsibility to ensure that individuals are treated professionally; in a way that is safe, respectful and informed by up-to-date theory.

People have come to expect a high level of professionalism when they become unwell, whereas, in the past, they might have thought they should take what they were given. Government policy, more widely available information, media, and service-user-led campaigns have led to higher expectations. To meet these expectations, we must ensure that our practice is governed by high standards. There have been many developments in care and treatment but, unfortunately, there has also been an increase in many of the challenges to good care and treatment; for example rises in violence to healthcare staff and in hospital-acquired infection.

Poor standards should not be tolerated wherever care is being given, and legislation exists to prevent this. This states that nurses, as well as other healthcare staff, must be made aware of the dangers to themselves and the people in their care and must be trained to tackle these dangers.

All nurses, nationally and internationally, are required to satisfy professional standards to register as a nurse. For example, to register as a nurse in the UK, a student must first satisfy the Nursing and Midwifery Council Standards of Proficiency, one of which is to:

Practise in accordance with an ethical and legal framework that ensures the primacy of patient and client interest and well-being and respects confidentiality.

There are many such legal and ethical frameworks that govern the practice of nursing; including the NMC Standards themselves. Others include the NMC Code of Professional Conduct and the Health and Safety Executive's Manual Handling Operations guidelines. The reason for this legislation is the protection of the patient.

Communication

Good communication is central to these skills; in fact, it is central to nursing. Nursing teams cannot operate without effective communication. Patient assessments cannot occur without communication with the client. Quality care cannot be given without communicating with the patient and gaining **consent**. The ongoing professional development of staff cannot go ahead without effectively communicating concepts, theories, and information. Effective communication can be learned, practiced, and developed—it is one of the essential skills of good nursing.

Moving and handling

This is a skill that the nurse uses almost every day and is integral to many other skills. It is also a health and safety issue for nurses themselves, with many becoming injured as a result of poor manual handling techniques. Back injury is the largest single cause of long-term sickness in the United Kingdom and costs the National Health Service about £300 million a year. The reasons behind this include lack of education, illness, poor practice, stress, and lack of resources.

Violence and aggression

These are of growing concern in healthcare. In 2000, the International Labour Office (ILO), the International Council of Nurses (ICN), the World Health Organization (WHO), and Public Services International (PSI) launched a Joint Programme to develop sound policies and practical approaches for the prevention and elimination of violence in the health sector (this can be found at www.who.int/

violence_injury_prevention/violence/activities/work-place/en/). This document states:

> *While workplace violence affects practically all sectors and all categories of workers, the health sector is at major risk: more than half of all workers in this sector may have experienced violent incidents at some point. Ambulance and pre-hospital emergency staff are reported to be at greatest risk. Nurses are three times more likely than other occupational groups, on average, to experience violence in the workplace.*

Violence remains a concern but, despite the worrying figures given above, there is much we can do to prevent this danger; healthcare workers can take measures to avoid being victims of violence and aggression in the workplace. Section 2.3 gives guidance into how this can be achieved, and how potential conflict can be recognized and avoided. *However, it should be recognized that full training in the skill is also required*.

Infection control

To prevent and reduce levels of hospital-acquired infection, nurses (and all other healthcare workers) must learn the principles of cleanliness and infection control. Bacteriology is an essential part of the syllabus in life sciences. However, in nursing theory this science is adapted and exploited to provide principles that govern nursing practice and give guidance on aseptic technique and the practice of cleanliness.

Resuscitation

In any care setting, witnessing the struggle to revive a dying patient can be an upsetting and emotional experience. It is, therefore, helpful to gain competence in the skills involved in basic life support in order to maintain the patient until expert help arrives. Section 2.5 provides details on the skills involved for both children and adults.

Safe administration of medicines

This is a fundamental nursing skill and is essential for patient safety. Section 2.6 discusses the correct administration of medicines as well as the different routes of administration.

UK competencies in mandatory skills for first-year nurses

The following extracts from the NMC Standards of Proficiency and the Essential Skills Clusters illustrate the need for education and the level to which a nurse should be skilled in the areas covered in this chapter. Non-UK readers can skip this section.

Communication (SECTION 2.1 AND CHAPTER 4)

When working with patients, the NMC Standards say that the nurse must:

> *6. Listen, and provide information that is clear, accurate and meaningful at a level at which the patient or client can understand.*
>
> *7. Protect and treat as confidential all information relating to themselves and their care.*

Moving and handling (SECTION 2.2 AND CHAPTER 10)

In relation to this, the NMC Standards state that the nurse should:

> *18. Identify and safely manage risk in relation to the patient or client, the environment, and others.*

Violence and aggression (SECTION 2.3)

The NMC Standards state that the nurse should:

> *19. Work to resolve conflict and maintain a safe environment.*

Infection control (SECTION 2.4)

The NMC Standards state that the nurse should:

> *20. Select and manage medical devices safely.*

21. Be confident in using health promotion strategies, identifying infection risks, and taking effective measures to prevent and control infection in accordance with local and national policy.

22. Maintain effective standard infection control precautions for every patient or client.

23. Provide effective care for patients or clients who have infectious disease including, where required, the use of standard isolation techniques.

24. Fully comply with hygiene, uniform, and dress codes in order to limit, prevent, and control infection.

25. Safely apply the principles of asepsis when performing invasive procedures and be competent in aseptic techniques.

26. Act to reduce risk when handling waste (including sharps), contaminated linen and when dealing with spillages of blood and body fluids.

Resuscitation (SECTION 2.5)

The NMC Standards state that the nurse should:

17. Work safely under pressure.

Safe administration of medicines (SECTION 2.6)

The NMC Standards state that the nurse should:

33. Correctly and safely undertake medicine calculations.

34. Work within the legal and ethical framework that underpins safe and effective medicines management.

35. Work as part of a team to offer a range of treatment options of which medicines may form a part.

36. Ensure safe and effective practice through comprehensive knowledge of medicines, their action, risks, and benefits.

37. Order, receive, store, and dispose of medicines safely in any setting (including controlled drugs).

38. Administer medicines safely in a timely manner, including controlled drugs.

40. Work in partnership with patients or clients and carers in relation to concordance and managing their medicines.

41. Use and evaluate up-to-date information on medicine management and work within national and local policies.

The above represent some of the policies that make the skills in this chapter mandatory. The following sections in this chapter will give you further insight into the need for these skills but will also give details of how this best practice should be carried out. It is that practice that will fix these principles in your mind but they should be constantly updated.

2.1 **Communication**

Introduction

The aim of this section is to begin to explore the communication skills that are of particular relevance within the full range of nursing environments, whether inpatient based or in a community setting. Communication is an important part of all that we, as nurses, do and that is why we have chosen to begin discussing it in this chapter on mandatory skills. Do it well, and you are likely to enhance significantly both patient care and your effectiveness as a nurse. However, when communication is poor, the resulting misunderstanding, confusion, or lack of awareness can result in problems that range from inefficiency and embarrassment to the threatening of life itself.

While some individuals appear to be more naturally gifted communicators, the good news is that communication skills can be improved and developed. This can be done by raising your awareness and understanding of the various aspects that influence communication, and by using this knowledge to practise ways of enhancing your communication in your professional and personal life.

The term 'communication,' however, encompasses a range of perspectives and skills that are too numerous and complex to discuss in this section alone. The information presented in this section has been chosen to reflect the aspects of communication that we believe will be most beneficial in your early experiences in clinical settings. These communication skills apply equally to all branches of nursing and in all clinical settings, whether you are working in hospital or community services. Having said that, to gain the most benefit from this book, we advise that you read this section in conjunction with Chapter 4 of this book, to provide you with more complete guidance on this subject.

The skills included in this section are: verbal and non-verbal communication skills, the communication of feelings, the variety of modes of communication, for example, written word, electronic media, and examining interpersonal interaction across the lifespan.

We cannot overemphasize how important communication is as an integral part of every nurse's role. Whether as an adult nurse providing information to a frightened pre-operative patient, a children's nurse supporting the parents of a child due to be admitted for inpatient care, a learning-disability nurse adapting nonverbal methods of communication to engage with clients who are unable to express themselves verbally, or a mental-health nurse assessing the level of risk in a person expressing suicidal thoughts, effective communication skills are an essential part of all that nurses do in each branch of nursing.

A transferable skill

Remember, too, that people with learning disabilities can become physically unwell, and children can experience mental-health problems, so if you examine the communication skills that are discussed in this book within the confines of any one branch, you will be ignoring the transferable nature of these skills in relation to the variety of clinical settings and experiences that you are likely to encounter as a nurse. This section will, therefore, explore the type of skilled behaviour required from and expected of all professional nurses (Sully and Dallas 2005). By developing understanding and employing effective communication skills, practitioners should be empowered to improve the quality of all of their professional interactions with patients, carers and families, colleagues, other professionals, and the public.

Communication is a fundamental activity that most people regularly participate in throughout their daily lives (Ellis *et al.* 2003). In today's society, we frequently encounter situations that require us to engage in some form of communication with others. This can range from a passing nod to a stranger in the street, or discussing shared interests with a friend, to a life-saving connection and exchange of ideas and feelings between individuals. As nurses, communicating with a range of individuals and groups is a central part of almost everything we do within our professional role. It is, for example, the means that we use to establish, maintain, and terminate the **therapeutic** interactions and relationships with those in our care (Grover 2005).

Therapeutic relationships enable us to engage with people in a professional, planned way, and focus on the individual's needs, not the nurse's. Such relationships promote personal growth in clients, as nurses support them in developing their skills to identify, consider realistically, and resolve problem issues. The three stages of a therapeutic relationship are:

1   Orientation, when the parties get to know one another,
2   The working phase, when problems are identified and solutions sought, implemented, and evaluated,
3   The termination phase, when **resolution** is reached (Videbeck 2006).

Owing to the high level of contact with patients and the pivotal role that nurses play within a multidisciplinary approach to care delivery, nurses are required to possess well-developed, efficient, and effective communication skills. Acquiring and utilizing such skills enables us not only to participate in the planning and delivery of high quality care, but also to fulfil our role in relation to health promotion and education. The Nursing and Midwifery Council (NMC) highlights the importance of effective communication for nurses in its Code (NMC 2008) and the Essential Skills Clusters (ESCs) for Pre-registration Nursing Programmes (NMC 2007), in particular in ESCs 1 to 8. You should take some time to read these ESCs to help you understand why effective communication is so crucial to successful nursing practice. They are available at www.nmc-uk.org.

We acquire communication skills from an early age and develop these as we grow, often being unaware of the complex relationship between the verbal and nonverbal aspects of our interactions. Over time, communication can become practised at a level that requires no conscious thought of the skills that are involved or indeed the skills that we are employing at any one time. In our daily lives, we often use complex combinations of verbal and nonverbal communication skills with little awareness of what we are doing to enhance our engagement or interaction with others. Howell (1982) suggests that we move through levels of ability from 'unconscious incompetence' to 'unconscious competence' as our awareness and our skills develop (see **Box 2.1**). Our development through these levels enhances our ability to work most effectively within the complete range of professional roles expected of nurses today.

Learning outcomes

These outcomes relate to numbers 6 and 7 of the NMC's Essential Skill Clusters and specifically to Care Domains 2 and 3 of the NMC's Standards of Proficiency for Pre-registration Nursing (outcomes to be achieved for entry to branch).

On reading the chapter and associated web pages and undertaking supervised activities, the student will be able to:

- Understand underpinning theories of communication
- Recognize and discuss the main components of basic communication skills
- Demonstrate an awareness of factors that influence meaning and significance
- Understand the role of communication in nursing interactions
- Comprehend communication skills in relation to multidisciplinary working
- Demonstrate an understanding of behaviours associated with **assertiveness**

Box 2.1 Levels of competence	
Unconscious incompetence	The nurse is inexperienced and lacks awareness of what to know and do. This results in the nurse being unable to identify or recognize individuals' specific needs and, therefore, being unable to support patients most effectively.
Conscious incompetence	As experience and understanding develop the nurse becomes more aware that patients require specific support and recognizes how that support may be given. The nurse still lacks the communication skills necessary to effectively provide this, however.
Conscious competence	At this stage, as well as being aware of the needs of patients, the nurse also has the communication skills necessary to consider, plan, and deliver support effectively.
Unconscious competence	As the nurse develops more expert communication skills, decisions about care and its delivery can be made quickly, accurately, and with less conscious thought.

(Howell 1982)

Prior knowledge

As human beings we use a range of skills to try to achieve our desired outcome in any given situation. The knowledge, understanding, and communication skills required to do this are developed over time and in a variety of settings. In your personal life you are likely to have already

developed some very effective and complex methods of communicating, which you adapt, depending on particular circumstances. Everyone reading this text for instance is demonstrating a level of prior knowledge of written language, which you acquired when you learned to read.

To be able to integrate fully into contemporary society, individuals need to acquire a similar understanding of a range of modes of communication and the skills associated with each of these. It is likely that technology and trends in communication will continue to develop and evolve, so maintaining updated knowledge and keeping abreast of these is necessary to enable the best use of any advances, and enable their effective integration into practice.

The increased popularity and availability of mobile phones, interactive television, and the Internet have made it easier than ever for us to communicate with each other using a variety of media (Cleary and Freeman 2005). However, the methods and language that we use to communicate with our close friends or family are likely to be very different from the ones we would employ in a formal interview or case conference involving a range of our colleagues.

We must also be aware of the professional boundaries that exist, as stated in the Nursing and Midwifery Code (NMC 2008), which aim to ensure that the relationship between ourselves and our patients remains a professional one. The Code states that as nurses we must ensure that we do not accept any gifts or favours from patients, as these may be viewed as a way to gain preferential treatment; we must not request loans from patients or their families; and we must clearly establish and maintain sexual boundaries with patients, families, and carers. It is important to have an understanding of the difference between the more casual, familiar approach of the former exchanges and the specific responsibilities nurses are required to demonstrate when fulfilling their professional role.

Different styles of communication

The use of **colloquial** terms may be fitting for some social situations, but in professional settings nurses are likely to be expected to use more appropriate terminology. It is worth considering, however, that there may be individual circumstances where the use of more informal language during a nursing interaction may actually help someone understand their situation more clearly. Deciding about when it would be appropriate to use this or not is a skill that can be developed through experience and assessment of each separate set of circumstances. By doing this, nurses can more easily identify the expectations of the individuals with whom they are communicating while adopting a flexible approach to interpersonal relationships.

It is also very important to be aware of when to use professional language appropriately. While some terminology

and abbreviations, for example ECG (electrocardiogram), may be recognizable and familiar to you and your colleagues, it may mean nothing to your patients. This can result in you believing that you have explained a situation or procedure to a patient, but by using terms and professional jargon that they do not fully grasp, you may actually have increased their levels of misunderstanding and anxiety. The more exposed we are to professional jargon and abbreviations when communicating with colleagues, the more familiar they become to us, and it can be very easy to slip into their use without realizing that others may not comprehend our meaning.

Some people, perhaps a patient who is also a nurse, may be comfortable with nursing terminology, and you should always try to assess the individual needs of those with whom you are communicating and adjust your language and approach accordingly. One way to do this is by 'checking back,' which involves asking the person to repeat their interpretation of the circumstances back to you. This technique is discussed more in Chapter 4.

Communication is irreversible, however, and once spoken or written, our words cannot be taken back. There is a need, therefore, for nurses to consider the consequences of what they say and to assess the likelihood that their messages may be perceived differently from what was originally intended when transmitted. By developing the skills to raise personal awareness of the possible alternative interpretations of our communications, and by trying to gauge accurately the possible impact of what we are about to say, we can increase the probability that our messages are expressed unambiguously. By demonstrating high levels of understanding of communication skills, along with excellent awareness of the alternative **perceptions** that others may have of their messages, nurses can function effectively in liaison between all formal or informal members of the multidisciplinary care team, including patients, their families, and carers.

Take a few moments to list the different situations in which you communicate with others, both in your personal life and as a professional. What forms of communication do you use? What methods do you utilize to send your messages? How do you evaluate how effective your communication has been? How does communication in your personal life differ from that in your role as a nurse? What might the reaction be if you communicated with people in your personal life as you do with those in your professional life and vice versa?

2.1.1 **Basic communication skills**

Definition

As nurses, we are often in the very privileged position of caring for people when they are most vulnerable and **dependent** on help. Having and demonstrating an appreciation of this can often be the difference between presenting oneself as a truly caring nurse, rather than someone who is perceived as merely doing a job.

An important part of communication is listening (Stickley and Freshwater 2006) and we must be careful that our interactions with others are not used solely as a means for us to transmit information to our patients. We must be equally aware of the different messages that people may be intentionally or unintentionally sending to us, and the vital role of **active listening** is discussed in detail in Chapter 4. Communication is the medium through which we endeavour to understand others, while conveying to them our own thoughts, feelings, ideas, and opinions (O'Carroll and Park 2007). Some of the purposes of communication in nursing are listed in **Box 2.2**.

Communication can happen at any time and in any situation or set of circumstances. As nurses, it is often an unplanned interaction that provides us with the opportunity to offer reassurance, support, or education to people in our care. For example, anxious patients may feel more able to ask about a pending operation when someone approaches them to assist with their hygiene or diet. This may be because nurses can often appear busy and patients may feel that, in the bigger scheme of things, their concerns are trivial or of little importance, therefore, they only voice these when the nurse is already with them performing another task. In such situations, the response we give to anyone attempting to engage with us can have a significant effect on the individual.

If we are dismissive or abrupt in our response then patients can feel devalued or believe that they are being seen as troublesome. This is likely to discourage some patients from initiating interactions and may result in unnecessary distress for the patient and missed opportunities for nurses to update information that may inform treatment options and care planning. Even when busy, it is

Box 2.2 Goals of communication in nursing	
Therapeutic relationship building	Communication is the main tool in establishing, maintaining, and terminating therapeutic relationships
Patient-centred care	Enables the identification of key issues and concerns from the patient's perspective
Facilitate patient's views	Assists patients to express their emotions, views, and opinions clearly, and to have these understood by others
Assessment and identification of needs	Enables a more accurate appraisal and interpretation of patient needs from different perspectives, for example, the individual, carers, and service providers
Education	Provision of information that may deepen understanding, alleviate anxiety, empower the individual in decision making, and develop coping strategies and self-care
Planning, implementation, and evaluation of care	Enables the effective planning and delivery of care to meet the specific needs of individual patients
Guidance and support	Provides some appropriate direction while ensuring that patients make their own decisions to the best of their abilities, and offers realistic comfort and reassurance
Sharing information	Allows the sharing of appropriate information between relevant participants in care planning and delivery, which minimizes the risk of duplication and makes better use of available resources

by being courteous in our explanations, or by arranging a more suitable time to talk with our patients, that we can alleviate much of the feelings of anxiety and trepidation that some patients experience. Communication can involve the aspects shown in **Box 2.3**, all of which are discussed fully in Chapter 4.

Box 2.3 Aspects of communication

Spoken word	Either face to face or over a telephone
Nonverbal cues	For example, through facial expressions, **gestures**, or touch
Empathic linkages	These are the direct connection of feelings
Written word	In case notes and, increasingly, using electronic sources

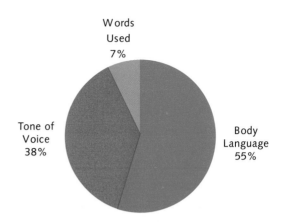

Figure 2.1 Factors that influence the interpretation of meaning

In any process of communication, first impressions provide a basis against which subsequent interaction is judged. The person with whom you wish to communicate is likely to make assumptions based on their perceptions of your approach and how you present yourself, your attitude towards both the situation and themselves, and your appearance and attire. In addition, research by Birdwhistell in 1970, which is still significant today, suggested that when communicating, people interpret meaning based on the following factors: 55% is taken from body language, 38% is taken from the tone of voice, and only 7% is based exclusively on the words used (as shown in **Fig. 2.1**). This research then implies that the way we say the words that we choose, rather than the words themselves, is more influential on how our messages are interpreted and understood.

When to use these communication skills

It is important to ensure that in every professional encounter with others, your initial contact demonstrates the standards of expertise and efficiency required of nurses in their professional role. The expectations of what this may entail will vary from individual to individual and some skill is involved in assessing your patients' particular views of what that might be. You should consider patients' potential views based on your initial observations, and then modify your approach to meet individual need, once you have completed a fuller assessment (Thompson 2002). While the initial contact provides the foundation for our interactions it is also necessary for nurses to bear in mind that they must continue to display high levels of professional behaviour throughout any communication process.

As has been mentioned, nursing is now carried out in an ever-increasing and diverse range of environments. Some branches of nursing, mental-health and learning-disability nursing, for example, frequently happen in patients' own homes, as more care provision has moved away from hospital settings. You should consider the specific impact that the environment in which you practice or deliver care is likely to have on communication. When in someone's home, we are there as guests and we should show the levels of courtesy, respect, and politeness that this entails. We should wait to be invited into someone's home, rather than behaving as though our position as nurses gives us exceptional rights. Remember, too, that while the information on communication provided in this book often only uses one example to demonstrate specific points, you should think of ways in which the skills described would apply in any of the environments in which nurses work.

Take time to consider the aspects of particular environments, for example, a house, busy with family members and a television blaring in the corner; a bed bay with only curtains between patients; or an older person, living alone and with visual and hearing impairment. Take some time to think about the effect that these may have on your own or your patient's ability to communicate effectively. Are there other examples that you can think of from a specific branch of nursing or that may occur in a particular care setting? How might you try to address such difficulties to enhance communication for yourself and your patient?

While nurses should attempt to optimize the opportunities afforded by any impromptu contact, communication in a nursing context should, where possible, happen as part of a planned interaction. There are a range of potential purposes of communication within nursing, which can affect our assessment of how we decide to transmit our messages to others. By identifying the purpose of each interaction we intend to participate in, the necessary components of the activity can be considered, and the most suitable skills employed for each situation. This should also minimize any potential barriers to successful communication and promote the likelihood of the interaction effectively achieving its goal.

Basic communication skills

Before engaging in any communication it is advisable to take a moment to reflect on the key aspects relating to that particular interaction. For example, who are you trying to communicate with? What is the purpose of the communication? What information are you particularly trying to communicate or obtain? Are there circumstances specific to the individual or the situation which you must consider to minimize the likelihood of communication difficulties? Are there any aspects regarding their physical or mental health that may make communication with particular individuals more difficult? These might include **sensory impairment**, disorientation, and inability to speak. If so, how might you best address these? Examples might be using an interpreter, simplifying your language while being careful not to patronize, or the use of sign language or picture boards.

Answering these questions and identifying potential barriers to good communication can enable actions to be planned that allow practitioners to compensate for such obstructions, and minimize their negative impact on the process. For example, if you know that someone is hard of hearing, ensuring that they have their hearing aid in place and that it is switched on increases the likelihood of a more successful exchange. While this may appear an extremely obvious thing to do, it is the type of action that is often overlooked, sometimes with very detrimental effects. It is also often such simple actions, like closing a door to reduce noise and distraction, or positioning yourself to enable good eye contact, that can have a significant effect on the impact of the interaction. Having said that, less obvious errors can be equally troublesome, for example, sending out case conference invitations with inaccurate date or venue details, or failing to alert people that a

meeting has been cancelled or rescheduled. It is important, then, to consider all of the aspects that may affect any interaction. These include features that are likely to have a more immediate impact, as well as those that may not have a bearing until a later date.

Aftercare

It is important for you to recognize that some people may need support beyond a specific interaction. You should try to assess when someone displays behaviour that might suggest a need for additional input, for example, by appearing agitated, afraid, or confused. This should be addressed by returning at appropriate intervals, offering reassurance, checking that what you have said has been understood, and asking if clarification or more information is required. Some people may simply require the presence or contact of another person to alleviate their distress. As it may be impractical to spend an indefinite time with someone, communication skills should continue to be used to try to explore the underlying reasons for their behaviour and emotions. This can enable the implementation of a support plan that is better suited to meet the individual's needs.

It is important that nurses take the time to assess each situation prior to engaging in any communication, and check the accuracy of the information being transmitted and received. In doing so, nurses can optimize the likelihood that the interaction will successfully achieve what it was initially planned for. In addition, a period of reflection following an interaction is equally important as this can provide the necessary insight into what was successful about the process, or what aspects could be improved on for similar circumstances in the future. In doing so, you will not only develop your own communication skills, but you will also raise your awareness of potential communication difficulties for your patients, and extend your knowledge of ways to pre-empt these, or successfully manage them, should they arise.

Developing your skills

In a work environment, decisions and actions are often constrained by time and other competing demands, and it can be easy to overlook the importance of the communication process in every aspect of what we do as nurses. By being

Basic communication skills

Action	Rationale
Generally be friendly and approachable	In most cases this should help people feel more able to engage with you, but be aware of circumstances where a more solemn or serious approach may be needed, for example, giving bad news, or following bereavement.
	Remember that individuals will have specific needs relating to how you communicate with them, so take time to assess what these might be and adapt your approach accordingly.
Speak clearly: be aware of rate and tone	Enables receiver to hear and interpret your message.
	Talking too quickly, too softly, or using an inappropriate tone, for example, being patronizing, can hamper effective communication.
Introduce yourself, stating your name and position	Identifies you to the receiver and may allay anxieties about who is interacting with them and what your role may be.
Ask how the person would like to be addressed	Empowers the individual, encouraging him or her to identify the most comfortable approach: for example, some people prefer being addressed by a first name or nickname, others may not like such familiarity, preferring to be addressed by their title and surname, for example, Mr Crabbe or Miss Smith.
Explain the purpose of the interaction	This should help the person understand the reason for the interaction and may alleviate some of his or her anxiety.
Choose language that is appropriate for the individual, for example, jargon free	To ensure that they understand what you want to communicate.
Explain what you are going to do	Provides the individual with information about a flexible structure of a planned procedure. It is worth highlighting that this can be adapted according to the changing needs of the individual.
Offer the opportunity to ask questions	Gives the person the chance to seek clarification of pressing concerns and enables the person to lead the direction of the discussion.

continued

Be honest if you are asked something to which you do not know the answer	It is better to offer to discuss this with others and return with the correct information than to give information that might be incorrect.
Give advice on how you may be contacted	Equips people with the information of how and when it may be appropriate to contact you again and prevents them from feeling uncertain or apprehensive about this.
Draw the interaction to a close	Demonstrates closure of the interaction and prevents the person from being unsure whether you have finished or intend to return.

continually attentive to how we are communicating at any given time, and maintaining an awareness of the skills that we can employ to enhance our interactions with others, we are likely to maximize the efficiency and improve the quality of all of our nursing interactions. Remember, too, that the factors that influence the potential success or failure of our own communications, apply equally to our patients. Be ever mindful of potential barriers for them to participate in communication, and implement strategies to minimize any difficulties that you identify.

Other factors to consider

Meaning and significance

Words are the verbal symbols we use to express our meaning and understanding, and to convey our thoughts, ideas, and opinions to others. Remember, however, that the significance and meaning that we assign to the words we say may not be the same as the meaning understood by those hearing them.

The same words can mean different things to people from different generations, cultures, or locations. The traditional meaning of the terms 'wicked' and 'bad,' for example, have more recently come to have the opposite meaning among younger people, but are likely to have retained their initial negative connotation for many older adults. Similarly, confusion can arise from the use of terms having specific meanings in one region that may be completely unknown in others, for example, 'pogged' is used in parts of Yorkshire, England to mean 'full up'. You should also take care when using abstract statements or figures of speech, as their meaning may be taken literally by

people who are not accustomed to their alternative use. For example, if you are not familiar with the term, and someone tells you to 'pull your socks up,' you might act on this literally by pulling up your socks, rather than increasing your effort, which is what you were likely to have been requested to do.

You can reduce the likelihood of any misinterpretation or confusion by assessing the person receiving your message, and adapting the words, phrases, and terms you use to best meet their needs. Whilst you are unlikely to be accurate in your assessment all of the time, there will be many occasions when you improve the efficacy of your communication by taking the time to consider this important element.

Confidentiality

As nurses we have the responsibility to treat information about and from the people that we care for as confidential. This means that we are obliged only to disclose to others involved in someone's care, information that specifically relates to that care (Arnold and Boggs 2007). Similarly, we are only entitled to healthcare information relating to those patients with whom we have a legitimate professional relationship.

Literal meanings of the term 'confidential' define it as information intended to be kept secret or as private information that is entrusted to another. Many patients are likely to expect that the information they give to you as their nurse will remain exclusively between you two unless they give you expressed permission to share it. While it is important that patients are confident that they can trust us to manage discreetly, in accordance with NMC requirements, the information that we obtain about them, there are occasions when we may be required to disclose some information to others. If, for example, patients tell you that they intend harming themselves or others, or that they are planning to carry out some unlawful activity, then you are duty bound to report this to a more senior member of staff. It is useful, therefore, to inform patients of this at an early point in any discussion, before you engage in deeper dialogue with them. The NMC Code (NMC 2008) provides clear advice in relation to confidentiality and you should take the time to familiarize yourself with this.

Maintaining confidentiality demonstrates respect for patients' privacy. If a patient has explicitly requested you not to discuss particular aspects or circumstances outside of the care team, then you must be careful that you do not breach confidentiality, even inadvertently. It can be easy to forget, while talking to their relatives, for instance, that a patient may have asked, or may not want, care details to be disclosed. It can help to ask what someone has already been told about the patients or their planned care. This enables you to assess current levels of understanding and provides you with a starting point from which you can decide what information is appropriate for you to discuss. In situations where you are unable to discuss matters openly, it is important that you use your communication skills to explain this in a diplomatic way. Remember that some people can feel rejected, excluded, or distressed by this, and you need to ensure that you are not abrupt, patronizing, or condescending when explaining the position to them. Finally, if you are in any doubt about whether you may be breaching confidentiality, it is wise to err on the side of caution and seek advice from an appropriately experienced colleague before engaging in discussion.

As well as being insightful regarding our own methods of communication, we need to remain mindful of the ways that our actions and communications may be perceived or interpreted by others. Similarly, we must bear in mind that our interpretations of others' communication with us may be different from the way that they intended when sending their message. But by heightening our awareness of the skills that we use when we communicate, and of how other people may use these skills in their contact with us, we can develop our expertise and utilize our understanding in our efforts to function most effectively, thereby enhancing all of our communication and interactions with others.

2.1.2 **Interprofessional communication**

Definition

It is important to acknowledge that while communication between nurses and patients or their families or carers is imperative in providing high quality, patient-centred care; communication must also be considered in a wider context. Contemporary healthcare requires nurses to liaise with practitioners from a range of disciplines, including medical staff, allied health professionals (for example, physiotherapists, occupational therapists, dieticians, podiatrists, psychologists, social workers, housing staff, police, voluntary agencies, and religious leaders) (Arnold and Boggs 2007).

This list by no means includes everyone who may play a part in a person's care and there may be other local and national organizations or contributors who should be considered, depending on each individual's needs. Multidisciplinary communication can range from interpersonal communication to group or even mass communication. As with many other forms of communication it can extend from an informal conversation between professionals to formal meetings, for example, case conferences and reviews.

When to share information with other healthcare professionals

Sharing information with other healthcare professionals can enable the more effective use of resources, allowing speedier access to services and facilitating the planning and delivery of the most appropriate care. However, you must bear in mind issues of consent and confidentiality. Take a few moments to think of the different disciplines, individuals and organizations who may contribute to the care of patients in your branch:

- How is information shared with them?
- What do you need to consider when sharing information with other professionals, statutory organizations, or voluntary services?

Interprofessional communication

Action	Rationale
Demonstrate professional respect and awareness by understanding other disciplines and their roles and identifying professional responsibilities and boundaries.	It is important to acknowledge and value the contribution that each member of the multidisciplinary team can offer to foster mutual respect, reduce the risk of services overlapping, and enable more efficient use of resources.
Demonstrate assertiveness skills (see Section 2.1.3) if there is an imbalance of power and responsibility among team members.	To ensure that your contribution is valued and effective.
Show an awareness of differing professional jargon.	Terminology used within one discipline may not be understood by others.
Take time to check and make sure that your contribution has been understood and that you understand the information being provided by other contributors.	Reducing the risk of misunderstanding and confusion.
Become familiar with local channels of communication between disciplines, through paper, electronic and telephone systems.	The effective timely flow of information enables speedier, more accurate decision making and care planning. Using the correct channel increases the likelihood that intended information will reach the correct participants.
Share information appropriately. It is essential that consent to share information is deemed to be informed and given freely, and that patients understand the potential benefits and risks involved.	While sharing information can improve the efficacy of planned care you must be familiar with and abide by professional guidance and legal requirements.
Information regarding consent must be recorded accurately and in the appropriate place within records.	Provides a permanent record and meets professional requirements.

- How do you exchange information regarding your findings?
- What are the benefits of sharing information in this way?
- What are the risks involved and how is patients' consent sought, recorded and included in decisions?

The sharing of information is usually very complex and it is impossible to advise on all of the specific circumstances and factors that you will need to consider when making decisions about information sharing. To help prepare yourself, take time to become familiar with the local policies and procedures in the areas you are working, as well as NMC guidelines, and discuss this topic with appropriately qualified colleagues from nursing and other professions.

2.1.3 **Assertiveness skills**

Definition

In general, assertiveness relates to acting in a clear and consistent way to set clear goals, successfully achieve them, and accept responsibility for the consequences of chosen actions. According to Hargie and Dickson (2004) it is a skill that can be learned and developed, and in keeping with the focus of this chapter, assertiveness is considered here in relation to communication.

When engaging in communication it is important that the views and opinions of all parties are heard (McRae 1998). For this to happen, nurses need to demonstrate assertiveness, as our role involves not only presenting our personal thoughts and views, but often those of our patients too. It is vital, therefore, that nurses feel confident in their position, are aware of the evidence to support their points of view, and are able to present these in an articulate, professional manner in a variety of settings.

At times, this may seem difficult and intimidating, but with practice you can develop assertiveness skills that will support you in your professional role and enable you to fulfil your professional responsibilities. **Table 2.1** highlights the differences in using passive, **aggressive**, and assertive approaches.

When to be assertive

Nurses are regularly required to demonstrate skills of diplomacy and they are often involved in interactions where the participants have very strong but opposing views. Conversely, nurses also frequently engage with individuals

Table 2.1 Passive, aggressive, and assertive communication approaches

Passive communication	Assertive communication	Aggressive communication
Speech is more timid, soft, and halting	Speaks in a clear, firm voice	Raised voice, often with **covert** or overt threat
Does not make eye contact, often looks downward, avoiding others' gaze	Ensures that verbal and nonverbal messages are congruent	Nonverbal messages can include body tensed and threatening, staring-out other parties, and impinging on their personal space
Body posture is closed, may be agitated and restless	Body posture is more open	Body posture may be invasive or appear threatening
Contribution may be vague and the meaning unclear	Makes clear, unambiguous statements	Can be demanding, threatening, and hostile
Is afraid or unwilling to contribute personal thoughts, feelings and views	Expresses position using 'I' statements, for example, 'I feel uncomfortable when you use that tone of voice'.	Dominates discussion and does not show consideration of others' views
If unable to contribute effectively to the focus of the discussion	Maintains the focus of the discussion, doesn't bring up issues that are unrelated to the immediate situation	Uses arguments outside the scope and relevance of the current discussion, for example, when discussing arriving late for work, 'Well, you always let other people get first break!'
Does not challenge views which they think are wrong or with which they disagree	Demonstrates awareness of others thoughts, feelings and views, challenges in a diplomatic, non-threatening way	Demanding and inflexible
Allows others to have their own way without compromise	Seeks workable compromise	Insists on getting their own way

Communicating assertively

Aspect	Rationale
Make clear, unambiguous statements	Provides others with a clear indication of your views
Speak in a clear, firm voice	Demonstrates confidence, clarity, and purpose. Ensures that other people hear and understand what you say
Express your position using 'I' statements, for example, 'I feel uncomfortable when you use that tone of voice.'	Enables you to challenge views in an unthreatening way
Ensure verbal and nonverbal messages are congruent	Communicates your views clearly in both a verbal and nonverbal way
Maintain the focus of the discussion: don't bring up issues that are unrelated to the immediate situation	Keeping to the focus of an interaction enables appropriate decisions to be considered, without personalizing issues or distraction
Demonstrate awareness of others' thoughts, feelings and views	Acknowledges that the views of all participants are important and should be considered equally
Seek workable compromises	Enables participants to explore win–win solutions by not always expecting to get their own way, especially if this is at others' expense

who are unable or unaware of how to express themselves and ensure that their contribution to any debate is understood and acknowledged (Bateman 2000).

Remember also that at times you may wish to present yourself in a less threatening way, for example when **engaging** with someone who is potentially aggressive. By adopting a more passive role, you may be more likely to defuse a situation and avoid escalating any risk of attack or violence. Keep in mind, however, that you should not confuse being passive with being timid or subservient, as this may make you seem like an easier target for a potential aggressor and put you more at risk. Although there may be some exceptions, and we must assess each situation individually, as a rule we should, as nurses, strive to display the behaviours associated with being assertive, while avoiding those related to passive and aggressive communication styles.

Developing your skills

By being assertive, nurses ensure that their voice is heard and their contribution to debate is acknowledged and valued. An assertive approach also, however, requires that all participants are afforded the same opportunities and that each participant's view is recognized as worthwhile and can influence discussion. Take a few moments to think of situations in which you may have behaved or may be likely to behave in a passive, assertive, or aggressive way. What factors influence how you might behave? What effect might your level of knowledge, experience, confidence, or being in a position of power have on this? What communication skills could you employ to enhance your ability to approach your professional life in a more assertive way?

Summary

This section has explored some of the key issues relating to communication in your role as a nurse. Remember that, as stated at the beginning of this section, you should read it in conjunction with Chapter 4, which will provide you with a more comprehensive view of communication in nursing. Just as we need to raise our awareness of our own communication skills and the factors that affect our interactions with others, we also need to develop our understanding of the key issues that influence the way that other people may understand, perceive and engage in their communication with us. The sections of this book dedicated to communication skills should help you to becoming more expert and engage in communication that is professional, adaptable and effective.

 Scenario

Consider what you should do in the following situation, then turn to the end of the section to check your answers. Further scenarios are available at ◐ **www.oxfordtextbooks. co.uk/orc/docherty/**

This communication scenario describes a situation that may occur equally with any client group in any setting. Consider how the circumstances might vary in different placements. In a learning-disability setting it may be someone anxious about having to make a decision. In mental health, it may be a patient with an anxiety disorder. Children's nurses may want to consider a child who is anxious at being separated from the family. Adults' nurses might encounter such situations with patients who are anxious about an investigation or procedure they are about to experience. It is worthwhile reflecting on other circumstances to which this scenario could apply.

While passing a patient sitting room you see Alan. He is usually chatty and jovial but today you notice that he is staring blankly ahead and is wringing his hands.

- What are your first impressions likely to be regarding what you observe?
- What should you go on to consider about the situation?
- What communication skills might you use to address this situation?

- How might you approach Alan and what would you say to engage with him?

Website

◐ **www.oxfordtextbooks.co.uk/orc/docherty/**
You may find it helpful to work through our short online quiz and interactive scenarios intended to help you to develop and apply the skills in this section.

References

Arnold EC and Boggs KU (2007). *Interpersonal Relationships: Professional Communication Skills for Nurses*, 5th edn. Saunders Elsevier, St. Louis.

Bateman N (2000). *Advocacy Skills for Health and Social Care Professionals. Jessica Kingsley*, London.

Birdwhistell RL (1970). *Kinesics and Contex: Essays on Body Motion and Communication*. University of Pennsylvania Press, Philadelphia.

Cleary M and Freeman A (2005). *Email etiquette: guidelines for mental health nurses. International Journal of Mental Health Nursing*, **14**, 62–5.

Ellis RB, Gates B, and Kenworthy N (2003). *Interpersonal Communication in Nursing: Theory and Practice*, 2nd edn. Churchill Livingstone, London.

Grover SM (2005). Shaping effective communication skills and therapeutic relationships at work. *AAOHN Journal*, **53**(4), 177–82.

Hargie O and Dickson D (2004). *Skilled Interpersonal Communication: Research, Theory and Practice*, 4th edn. Routledge, Hove.

Howell W (1982). *The Empathic Communicator*. Wadsworth, Pacific Grove.

McRae B (1998). *Negotiating and Influencing Skills: The Art of Creating and Claiming Value*. Sage, London.

NMC (2007). *Essential Skills Clusters (ESCs) for Pre-registration Nursing Programmes*. Nursing and Midwifery Council, London.

NMC (2008). *The Code: Standards of Conduct, Performance and Ethics for Nurses and Midwives*. Nursing and Midwifery Council, London.

O'Carroll M and Park A (2007). *Essential Mental Health Nursing Skills*. Mosby Elsevier, London.

Sully P and Dallas J (2005). *Essential Communication Skills for Nursing*. Elsevier Mosby, London.

Thompson N (2002). *People Skills*. Palgrave Macmillan, Basingstoke.

Videbeck SL (2006) *Psychiatric Mental Health Nursing*, 3rd edn. Lippincott Williams and Wilkins, Philadelphia.

Useful further reading and websites

Check **www.oxfordtextbooks.co.uk/orc/docherty/** for changes and new developments. Updated research, guidelines, or equipment will be added every four months.

Answers to scenario

You should initially consider why Alan may be behaving as he is, remembering that there are likely to be several possible explanations for his behaviour.

- Consider physical explanations; for example, is he in pain or discomfort?
- What psychological factors may be influencing him? For example, is he upset, worried, frightened, or uncertain? Has he received distressing news?
- Are there any environmental factors to take into account? For example, is he in unfamiliar surroundings, does he know anyone else, or does he feel alone and isolated?
- Be wary of making assumptions, as these may be incorrect. It is important to assess Alan's situation accurately, using verbal, nonverbal, and observational skills to help you reach an informed decision
- By initially observing his nonverbal cues, you can assess levels of agitation or anxiety and plan the most appropriate way to engage with him
- Consider possible risks. Are you putting yourself in potential danger by approaching Alan on your own? What would your route of escape be if Alan's agitation develops into aggression?

- Assess the environment in general. Is it the most suitable place to talk? Are others present? Are there issues of privacy, confidentiality, or embarrassment for Alan? Are there too many distractions, for example, radio or television?
- You should approach Alan in a calm way, trying to make eye contact and speaking in a gentle, controlled, and steady voice. Avoid startling him by approaching too rapidly, brusquely or from outside his vision
- Ask him what is happening from his point of view, for example, 'Hi, Alan! I noticed you sitting here and wondered how you are doing. How are you today?'
- Use language and terms that you believe Alan is most likely to respond to. Be careful to avoid using jargon or being patronizing
- Be ready to offer support using all of your communication skills, for example, giving Alan your full attention, repeating or paraphrasing what he says to check and show him that you understand, nodding to demonstrate that you are listening and encourage him to continue talking
- If appropriate use touch, for example, by holding his hand or putting a hand on his shoulder
- By remaining calm and communicating in a professional and caring way you can demonstrate to Alan that you are able and willing to assist him to address his perceived difficulty
- Once you have formed an opinion of what is happening, discuss the possible solutions with Alan, as he should be involved in decision making, and keeping people informed can help alleviate anxiety for some individuals
- If you believe that you are unable to support Alan yourself you should discuss with a more senior member of staff how best to proceed
- You should always pass on the details of such interactions to ensure that the information is properly recorded and shared with appropriate members of the care team
- You should ensure that you or another member of staff continue to check back on Alan at appropriate intervals to reassess how he is progressing and how effective any interventions have been

2.2 **Moving and handling**

Introduction

The moving of patients is often referred to as manual handling. The UK Health and Safety Executive (HSE 2002) define manual handling as, 'the lifting, lowering, pushing, pulling, carrying, transporting, or supporting, by hand or bodily force, any object including a person.'

Nurses are involved in moving patients and inanimate objects as part of their daily routine. This often results in musculoskeletal damage, which can affect muscles, **tendons**, **ligaments**, **peripheral nerves**, blood vessels, joints, cartilage (such as intervertebral discs), or bones in the arms, legs, neck, back, or trunk. This damage can occur suddenly as a one-off injury due to unexpected movement, strenuous, or awkward handling, but is often as a result of **cumulative strain** over a prolonged period of time. Cumulative strain occurs after habitual, excessive muscular **contraction** and can lead to a progressive stiffening of the body tissues. This excessive tension in the tissues reduces their adaptability and means that they are more likely to become tired and injured.

Back injury is the largest single cause of long-term sickness in the United Kingdom and costs the National Health Service about £300 million a year. The reasons behind this include lack of education, illness, poor practice, stress, and lack of resources.

The aim of moving and handling should be that the nurse employs minimal effort to achieve efficient movement and that the patient suffers no discomfort.

It should be noted that the term 'lifting' is no longer used to describe moving and handling activities. 'Lifting' is no longer used because this gives the impression that the handler has to take the patient's full weight. If the patient's full weight needs to be taken, then equipment, such as a hoist, should be used be prevent injury to the patient and handler.

Learning outcomes

These outcomes relate to numbers 9 and 18 of the NMC's Essential Skill Clusters and specifically to Care Domains 2 and 3 of the NMC's Standards of Proficiency for Pre-registration Nursing (outcomes to be achieved for entry to branch).

On reading the chapter and associated web pages and undertaking supervised activities, you will be able to:

- Demonstrate knowledge of the legislation surrounding moving and handling
- Identify the five areas of risk assessment, perform this assessment and suggest or demonstrate ways to avoid or reduce the risk
- Understand the principles of efficient movement
- Identify unsafe practices and understand why these practices are unsafe

Prior knowledge

Before reading this chapter, you should be familiar with:

- The anatomy and physiology of the neuromuscular system
- The basic **biomechanics** (study of the application of mechanical principles to living tissue) of human movement
- The appropriate legal and professional guidelines in relation to manual handling. This can be obtained by reading:
  - *Health and Safety at Work Act* (HMSO 1974),
  - *Manual Handling Operations Regulations* (HSE 2002),
  - *Lifting Operations and Lifting Equipment Regulations* (HSE 1998),
  - *The Royal College of Nursing Code of Practice for Patient Handling* (RCN 2002),
  - *The Guide to the Handling of Patients* (Smith 2005).

Health and Safety at Work Act (HMSO 1974)

This Act first highlighted that employers have a legal responsibility to prevent work-related accidents and ill health, including musculoskeletal injury. It states that individuals have a duty to 'take reasonable care for their own health and safety and that of others who may be affected by their acts or omissions.'

Manual Handling Operations Regulations (HSE 2002)

These regulations were published to follow on from the Health and Safety at Work Act. These focus specifically on manual handling at work and highlight the importance of risk assessment as a mandatory requirement. These regulations state that manual handling should be avoided where practicable and if it cannot be avoided then the risks should be assessed and reduced to the lowest reasonable level. Employers, therefore, must provide suitable handling aids and training in their use.

Lifting Operations and Lifting Equipment Regulations (HSE 1998)

These came into force in 1998 and aim to reduce risk to people when using lifting equipment. In relation to nursing, this would include any equipment that is used to lift patients, for example, hoists and their accessories.

The Royal College of Nursing Code of Practice for Patient Handling (RCN 2002)

Further to this, the Royal College of Nursing (RCN), through the Advisory Panel on Back Pain in Nurses, published the *RCN Code of Practice*. This guidance advocates a 50 kg weight limit for a patient being moved by two nurses and sets out 'ideal conditions' that must first apply. It states that the nurse should not move a patient if he or she bears most or all of the patient's weight. It adds that hoists or other suitable handling aids should be used where appropriate and that education and training should be given to support their use.

The Guide to the Handling of Patients (SMITH 2005)

Further nursing guidance can also be found in the book entitled 'The Guide to the Handling of Patients' published in association with The National Back Pain Association and the RCN which gives advice on safe patient handling and has been credited with improved practice by removing certain 'banned' lifts from practice (these will be discussed later).

Risk assessment for moving and handling

Risk assessment is a mandatory component of patient care under various regulations (HSE 1998, 2002). Carrying out a risk assessment identifies risk to the patient and the handler and should prevent hazardous manual handling and reduce the risk of injury.

Before beginning any move, it is vital that the nurse checks the moving and handling assessment for the individual concerned. All risk assessments should be updated regularly to accommodate any changes and, legally, this information must be documented.

In assessing risk, the nurse should begin by asking, 'Do I need to do this task?' Following on from this, an assessment of what is to be moved and how it should be moved, along with an assessment of the handler (the nurse) and the surroundings should be undertaken. This risk assessment commonly falls under the acronym ELITE (environment, load, individual, task, equipment; see **Table 2.2**). It is important not only to assess all these areas, but also to see how they relate, and how one influences another.

Along with this risk assessment, there should be an individualized moving and handling patient assessment (see Chapter 10).

Once a risk assessment has been carried out it is vital that it is not filed away and forgotten about. It should be visible to all staff involved in the patient's care and continuously updated.

2.2.1 **Principles of efficient human movement**

Definition

This involves the safe and efficient movement of the nurse or carer and the patient or load. The practice of moving and handling involves principles rather than a step-by-step

Table 2.2 ELITE assessment

Assessment area	Areas to assess; questions to ask
Environment	Is there enough room?
	Are objects at a convenient height?
	Flooring, lighting, air currents, steps, loose matting, obstacles, variations in levels, temperature of area
Load (patient, object, piece of equipment)	Weight and height, bulk, stability
	Diagnosis of patient
	Ability to assist
	Physical constraints, pain, and fatigue
	Behaviour
	Clothing, footwear, prosthesis, orthosis
	Holding issues, stability, temperature, sharp, harmful, contours
	Communication issues
Individual (you, the nurse)	Capabilities, fitness for task, fatigue, health issues
	Experience with the client
	Clothing, jewellery
	Knowledge base
	Personal protective equipment
	Communication issues
	Stress, morale, attitude
Task (what it is that you need to do)	Does it need to be done?
	Is there a documented moving and handling assessment?
	Could the client move unaided?
	Purpose and duration of task
	Twisting, stooping, reaching
	Working while seated

Table 2.2 (*Continued*)

	Long carrying distances
	Strenuous pushing or pulling
	Unpredictable movement
	Repetitive handling, prolonged activity
	Insufficient rest or recovery
	Number of handlers (if there are not the required appropriately trained staff then the move should not take place)
	Is equipment required?
	Is the equipment appropriate to the task, environment, patient, and individual?
Equipment	Walking aids, wheelchair, other personal equipment
	Familiarity with equipment (are you trained to use it or are you working with someone else who is?)
	Maintenance of equipment (has it been checked prior to use?)

guide. Knowledge of these principles and the ability to apply them to practice are the tools that all nurses require. Efficient movement is the basis of good handling practice. A summary of these main principles, which can be applied to any handling situation, can be seen in The safe movement of a patient, p. 27.

Background

One of the principles of effective movement deals with the posture of the handler. The best posture should be one where the three curves of the spine are in their natural balances position (see **Fig. 2.2**). Poor posture can lead to muscle weakness and joint problems. Your posture can be improved by keeping your weight optimal and exercising regularly.

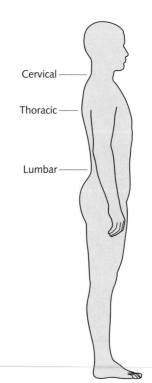

Figure 2.2 The spinal curves in their natural balanced position

The safe movement of a patient

Key point: The dignity of patients should also be considered at all times. It is, therefore, vital that the patient's wishes are taken into account along with effective communication skills to maintain patient compliance and comfort.

Step	Rationale
1 **Assess the task (see section on risk management)**	Identifies hazards or risks
Ask, 'Do I need to make this move?'	
Plan the move **Is equipment required?**	Enables the handler to select the most effective way to carry out the move
Prepare the area	To remove any hazards or obstructions
2 **Communicate; with any other handler involved, with the patient**	To ensure cooperation, maintain trust, and obtain consent Lack of communication with the patient can cause confusion and anxiety, especially if the patient is more vulnerable
'1, 2, 3,' should not be used as a command, as confusion might occur. Instead, the team leader can ask, 'Are you ready?' and then give an already agreed command that also reminds you of the movement, for example, 'Relax, knees, and head.'	To ensure the move takes place in a coordinated manner (this will reduce the risk of injury)
3 **Relax the muscles**	To prevent tension, which causes unwanted pressure
4 **Maintain a stable base**	To ensure balance
Position the feet slightly apart, with the lead foot pointing in the direction of movement	To prevent twisting or turning
During the move the feet should move to maintain this position	
5 **Lower your centre of gravity**	Relaxes the posture and provides stability

continued

	Loosen the knees (do not bend them too much, just squeeze them and then relax)	It is difficult to move your feet if your knees are locked
6	Keep your spine in line:	To prevent top-heavy or twisting movements
	Maintain the spine's natural curvature	Top-heavy positions are often adopted unconsciously and although immediate problems may not be felt, long-term effects and injury occur with recurrent **top-heavy movements**. They cause the spine to form a C shape. This weakens the back and increases the risk of injury
	Avoid twisting or bending sideways	
	When viewed from the side, the spine should show normal curves that form an S shape (see Figs 2.3 and 2.4)	To prevent spinal compression
7	Keep the load close to your body (centre of gravity)	To reduce strain or effort and increase efficiency and reduce risk of injury – the load becomes heavier the further away from the body it is and reaching makes the body unstable
	Points of contact with another person should be on their trunk where possible	To control the movement centres
8	Move your head in an upward direction when moving and hold your chin in	To initiate movement – the head leads the body in its movement and maintains good posture as it allows the spine to form its natural curves
This also raises the chest, which helps with breathing and allows you to see where you are going
9	Apply the force to the direction you want to move	Relates to forces – force should be directed in the direction of movement or else energy is wasted
10	Make the 'levers' of your arms as short as possible. Elbows should be close to the body and not jutting out	To reduce demand on muscles and ligaments
Brings the centre of gravity of the patient closer to your own centre of gravity
Hands are weaker if further away from the body
11	Maintain an appropriate hold depending on the size and weight of the client
You should use indirect, palmar holds, and stroking, that is, do not grip, see Fig. 2.5	To allow for easy release and patient and nurse comfort
To aid clients in their movement
12	Use your major muscle groups for effort	They are designed to bear weights, unlike minor groups of muscle further away from the trunk

Aftercare

It is important that you ensure that your patient is safe and comfortable before leaving. As assessment is a continuous process, any changes to the original risk assessment or moving and handling plan that were made during or after moving the patient should be documented in the patient's notes.

Developing your skills

As moving is a developed skill, a one-off training session is not enough. Competence in this skill takes practice and regular updates. These sessions should involve applying the above principles in practice, identifying risks, and developing solutions. Chapter 10 will demonstrate how to put these principles into practice when moving patients.

Healthcare organizations must have a manual handling policy with clear roles and responsibilities for employers and employees. When you are on your next clinical placement, ask to see this as part of your induction to the clinical area. Each organization has different risk assessment and patient moving and handling assessment forms, therefore, it is good practice to familiarize yourself with this documentation on each clinical placement. Each placement setting may also have different moving and handling equipment, therefore, it is essential that you do not use this equipment unless you are supervised or have been trained in its use by a qualified member of staff.

Other factors to consider

As well as looking after your posture, it is important to look after the rest of the muscles in your body. The abdominal muscles are important, as they work with the lower back muscles and, if strong, can reduce the stress on the intervertebral discs. You should take regular exercise, such as walking and swimming and start and end your shift with warm-up and cool-down

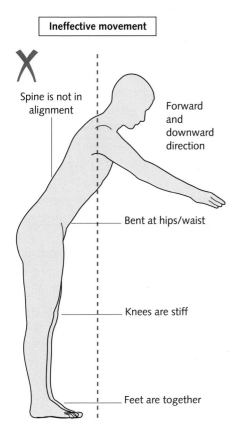

Figure 2.3 Inefficient movement

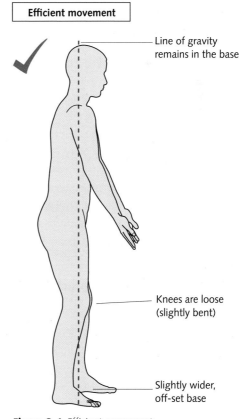

Figure 2.4 Efficient movement

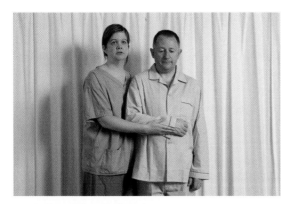

Figure 2.5 Indirect hold on patient

stretching exercises. As well as lessening back pain, this exercise can also improve fitness, well-being, balance, and posture.

Along with you looking after yourself, your employer has a legal responsibility for looking after you. There are many issues beyond your control, which can affect the way your patients are handled. The provision of equipment and training is one, and staffing levels is another. Inadequate staffing levels or a poor skill mix of staff affects staff performance and can, therefore, lead to accidents and injuries if they are tired or rushing. Risk assessments may be forgotten or care may be inappropriate, based on a poor assessment.

In the community, there may be difficulties in accessing appropriate equipment and fitting this equipment into confined spaces. There will also be differences in bed heights, toilet facilities, and many other environmental differences. A risk assessment is vital, therefore, and you should always be aware of maintaining your own safety and that of the patient. It is your responsibility to report any problems to the appropriate person and not take part in any practice you see as dangerous.

Banned moves and unsafe practice

You should not, under any circumstances, take part in unsafe practice as this may put the patient or you, yourself, at risk. Banned moves, as listed in **Table 2.3**, are included in this chapter so that you can recognize and avoid unacceptable practice. Alternative acceptable techniques are discussed in detail in Chapter 10.

The Royal College of Nursing has published guidance on lifting, moving, and handling patients. This guidance has been updated in further editions, the most recent being that edited by Smith (2005). This guidance is widely used. Along with health and safety legislation, and the concept of clinical governance, the subject of moving and handling has had widespread publicity in healthcare.

The evidence for banned moves is difficult to collect, owing to the danger in researching them; however, expert opinion suggests that these are dangerous moves and should not be used in practice, as they cause injury to nurses and patients. Ideally, before techniques are put into practice they should be researched. This would then prevent these moves being recalled as dangerous once injuries occur. Until further evidence is available, practice should be based on professional opinion. If you are in any doubt, you should seek advice from your mentor on placement or from your university.

As a student nurse, you may still observe some of these banned techniques used in practice. You should discuss this with your mentor, as undertaking banned moves could be seen as a form of abuse. Although any injuries caused to patients may not have been intended, poor handling techniques may result in preventable injuries.

Some physical indications of poor handling technique include bruising, particularly under the arms, around the lower leg, and around the rib area; however, patients may also show psychological and behavioural signs, such as an unwillingness to cooperate or aggression or distress when being moved or handled. If a patient behaves in this way, you should mention it to the appropriate person, although this is a very sensitive issue and may be unrelated to handling techniques.

There are other instances, particularly in children's nursing, where it may seem acceptable to pick up or carry a child, because they are lighter and, therefore, may not cause injury. This is not the case as, from the risk assessment information given earlier; it is not just the weight of the load (patient) that causes injury to the nurse and patient during a move. There is not a safe weight, as such, for carrying a child, as injuries can occur in relation to many factors and repetitive strain. A full risk assessment should be carried out as normal. Other complex needs of patients are discussed in Chapter 10.

Table 2.3 Banned moves and why they are dangerous

Technique name	Method	Danger to patient	Danger to nurse
Underarm or drag lift	The nurse's arms are placed under the client's axilla (see **Fig. 2.6**)	Shoulder dislocation Discourages patient from mobilizing Shearing forces can cause skin damage	Involves twisting Patient (load) is taken at a distance from the base
Orthodox (cradle) lift	Two nurses stand on either side of the bed and lift the patient on their clasped wrists under the patient's back and thighs (see **Fig. 2.7**)	Patient's head and limbs are unsupported	The nurse is bent, therefore, the nurse is unbalanced and twists at the end of the movement The weight of the patient is carried on a small part of the body
Shoulder (Australian) lift	Involves two nurses, carrying the patient on one shoulder each – uneven loading (see **Fig. 2.8**)	Nurses' shoulders press against the chest wall of the patient	Nurse is twisted and bent Nurse cannot see the patient and so there are potential risks for the nurse, for example, patient stiffening or using arms
Through-arm lift (two nurses)	Two nurses lift the patient on linked arms under the patient's thighs and around their back (see **Fig. 2.9**)	The patient's heels can drag on the bed and the patient's head is unsupported. Discomfort in the axilla area, as part of the pull is under the axilla	Nurse has back bent and is working a long way from the base of the spine
Three (or more) person lift	Three or more lifters lift the patient horizontally with their arms out straight under the patient. Often used to move a patient from bed to trolley or vice versa (see **Fig. 2.10**)	Patient may be dropped if one of the lifters stumbles	Weight can be displaced on to other lifters if one stumbles or is of a differing height (uneven shared load) May have to lower or lift the patient if the trolley or bed is at a different height
Poles and canvas	Involves a total body lift using two poles and a canvas (see **Fig. 2.11**)	Patient may fall from a height	A full lift is carried out using the arms and shoulders. The nurses cannot bend their knees and leaning over or twisting is often required to reach the bed

Table 2.3 (*Continued*)

Front-assisted transfer with one carer (pivot, bear-hugging, rocking)	Patient places arms on the nurse's waist or around the nurse's neck. Often the patient is rocked to build momentum of movement (see **Fig. 2.12**)	The nurse is in the way and is standing directly in front of the patient. This prevents natural movement and reaction from the patient	Risk of neck injury if the patient falls If the patient falls, the nurse may be pulled down too Lack of control over the amount of weight being carried

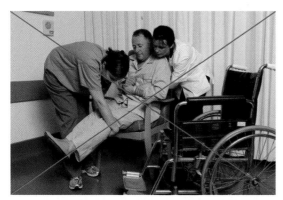

Figure 2.6 Underarm or 'drag' lift: this can damage the patient's shoulders and the nurses' backs

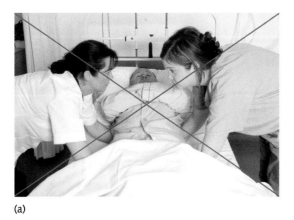

(a)

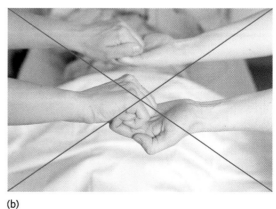

(b)

Figure 2.7 'Cradle' or 'orthodox' lift: (a) the patient's head and neck are unsupported; (b) the nurses are carrying the weight on their hands and wrists

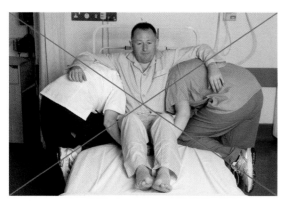

Figure 2.8 'Australian' or shoulder lift: this can damage the patient's chest wall and the nurses' backs

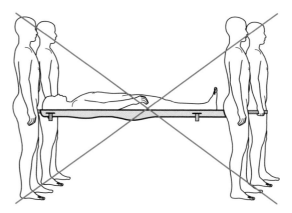

Figure 2.11 Pole and canvas lift: this could damage the nurses' shoulders or the patient could fall

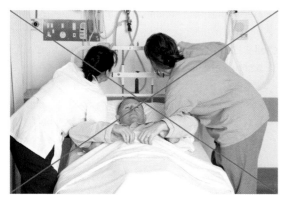

Figure 2.9 Through-arm lift: this can damage the patient's underarms and the nurses' backs

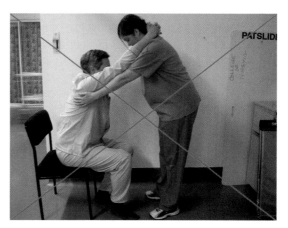

Figure 2.12 Front assisted transfer: this could damage the nurses' neck or either person could fall

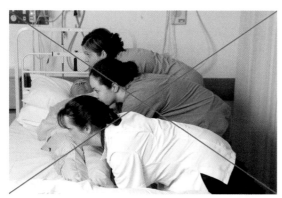

Figure 2.10 Three-person lift: the patient could fall, or if a nurse stumbles, uneven loads would be transferred

Nurses are responsible for their own practice and, as such, must keep up to date with current evidence-based guidelines on the moving and handling of patients. Employers must provide their staff with appropriate training, information and resources but it is the duty of the nurse to attend and comply with this guidance in order to practise safe and effective nursing care.

 ## Scenario

Consider what you should do in the following situation, then turn to the end of the section to check your answers.

Further scenarios are available at ⊕ **www.oxford textbooks.co.uk/orc/docherty/**

You are working in a residential care home for the elderly. You have been asked to assist a healthcare assistant in moving Mary from her chair to a commode. The healthcare assistant goes to put her arm under Mary's axilla and asks you to put your arm under Mary's other axilla and then lift Mary up.

1 What is this move called, and should you carry it out?
2 If not, what should you do instead?
3 If the healthcare assistant insists on moving the patient in this manner what should you do?

Website

⊕ **www.oxfordtextbooks.co.uk/orc/docherty/**
You may find it helpful to work through our short online quiz and interactive scenarios intended to help you to develop and apply the skills in this section.

References

HMSO (1974). *Health and Safety at Work Act. HMSO,* London.

HSE (1998). *Lifting Operations and Lifting Equipment Regulations.* HMSO, London.

HSE (2002). *Manual Handling Operations Regulations 1992. As amended 2002.* HMSO, London.

RCN (2002). *Code of Practice for Patient Handling.* Royal College of Nursing, London.

Smith J (2005). *The Guide to the Handling of People,* 5th edn. The National Back Pain Association and The Royal College of Nursing, London.

Useful further reading and websites

Blood R (2005). Safe moving and handling of individuals. *Nursing and Residential Care,* **7**(10), 439–41.
This article explains how to move individuals safely by preparing individuals, equipment and the environment and by promoting independence as much as possible.

Brown Wilson C (2001). Safer handling practice for nurses: a review of the literature. *British Journal of Nursing,* **10**(2), 108–14.
This article reviews the research on the moving and handling of patients. It states that safer handling practice has the potential to positively influence the mobility of older people.

Chell P (2003). Moving and handling: implications of bad practice. *Nursing and Residential Care,* **5**(6), 276–9.
This article explains how to avoid incorrect moving and handling techniques and the relevant legislation.

Department of Health (2002). *NHS Back in Work Back Pack,* Department of Health, London.
This pack contains practical guidance, key contacts, and useful publications, information brochures, and posters.

Health and Safety Executive website, www.hse.gov.uk/msd/index.htm.
This is a very good website. This link takes you directly to the section containing information about musculoskeletal disorders.

Hignett S, Crumpton E, Ruszula S, Alexander P, Fray M, and Fletcher B (2003). Evidence-based patient handling: systematic review. *Nursing Standard,* **17**(33), 33–6.
This article summarizes the findings of a systematic review of patient handling and supports the provision of equipment and multifactor intervention strategies based on risk assessments.

HSE (2004). *Manual Handling Operations Regulations 1992 Guidance on Regulations,* HMSO, London.

RCN (2001a). *Manual Handling Assessments in Hospitals,* Royal College of Nursing, London.

RCN (2001b). *Changing Practice—Improving Health: An Integrated Back Injury Prevention Programme for Nursing and Care Homes*, Royal College of Nursing, London.

This RCN document is based on a pilot project and discusses useful interventions that can be part of an integrated injury prevention programme for nursing and care homes.

Trew M and Everett T (2001). *Human Movement: An Introductory Text*, 4th edn, Churchill Livingstone, London.

This textbook, designed for healthcare professionals, discusses human movement and the assessment and rehabilitation of patients with impaired movement and function. It contains case studies and activities. Check **⚫ www.oxfordtextbooks.co.uk/orc/ docherty/** for changes and new developments. Updated research, guidelines, or equipment will be added every four months.

 Answers to scenario

1   This is called an underarm or drag lift and should not be carried out, owing to the risks to both patient and handler.

2   Instead, you should risk-assess the situation using ELITE and look in Mary's care plan to find her moving and handling assessment (this should let you know whether she can weight-bear, how much assistance she requires, etc.). You should then follow the principles of efficient movement. It will be important to explain to Mary what you are going to do as this may be the first time that she has been moved in this way. Further information can be found in Chapter 10.

3   You must approach this in a nonconfrontational way; for example, suggest an alternative by explaining the benefits, to both Mary and the healthcare assistant, of your alternative suggestion. You should not blame the healthcare assistant or appear condescending.

If the healthcare assistant still does not agree then you should state that you cannot take part in this move and that you will need to speak to your mentor.

This can be a very difficult situation to deal with as a student—remember that you have support at the university, or there may be a moving and handling coordinator linked to your placement area to whom you could speak; however, the priority when moving patients is that neither you nor your patient is put at risk.

2.3 The management of aggression and violence

Introduction

Aggression and violence are often thought to be the domain of the mental-health nurse and those adult nurses working in Accident and Emergency Departments, but either can be a facet of all branches of nursing and midwifery (almost 10% of adult nurses are assaulted in the UK each year, Wells and Bowers, 2002). It is not, however, a 'fact of life' or 'part of the job' that has to be tolerated. Aggression and violence can be anticipated, avoided, and prevented; in other words, they can be managed.

This section will not equip you to deal with a violent situation but it will help you understand the importance of:

● Beginning to recognize the potential for violence in situations (in other words—risk assessment)
● Allowing experienced staff to deal with violent or potentially violent situations
● Attending training sessions given by the university or placement

Key point: The skills shown here will help reinforce training but they will not replace it.

Some of the major skills in the management of aggression and violence will involve subjects already encountered elsewhere in this book; for example, observation, communication, and reporting. Observation and communication, in particular, are key parts of the process of **de-escalation**. This is the main 'skill' in the management of aggression and violence as its purpose is to reduce the level of actual or potential conflict.

In this section, we will look at some definitions of aggression and violence, some of the general causes of conflict in a clinical setting, how to recognize when someone is becoming aggressive or violent, and how and when to use the skills of de-escalation. When violence does occur, there are some skills that you can use to keep yourself safe and these will be dealt with later in the section.

These skills, however, will only keep you safe when you learn them fully; after reading this chapter and after taking some formal training. Some form of training is offered in many trusts and health authorities and may be locally developed or might be the Conflict Resolution Training offered by the NHS Counter Fraud and Security Services. You will find the website address for this and, in Scotland, the Flying Start website looking at conflict resolution, at the end of this section.

Learning outcomes

These outcomes relate to number 19 of the NMC's Essential Skill Clusters and specifically to Care Domains 2 and 3 of the NMC's Standards of Proficiency for Pre-registration Nursing (outcomes to be achieved for entry to branch).

On reading the chapter and associated web pages and undertaking supervised activities, the student will be able to:

- Discuss various concepts of aggression and violence
- Understand the difference between anger and aggression
- Recognize clinical situations where aggression and violence are possible outcomes
- Understand the role played by communication in management of aggression and violence
- Discuss the principles of de-escalation
- Demonstrate the 'protective stance' and the fundamental breakaway techniques

Prior knowledge

To use the skills of de-escalation it is important to understand the principles of communication and relationship building. This can be found in a range of texts but also elsewhere in this book.

Particular attention should be paid to:

- Nonverbal communication (including tone of voice and body posture)
- Eye contact
- Barriers to communication
- Respect for the individual

What are aggression and violence?

These are difficult to define. Some define them separately; often aggression is seen as the threat and violence, the act; whereas others use the terms interchangeably. Some people may see a situation as aggressive or violent, whereas others will not. There are many articles on violence for nurses, many stating the lack of clarity of definition or simply not attempting a definition.

Here, we will use aggression (which can be either verbal or physical) to mean the threat of violence, which is an action intended to cause harm or injury—although it can be any action that is 'perceived by the victim' to be intended to cause harm, either physical or psychological.

Recognizing aggression

It is easier to recognize changes in behaviour in someone you know. You will know when someone with whom you have a relationship is becoming angry. You might have seen the signs before. However, many people, whether they are patients, relatives, or other visitors to your clinical area will not be known to you. Each will have a unique way of expressing anger or aggression. Any unusual behaviour should be noted.

The following are common signs that might be noticed when someone is becoming aggressive (Luck *et al.* (2007).

- Person may be flushed
- Angry facial expression
- Voice volume might increase or person might become unusually quiet
- Speech content becomes more aggressive or sarcastic
- Increased eye contact
- Increased body tension
- Erratic or quick movements

- Threatening behaviour—physical or verbal
- Restlessness and pacing

Anger

Anger is OK. While we do not want anyone to be angry at us and we do not want to be angry, it is a normal emotion and is a reaction to a set of circumstances, which will be unique to the individual. People can become angry for a number of reasons; they may be dealing with something that is not being resolved, they might feel that they are being treated unfairly or they may think that someone has been rude to them or otherwise disrespectful. Anger is a feeling—it is not an action (and it is not aggression).

Can we control anger or is it something that must take its course?

It is usually healthier that anger is let out and not 'bottled up'. However, unexpressed anger will not necessarily cause problems later unless this is your usual way of dealing with it. People have different ways of dealing with their anger. They might express it, letting others know that they are angry and why, or they might suppress it and try to hide it from others (and perhaps themselves).

Letting someone know you are angry at something they have done is usually useful, if done in a calm, respectful way. Raising your voice to let everyone know you are angry is not usually a useful way of doing it (the first may be seen as assertive, the other, aggressive).

(Slamming doors and 'stamping off' is seldom useful and kicking the cat never is—especially not to the cat... It does not solve anything—it's better to let your anger out in some constructive way, exercise, work, and so on—or destructive, but only if you have something you want broken, like an old garden shed.)

It is important to recognize the difference between anger and aggression.

Anger exercise

This exercise can be a group, paired or individual task. If done with a partner or group, fill in your own table first and then discuss the result. This exercise should take about 20 minutes to complete.

Think of an occasion recently where you have been angry (nothing too serious—perhaps a shop assistant was rude to you or someone did not do something you had asked them to and preferably something you are not still angry about). Write the situation in a table (such as given in Table 2.4).

Now ask yourself the following questions:

- Was the situation resolved?
- If it was resolved, was it in a positive way?
- What was the most useful thing to do in its resolution?
- How easy is it to describe feelings without talking about thought or actions?
- Did you allow yourself to feel anger?
- After thinking about it or discussing it, was the anger reasonable?

Spend a few minutes discussing the exercise with your partner or in a group. Do the feelings of anger resurface when you speak about it?

Ethical and legal considerations

The NMC Code of Conduct states:

Make the care of people your first concern, treating them as individuals and respecting their dignity.

Table 2.4 Anger exercise

I was angry because	I felt (describe the actual feelings)	I resolved the situation by

The law requires that a person:

... may use such force as is reasonable in the circumstances for the purposes of:

- Self-defence; or
- Defence of another; or
- Defence of property; or
- Prevention of crime; or
- Lawful arrest

In assessing the reasonableness of the force used, prosecutors should ask two questions:

- Was the use of force justified in the circumstances, i.e. was there a need for any force at all? and
- Was the force used excessive in the circumstances?

The courts have indicated that both questions are to answered on the basis of the facts as the accused honestly believed them to be.
(Crown Prosecution Service at http://cps.gov.uk/ legal/section5/chapter_d.html#04)

2.3.1 **De-escalation**

Definition

De-escalation aims to prevent violence developing in a situation where there are tensions and heightened emotions. It incorporates communication skills (see Section 2.1 and Chapter 4) and a range of protective measures, including assertiveness. Assertiveness would require a chapter on its own, however, it is an essential part of the process of de-escalation, and so merits further reading (for example, Dryden and Constantinou 2004).

Remember that, for the most part, people become angry because they are anxious, fearful, or frustrated, and often just want someone to listen to them and keep them informed. Relatives often only want to protect the person they have brought to hospital; so, a respectful, understanding, manner is often all that is required to help them remain calm.

De-escalation is about reducing the likelihood of violence taking place when someone is angry and becoming aggressive.

People, whether they are patients, relatives, or others likely to be encountered in clinical areas, should be dealt with in a reasonable and calm manner. Nurses must learn to control their own responses to anger and aggression. Don't meet aggression with aggression.

Always try to be aware of how you might appear or sound. It is your responsibility to avoid further **confrontation** (NICE 2005) and not to **provoke** escalation of the situation.

Background

If someone is shouting at you, the impulse might be to shout back at them. That's the key—impulse. If you do not exhibit impulse control, why should the other person? If you 'model' calm behaviour the other person is more likely to respond in that way.

What is your body doing during a confrontation? Does it look ready for a fight? Is your expression angry, your jaw tight, your hands clenched into fists; are you making prolonged eye contact? If so, try to let these be more relaxed.

Allow space and time to talk about what is troubling the person—listen and try to understand why he or she is upset. Acknowledge concerns and frustrations the person might have.

It may be useful to take the person to a quieter, perhaps less stimulating environment. Speak to the person in a measured way. Try to avoid large variations in tone, excitement, and body movement, especially hand gestures.

Be aware of the level of understanding the person is likely to have. Although you should not assume lack of understanding, especially in someone old, very young, or with learning disability.

Anger exercise

Remember a time when you were angry: do the feelings come back? If so, control them; relax your jaw, breathe more deeply and slowly, tell yourself, I do not need to be angry at the moment—relax—prove to yourself that anger is controllable.

When to use de-escalation skills

De-escalation is not the first step in the management of aggression, it follows where other measures have been insufficient or the situation was not anticipated. This can happen for a number of reasons; a normal situation can break down, there can be misinterpretations of events or stimuli, or mistakes can be made.

It is impossible to make sure every eventuality is covered but, if sufficient information is available to people, if nurses are courteous and treat individuals with respect, if the environment is reasonable, then there is less likelihood of aggression arising.

Procedure: a protective stance

Key point: When aggression cannot be avoided it is important to keep yourself and others safe. Get help immediately or get out of the situation. Normally, a more senior person will take control of dealing with a violent incident; a student should be supervised at all times to ensure that he or she is not left in a threatening situation.

If you have to wait for help to arrive and cannot, immediately, remove yourself from the area, *make yourself into a smaller target*. To adopt a protective stance, as shown in **Fig. 2.13**, you stand side-on to the person to present a smaller area as a target and protect your more delicate parts—abdomen, groin, and face. You have stepped away from the person, thus, increasing the distance between you.

It is important to have a more solid base. If your weight is evenly balanced between your two feet, then it is more difficult for an assailant to knock or pull you down. You can move forwards or backwards in this stance without making yourself more vulnerable.

In the protective stance you will also be using the larger muscle groups in your hips and legs to help propel you backwards or forwards. By bending your legs slightly, you have these muscles in a more 'ready' state.

Your right hand protects your face and upper body. Your arm should be, more or less, in line with your body and bent so that your hand is at shoulder height (do not allow it to block the line of sight between you and the other person).

Your hand should be open, with your fingers together and your thumb tucked in. Your left hand is also open and held across your abdomen, thus, it protects your abdomen and lower body.

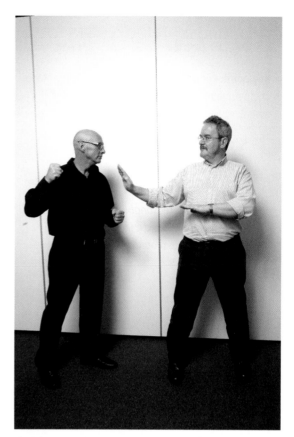

Figure 2.13 Protective stance

The protective stance is also central to some of the breakaway moves that follow.

Other factors to consider

Avoiding injury

The best way to avoid injury is to ensure that you are not there when someone takes a swing or a grab for you. Run away if you can (if you can't avoid being there in the first place). When you are dealing with someone known to be violent, someone unknown, or where you get a sense of escalating anger, do not get too close to the person. Stay one and a half to two paces away. This means that if the person tries to reach you, he or she must first take a step forwards. This gives you a little time to move away—either completely or into a protective stance. If you are closer than this, the person can simply strike out. Blows, whether they are slaps or punches, are generally very fast and difficult to dodge. Being further away means that you have time to react as the person moves forwards.

Adopting a protective stance

Key point: Remember that this is a 'protective stance' not a fighting stance. Continue to try to de-escalate the situation; continue to speak to the person, calmly. If the person moves towards you, do not raise your voice; be firm and assertive, asking them, for instance, to 'Back off, please,' or 'Stay where you are, please.'

▶ Step	Rationale
1 Turn (stepping back) so that you are side on to the person.	You present a smaller target and turn the more sensitive areas away from assault.
2 Lift your right hand to guard your face and your left hand to protect your middle.	Right hand forwards, because the majority of people are right-handed (if the assailant is left-handed – review the risk and take appropriate action – perhaps reversing the stance). Make sure that you don't cover your face or block your view of the assailant.
3 Keep your feet apart, knees slightly bent, and your weight evenly spread between both feet.	This gives a more solid, grounded base and means that your bigger leg muscles are in a state of readiness to move. Your equal balance means that you are less easy to knock down or be pulled off balance.
4 Keep your feet parallel to one another.	This means that you can move backwards or forwards easily without walking backwards, which would expose you to risk.
5 Continue to look at the person, maintaining good eye contact. You will be looking along your right shoulder.	You can see what the person is doing and he or she can see your face (especially your mouth while talking if the person has hearing difficulties) continuing to talk – de-escalation continues.

2.3.2 **Breakaway techniques**

Definition

This section will concentrate on three techniques:

1　An elbow lift (sounds odd but is very effective in many situations),
2　Dealing with wrist grabs,
3　Scratches.

These are three simple and effective methods of removing yourself from potential damage. When done quickly and effectively, they will give you confidence in dealing with an assailant. They also demonstrate to the other person that you are taking back control of the situation and that, in itself, might reduce the possibility of further violence

When to use breakaway techniques

When a situation has escalated to the point where an attacker has managed to get a hold of you. In this case, we are speaking about arm or clothing grabs and strangle holds and scratches.

Key point: If a patient is likely to be violent, do not approach alone. Make sure that you have support with

Using an elbow lift to free yourself

Step	Rationale
1 Step back into the 'protective stance'. As you do so, your right hand grasps the person's right wrist. This might take the person by surprise and affect his or her balance (try to reach over the assailant's two arms and use leverage by pushing your elbow down on their arms; if the person is too tall for you to do this, reach between the arms) (see Fig. 2.14).	Moving into the protective stance turns you away from the person and protects more sensitive areas. It might also dislodge the person's grip
2 Now, bring the lower, left hand up to lift the person's elbow and step forwards, in front of the person, continuing to push the elbow. This will force the assailant to turn away from you.	This has the effect of turning the person away from you, changing his or her centre of gravity – the person will have to move away in order to keep balance. (it is important that you push the elbow from below – if you push from the side there is a danger of damaging the person's arm – pushing against the joint.)
3 Then you move away from the assailant.	Get out of reach of the person – especially if you have no support. Move to a safe place.
4 If your chest hair or skin is gripped or in a hair pull; rather than gripping the wrist, grip the side of the person's hand, under the little finger, and prise the hand up before continuing with the manoeuvre. This might force them to loosen their fingers slightly and ease their grip.	This also helps to turn the arm so that the elbow joint, when pushed from below will force the person away.

you to help deal with any situation that might arise. A student nurse should always be observed by more senior, experienced staff and not put in positions of risk.

Procedure: the elbow lift

This is a useful manoeuvre when someone grips your hair, neck or clothing.

It is, of course, better to avoid being grabbed at all but, when it does happen, this is a quick and effective method of freeing yourself. Someone has a grip on your clothing at your neck. He or she is likely to be angry and, perhaps, intent on injuring you so move fairly quickly (this is sometimes called inward **rotation**).

Procedure: wrist grabs

It is not uncommon to be grabbed by the wrist, sometimes by confused, elderly people; in which case, make a judgement about the strength of the grip, and the frailty of the hand behind it. Your wrist may also be grasped by others, who are simply intent on keeping your attention.

A wrist grab can be surprisingly easy to get out of, even if the person is quite strong. Remember, the thumbs are the weakest part of this grip—even when two hands are used. You would not, normally, have to adopt the protective stance in this unless you consider the intent to be very threatening. You would find it difficult to do this anyway, if your wrist was being held.

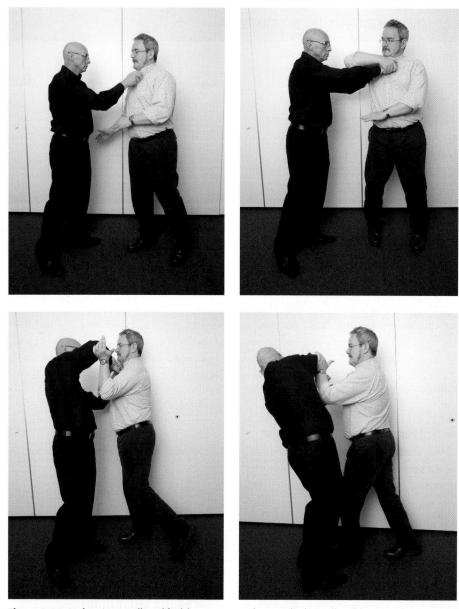

Figure 2.14 Performing an elbow lift: (a) aggressor grabs nurse's shirt collar; (b) nurse adopts protective stance and uses right hand to grab aggressor's right wrist; (c) nurse uses left hand to push aggressor's right elbow upwards; (d) the aggressor is forced to turn;   (*Continued*)

Breaking away from wrist grabs

Step	Rationale
1 If held in this way, check where the person's thumb is in the grip and push against it	The thumb is the weakest part of the grip and, if the person's hand does not completely encircle your wrist, there will be a gap.
2 If the thumb is down – push your arm down (see Fig. 2.15), if it is up, raise your arm by bending your elbow (rather than lifting your shoulder, see Fig. 2.16)	The elbow only bends in one way and that is a powerful action – the flexibility of the shoulder reduces its strength.
3 If the grip is strong, or where two hands are gripping, clench your fist. This will strengthen your wrist and makes the extraction easier. You might even grab your own, gripped, hand and pull it out of the grip	If your hand remains 'soft' and you try to pull it through against a strong grip, you might injure yourself. Clenching your fist tenses muscles in the forearm and hand.
4 The element of surprise is also useful here, especially against a strong grip. 'Feinting' in one direction may make the person attempt to change their grip and gives more time for you to remove yourself	The person will normally, momentarily change their grip making it easier for you to break free.

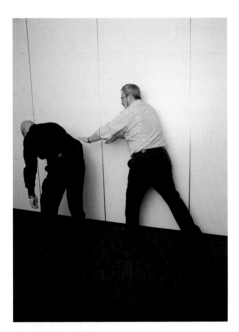

Figure 2.14 (e) the aggressor moves away to correct balance

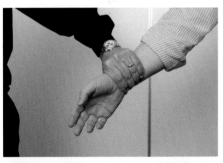
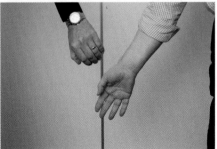

Figure 2.15 Wrist grab: the aggressor's thumb is down; the nurse breaks away by pushing the arm down and out of the grab

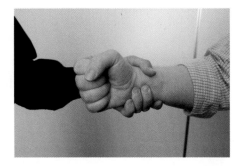

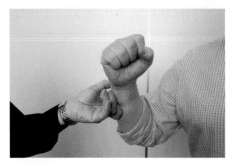

Figure 2.16 Wrist grab: the aggressor's thumb is up; the nurse breaks away by bending the elbow to raise the arm out of the grab. Note the nurse's clenched fist; this gives the movement more strength.

Procedure: scratches

Scratches can be unpleasant, painful, and potentially open cuts up to infection from dirty fingernails. You will want to avoid the skin being broken or broken further if already pierced.

Aftercare

If possible, see to the person who carried out the attack as soon as possible. You would not do this if the person is still very angry or aggressive: in this case de-escalation should continue, but after an attack, the person will have settled and may be shocked or upset that he or she has assaulted someone. Reassure the person and, if possible get them to talk about the problem. Try to find out the reasons for their anger. This will not be done immediately if the attack has been violent and, particularly, if someone has been injured.

Police might be involved and they will take the lead in potentially dangerous situations.

Developing your skills

There will be times in your nursing career when you will be dealing with the unknown. When you first visit a patient at home and you don't know the family; when you are receiving a new admission; when you go to work in a new unit or community team. You will have to gain a knowledge and understanding of new patients and their behaviours and the likely behaviours of others around them. If you know the patients you are working with, you are less likely to be taken by surprise. It is always worthwhile to consult others and read nursing notes.

If you work with patients who have a history of aggression, find out the triggers to this aggression and try to avoid them. Be aware of how you approach the person; perhaps directly if the person is suspicious, more obliquely if you know that the person is likely to lash out (though being careful not to 'surprise' them).

Other factors to consider

Children and young people

When dealing with children and young people your approach will vary according to their size, level of understanding, and degree of arousal. Different techniques might be used in breakaway and control, including de-escalation; there will be local policy on dealing with violence in young people. Your awareness and arousal will also be heightened in the face of violence, so it is important that you look at the context in which the aggression is taking place, and it is very important to risk-assess each incident. Children may be small but, if highly aroused, can cause a lot of injury to themselves or others.

Older people

Violence in old people can occur for all the same reasons as in any other adult but might also arise because of

Dealing with scratches

Step	Rationale
1 To prevent damage – fix the scratching hand by holding it across the fingers. This will prevent the scratch from going any further.	Hold the scratching hand across the fingers ensuring carry on the scratch.
2 Now lift the hand away from the direction of the scratch (see Fig. 2.17).	Prevents fingernails lifting the skin or digging further in.
3 Do not lift straight up from the skin	Lifting straight up when nails are embedded would simply lift the skin and open a wound.

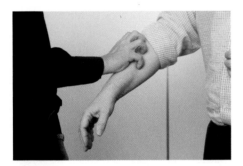
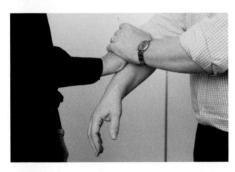
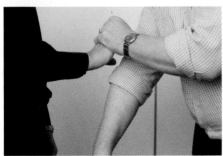

Figure 2.17 Scratches

confusion. Working with older, perhaps more frail, people (remember however, that a 75-year-old ex-boxer is still an ex-boxer) will require a more gentle approach. Frailer bodies and unsteadiness should also be taken into account in your risk assessment.

(S) Scenarios

Consider what you should do in the following situations, then turn to the end of the section to check your answers.

Further scenarios are available at 🌐 **www.oxford textbooks.co.uk/orc/docherty/**

(S) Scenario 1: an angry parent

A woman brings her young son to A & E. He has had a fall and sustained extensive bruising to his leg and both he and his mother are distressed by this. He has been seen by the triage nurse and has been assessed as being nonurgent. Because there are several more urgent cases they have to wait for some time. The woman thinks that her son is more seriously injured and is angry at having to wait as she has another child to pick up from school and expresses this to anyone within earshot.

What would you say to this woman?

1   Please be quiet, you are upsetting other patients.
2   Your son is not seriously injured and will just have to wait.
3   We're sorry you are having to wait. Your son will be seen as soon as possible.
4   The doctor will see your son in the next ten minutes.

 ## Scenario 2: the assertive nurse

You are in a room with your mentor, going over your learning outcomes, when a patient walks in and sits down. She says loudly to your mentor, 'I've got a bone to pick with you. You promised you'd speak to my social worker to sort out my housing benefits. I saw you sitting in here—are you avoiding me?' The patient appears to be very angry.

Your mentor, a staff nurse, replies quietly, 'Can I ask you to come back in ten minutes when I'll be finished speaking to this student and I'll see you here to discuss what I've done so far.'

The patient stands but says, 'I'm being fobbed off again, you people never do anything for me!'

What should the staff nurse do?

1   Ask you to wait while she goes and deals with the patient.
2   Repeat what she has just said.
3   Say more forcefully to the patient, 'Wait just ten minutes and I'll see you!'
4   Say to the patient, 'I will not speak to you while you're in that mood.'

Website

🌐 **www.oxfordtextbooks.co.uk/orc/docherty/**
You may find it helpful to work through our short online quiz and interactive scenarios intended to help you to develop and apply the skills in this chapter.

References

Dryden W and Constantinou D (2004). *Assertiveness Step By Step.* Sheldon Press, London.

Luck L, Jackson D, and Usher K (2007). STAMP: components of observable behaviour that indicate potential for patient violence in emergency departments. *Journal of Advanced Nursing,* **59**, 11–19.

NICE (2005). *Violence: The Short-Term Management of Disturbed/Violent Behaviour in In-Patient Psychiatric Settings and Emergency Departments,* Clinical Guideline 25. National Institute for Clinical Excellence, London.

Wells J and Bowers L (2002). How prevalent is violence towards nurses working in general hospitals in the UK? *Journal of Advanced Nursing,* **39**(3), 230–40.

Useful further reading and websites

These contain useful guidelines for the management of aggression and violence and often are, or form part of, national and local policies on the management of violence.

CRAG Working Group on Mental Illness (1996). *The Prevention and Management of Aggression. A Good Practice Statement.* HMSO, Scotland.

CRAG was established in 1989 and is now clearly identified as the leading body within the Scottish Executive Health Department, shaping clinical effectiveness policies in Scotland (www.crag.scot.nhs.uk/).

Di Martino V, Beaulieu J, and Gentizon C-P (2005). *Framework Guidelines for Addressing Workplace Violence in the Health Sector. Training Manual.* International Council for Nurses, Public Services International, World Health Organization, and International Labour Office, Geneva, Switzerland, www.icn.ch/SEW_training_manual.pdf.

www.cfsms.nhs.uk/training/crt.html.
This is part of the website of the NHS Counter Fraud and Security Management Service. The section on Security Management provides courses on the management of violence and also how to keep safe in a number of different situations. Much of the advice and training offered is in nonphysical, therapeutic approaches.

www.flyingstart.scot.nhs.uk/ConflictResolution.htm.

Flying Start NHS is a national development programme for all newly qualified nurses, midwives, and allied health professionals in the NHS in Scotland. It has been designed to support the transition from student to newly qualified health professional by supporting learning in everyday practice. It is a very useful site for instruction on many aspects of nursing.

Check ◉ **www.oxfordtextbooks.co.uk/orc/docherty/** for changes and new developments. Updated research, guidelines, or equipment will be added every four months.

 Answers to scenarios

Scenario 1

Answer 3 is correct. This woman is anxious about her children and although this does not solve her immediate problem, it lets her know you are still aware of her. Answers 1 and 2, while basically correct, are not respectful and do not help reduce her anxiety. They are probably more likely to make her angrier if she is in an aroused state. Answer 4 is not true—you don't know whether the doctor will definitely be able to see her in that time (what happens after the 10 minutes are up?).

Scenario 2

Answer 2 is correct. The patient is already standing to leave, but is getting a last word in. This is the assertive response. There is no need to add to what has been said. Answer 1 might seem to the patient that her approach has worked and the staff nurse is intimidated by her. Answer 3 is becoming more aggressive and there is no call for it. You can speak firmly to people, in an assertive way—that is, making a point but still being respectful. Answer 4 is one you might use with the person when you are discussing, in private, her behaviour, but only in certain circumstances, for example, during **socialization** training.

2.4 Infection prevention and control

Introduction

The danger of introducing or transmitting infection when working in the healthcare environment must be recognized and steps implemented to minimize this risk where possible. To engage with this process, however, it is important to understand what infection is.

Infection has been defined as the failure of the body's defences to respond to the invasion and multiplication of microorganisms. Some infections are asymptomatic, that is, the patient does not experience any signs or symptoms of that infection. Another possible outcome of the infection process is an *immune response*. In this situation, signs and symptoms will be evident and may include elevated body temperature, inflammation, pain, or localized tenderness and loss of function of the affected tissues.

Whatever the body's response to becoming infected, it is widely recognized that reducing the risk of transmission or spread of infection is a key nursing role when providing healthcare.

Learning outcomes

These outcomes relate to numbers 20 to 26 of the NMC's Essential Skill Clusters and specifically to Care Domains 2 and 3 of the NMC's Standards of Proficiency for Pre-registration Nursing (outcomes to be achieved for entry to branch).

On reading the chapter and associated web pages and undertaking supervised activities, you should be able to:

- Be aware of the professional, legal, and ethical issues surrounding infection control
- Demonstrate a knowledge of the principles of infection control

- Identify potential sources of infection when caring for clients
- Recognize possible routes of transmission
- Apply this learning to minimize the spread of infection, reducing the risks for clients, visitors and healthcare providers

Prior knowledge

When attempting to minimize the risk or transmission of infection, nurses must have a sound knowledge of their related professional, legal, and ethical responsibilities. Furthermore, a basic knowledge of the pathophysiology associated with infection will help the nurse to recognize any indicative signs and symptoms of infection.

Professional and ethical responsibilities

The following texts will provide the necessary background reading:

- *The Code: Standards of Conduct, Performance and Ethics for Nurses and Midwives* (NMC 2008). This document highlights the key principle of protecting the client from harm
- *An NMC Guide for Students of Nursing and Midwifery* (NMC 2005a). This document provides general guidance for students when in clinical placement including client confidentiality and student accountability
- *Guidelines for Records and Record Keeping* (NMC 2005b). Communicating information to the appropriate person is a key element of infection control— this will allow the necessary action to be taken. This document addresses communication and documentation

Legal and health authority

It will be necessary to consult the following sources of information:

- *Local infection-control policies*. Local service providers produce infection-control policies to guide healthcare staff when caring for clients; copies of this documentation should be available in clinical areas
- *The Health Act 2006: Code of Practice for the Prevention and Control of Healthcare Associated Infections* (Department of Health 2006). This sets out the criteria on which NHS service providers base local infection control policies
- *Uniforms and Workwear: An Evidence Base for Developing Local Policy* (Department of Health 2007). Provides the evidence underpinning local staff uniform policies in relation to infection control. Those working in the community, mental-health and learning-disability areas may not wear uniforms: refer to service-specific policies for further guidance

Pathophysiology and clinical features of infection

Attainment of the skills within this chapter should be underpinned by a sound knowledge of the clinical features that may be exhibited by the client when infection is present. As such, a basic knowledge of the pathophysiology of the infection process is beneficial. It is important to remember that the presence of these indicators of infection will provide the nurse with the opportunity to initiate interventions that, if effective, can contribute to both the minimization of infection spread *and* overall eradication of the causative microorganisms.

There are many texts, professional journals, and online resources where this information is located; a keyword literature search may also be useful.

Background

Rationale for infection prevention and control

The nurse will come into contact with clients from various backgrounds with differing healthcare needs; these

Table 2.5 Universal precautions to prevent infection

Precaution	Rationale
Effective hand hygiene	Reduces the transmission of microorganisms
When in contact with body fluids and spillages, treat as a possible source of infection; wear protective clothing and disinfect the area following local infection control guidelines	Some infections may be undiagnosed and can be transmitted in body fluids or spillages
Cover any broken skin with a waterproof dressing	Broken skin is a direct route of entry for microorganisms
Dispose of sharps safely	Sharps pose a health and safety risk; they can puncture the skin and can also transmit microorganisms
Dispose of waste safely; follow clinical waste policy	Clinical waste is a source of microorganisms; inappropriate disposal can increase the risk of infection spread
Decontaminate equipment.	Equipment is often used by more than one patient; correct cleaning during use and before transfer to another patient can reduce the spread of infection

ever-changing demands increase the risk of cross-contamination for clients, visitors, and healthcare staff. Therefore, when providing care, the nurse must be aware of both the *potential for infection* and the possibility that harmful microorganisms may be present but that the client might be asymptomatic. As such, adherence to procedures designed to prevent the introduction of infection and the control of pre-existing infection will contribute to ensuring the best possible care for all clients. This awareness and adherence to protocol will also provide protection for both visitors and healthcare staff.

Transmission of infection can have a detrimental effect on the clients' physical and psychological wellbeing. In addition, their stay in hospital may be elongated, as the presence of harmful microorganisms can delay the healing process and exacerbate existing medical conditions.

Therefore, when caring for clients and considering the prevention and control of infection, the nurse should not make assumptions regarding the infection risk posed and,

instead, should adopt precautionary infection control practice in all healthcare situations; these are often referred to as **universal precautions**.

Universal precautions

It is possible for the infection status of a patient to be unknown or in a state of change, therefore, precautionary measures that should be adopted by all healthcare staff to safeguard; clients, visitors, and fellow colleagues should an undiagnosed infection be present. The key principles of the *universal precautionary* approach are given in **Table 2.5**.

Factors that increase the risk of infection

The large variety of clients presenting with healthcare needs increases the likelihood of infection already being present and, thereafter, transmitted to others.

There are additional factors, however, that are known to further increase the risk of infection. These include:

- The presence of invasive devices
- Surgical wounds
- Extremes of age—newborns and the elderly are more susceptible to infection
- Immunosuppressant drugs, such as **chemotherapy**
- The presence of underlying disease
- Poor hand-washing techniques

The nurse must be aware of these predisposing factors, as they increase the risk of infection for the client (Storr *et al.* 2005). As with all clients, an individualized care plan should be undertaken to ensure that the care given minimizes the risk of infection.

When considering the clinical skills relating to infection control, the key elements are (ICNA 2005):

- Hand hygiene
- Personal protective clothing and equipment
- Cleaning of equipment
- Clinical waste and linen disposal
- Source isolation
- Protective isolation
- Safe management of accidents and spillages

Each of these areas, if addressed effectively, can reduce the risk of cross contamination with harmful microorganisms. One key principle that applies to all aspects of infection control, however, is *hand hygiene*. The student nurse must be fully aware of the correct technique for both hand washing and application of hand gel.

2.4.1 **Hand hygiene**

Definition

Hand hygiene is widely acknowledged as the single most effective intervention when attempting to reduce the spread of microorganisms (Storr and Clayton-Kent 2004). As such, if the skill is performed effectively, it will contribute to both the eradication of microorganisms and the transmission of infection between clients, visitors, and healthcare staff.

When to use soap and water or hand gel

There are many different ways to wash your hands in the clinical area. Each is dependent on the task or clinical activity being undertaken. However, hand washing with plain soap and water should always be performed before *and* after patient contact and sometimes during the task if hands have become soiled. Student nurses are morally and legally accountable for their own actions and should base their hand washing practice on these guidelines.

Nurses are also responsible for their own practice and must decide whether hand washing or application of hand gel should be carried out. As a student, however, you may not be sure which is the most appropriate; your mentor can provide guidance in these situations. It is important to remember, however, that hand gel is ineffective in the presence of organic material and should therefore only be carried out in the absence of any visible soiling. If your hands are dirty then you must wash them.

Aftercare

After washing hands ensure that you leave the sink clean and dry and that all waste is disposed of according to local policy guidelines.

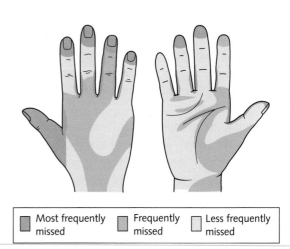

| ■ Most frequently missed | ■ Frequently missed | □ Less frequently missed |

Figure 2.18 Areas of hands most frequently missed during washing

Hand washing and aseptic hand washing

- Sink with elbow or foot-operated taps,
- Liquid soap for hand washing,
- **Antimicrobial** soap for aseptic hand washing,
- Disposable towels,
- Waste disposal bin operated by a foot pedal.

Key points: This procedure should be followed regardless of which detergent is used. Being organized will both save time and contribute to the effectiveness of the procedure.

▶ Step / Rationale

	Step	Rationale
1	Remove any jewellery and wristwatches.	These checks will help to ensure that all surfaces of the hand and wrist are exposed to detergent and water.
2	Securely cover any breaks in your own skin with a waterproof dressing.	All areas of the hand and wrists can be dried thoroughly.
3	Make sure you are not allergic to the detergent to be used.	Seek advice from your senior colleagues if you think you have an allergy to any of the commonly used hand-cleansing preparations and take appropriate action.
4	Turn on the taps – adjust the water flow until a comfortably warm temperature is achieved and the splashing of water to surrounding areas is minimized.	Care during this initial phase will reduce the risk of scalding and will also minimize splashing of water.
5	Wet both hands thoroughly.	Lathering of soap will be easier.
6	Apply the chosen detergent solution and rub the hands together to create a soapy lather.	Lathering of soap will help to dislodge microorganisms from the hands.
7	Continue to rub hands together briskly, paying particular attention to the areas highlighted in Fig. 2.18, and following the method shown in Fig. 2.19.	Rubbing hands together briskly will help to dislodge microorganisms. Also, the likelihood of missing the areas highlighted in Fig. 2.18 can be reduced if the approach advocated in Fig. 2.19 is followed.
8	A nailbrush should only be used if the nails are dirty – it should not be used on the skin.	Using a nail brush on the skin is not recommended as it can cause small abrasions.
9	Continue to wash hands, as directed in Fig. 2.19, for a minimum of 15 seconds.	The duration of washing is directly proportional to the number of microorganisms dislodged.
10	Rinse hands thoroughly under the warm water, again being careful not to splash the surrounding area. There should be no visible trace of detergent remaining on the hands.	Rinsing the hands is part of the microorganism dislodgement process and must be thorough in nature. If detergent remains visible after rinsing then rinsing should be repeated.

continued

11 Turn off the water using either the elbow or foot depending on the taps. If the taps do not operate this way, leave the water running until drying of the hands is complete, when the taps can be turned off using a clean paper towel.

At this stage the hands should be clean; therefore, it is essential that the hands do not touch the taps as they may then become recontaminated with microorganisms.

12 Disposable paper towels should be used to pat the hands dry; it is recommended that drying should be initiated at the fingertips and proceed upwards to the wrists.

Disposable towels are recommended as they are for single use only and will reduce the risk of recontamination of the hands after washing. Remember: warm damp areas, such as ineffectively dried hands, are optimal for the growth of microorganisms.

13 Used paper towels should be disposed of according to the local infection control policy.

Local policies for waste disposal form part of the infection control procedures in healthcare.

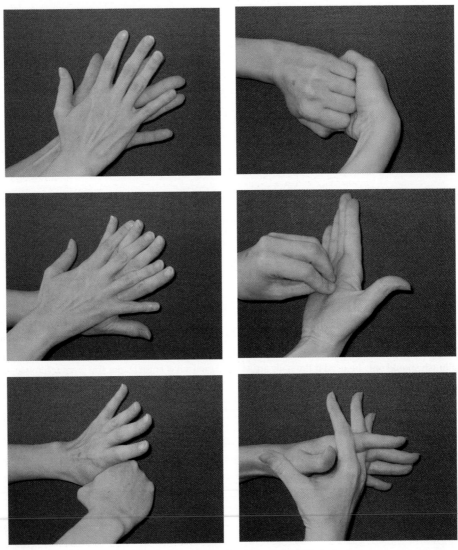

Figure 2.19 Hand washing technique. Courtesy of Debbie King and Katie Burke.

Application of antiseptic hand rub

PREPARATION

You will need alcohol-based or antiseptic rub, preferably from a pump dispenser. Utilizing a pump dispenser reduces the risk of further contamination when coming into contact with the container.

Key point: The use of either alcohol or antiseptic rub will make this procedure effective.

Step	Rationale
1 The hands should have been washed previously and must be visibly clean.	Hand rub will reduce the number of microorganisms on visibly clean hands. However, it will be completely ineffective on hands that are soiled to begin with.
2 All jewellery and wristwatches should be removed.	Removing jewellery and wristwatches will ensure that all areas of the hands are exposed to the hand rub solution.
3 Any breaks in your own skin should be securely covered by a waterproof dressing.	As some hand-rub solutions are alcohol-based they can cause irritation or pain if the skin is broken.
4 Make sure you are not allergic to the hand rub to be used.	Allergy can lead to broken skin; this can be painful and increases the risk of infection for both the nurse and the patient.
5 Dispense the hand rub from the container, ensuring enough is obtained to cover all areas of the hands.	All areas must be covered with hand rub to promote effective microorganism removal.
6 Rub hands together briskly, as for hand washing. Continue until the hands are dry.	The rubbing action will contribute to microorganism removal by spreading the hand rub over all aspects of the hands.

Developing your skills

Remember the importance of continual assessment of hand hygiene; it may be necessary to wash your hands during tasks or procedures.

Other factors to consider

In a patient's own home

When caring for patients in their own homes in the community setting, you should ask permission to use the sink or hand basin. The method of hand washing will depend on what is available to you in the home (Jenkinson *et al.* 2006). Patients will usually have soap and water although they may not have taps that can be operated by elbows; in these situations consider applying hand gel after washing (Gould *et al.* 2000). Most community staff carry portable hand gel dispensers; you should make sure that you are provided with this when working in the community setting.

2.4.2 **Personal protective clothing and equipment**

Definition

This is clothing that is worn when practising in the clinical area or when working with clients requiring healthcare interventions in the community.

Selecting appropriate clothing

You must develop the ability to assess each situation as it arises. This assessment will form the basis for the decisions made in relation to protective clothing and equipment.

Key points: The term workplace uniform refers to clothing as dictated by local workplace guidelines.

Personal glasses are not considered as suitable eye protection if splashing is a risk.

Nursing situation	Clothing/equipment and appropriate actions	Rationale
No direct client contact For example: ● Answering the telephone ● Writing client notes ● Communicating with colleagues	Workplace uniform or clothing as directed by local policy guidelines	In the absence of direct client contact the risk of cross contamination of microorganisms is greatly reduced. Therefore, it is acceptable to wear workplace uniform without additional protective clothing or equipment (Leggatt and Watterson 2005).
Possible contamination: blood, body fluids or microorganisms. For example: ● Bed making ● Collection of specimens ● Disposal of domestic or clinical waste ● Cleaning of contaminated equipment	Workplace uniform Plastic apron Disposable gloves Remember: ● Wash hands before donning protective clothing/equipment. ● Gloves are available in various sizes; choose a size that fits securely. ● After the procedure/activity dispose of apron and gloves as per local infection control policy guidelines. ● If there is a risk of splashing then eye protection and a face mask should also be worn. ● Personal glasses are not considered as suitable eye protection if splashing is a risk.	Everyday clinical activities carry the risk of microorganism transmission. Whilst the risk is apparent in relation to blood and bodily fluids, it is important to remember that microorganisms are invisible to the naked eye. As such, direct contact with clinical or domestic waste, dirty linen, or contaminated equipment poses a significant risk. Plastic aprons and disposable gloves are quick and easy to apply. These items can be renewed when necessary, reducing the risk of microorganism transmission when in contact with clients. Securely fitting protective clothing and equipment further reduces the risk of microorganism spread as it can be disposed of and renewed when required. Local infection control policies provide detailed guidelines for the disposal of this equipment. Adherence to these guidelines reduces the infection risk for staff disposing of this clothing or equipment.

Selecting appropriate clothing

Workplace uniforms

These garments serve for staff identification and contribute to minimizing the spread of infection. They may be considered unnecessary and may not be worn in some areas, so please refer to local policy for further guidance.

Protective equipment

There are a number of items designed specifically to reduce the risk of spreading microorganisms. These are worn in conjunction with the workplace uniform or over personal clothing if necessary.

When to use personal protection clothing and equipment

Personal protective clothing and equipment are recommended to help reduce the spread of microorganisms when in contact with clients, visitors, and fellow colleagues (Health Protection Scotland 2008). Whilst the wearing of the workplace uniform is compulsory in some areas, nursing students must develop the skill of understanding when, where, and how to use protective equipment. Attainment of this skill will help to reduce the risk of transmission of microorganisms when practicing clinical skills.

Aftercare

It is important to remain vigilant whilst using personal protective clothing or equipment; the nurse must ensure that there has been no breach. Should a breach occur, the nurse should ask a colleague to relieve them of the task; this will allow retrieval of new clothing or equipment.

Personal protective clothing should be removed following completion of the identified task and disposed of according to local policy guidelines; this will further reduce the risk of transmitting an infection.

Developing your skills

You should ensure that you wear the correct apron depending on the task to be undertaken; local infection control policies will provide this information. Wearing the correct clothing identifies the nature of the task you are undertaking to other members of staff. Whilst personal protective clothing is viewed as an essential aspect of reducing transmission of infection, the patient or visitors may feel increased anxiety; the nurse should, therefore, always explain at the outset why this precaution is necessary.

2.4.3 **Nursing a patient in isolation**

Definition

This skill involves providing nursing care for a patient who has been isolated from others in the ward environment. This may be because the patient is at risk of catching an infection, or because that patient has an infection that is at risk of being transmitted to other patients.

When to nurse a patient in isolation

Nursing a patient in isolation is recommended for either of the following:

- **Patient protection** In this situation, the patient may be immunocompromised and, subsequently, has increased risk of contracting infection. Nursing the patient in this situation is often referred to as *protective isolation*
- **Isolating the source** Here, a patient may have been diagnosed with a particular infection that is either high risk or highly transmissible to others. Nursing the patient in isolation in this situation is often referred to as *source isolation*

Procedure

The patient will be allocated a single room with bathroom facilities. All nursing care will be provided within the confines of the room; the patient is not permitted to go outside this area unless to undergo investigations that require transportation to another area of the hospital. Whilst similar principles apply to both *protective* and *source isolation*, it is important to remember that local policies will provide further guidance in relation to more specific nursing actions. In particular, if nursing the patient in *source isolation*, the guidelines vary depending on the infection type.

Preparation

Remember, before entering an isolation room it is important to collect all equipment necessary to undertake any tasks to be performed while there. This will reduce the need to enter and exit the room unnecessarily.

When preparing to nurse a patient in source isolation you will need to arrange:

- A single room with bathroom facilities—this will act as a physical barrier to infection
- A supply of soap, water, alcohol gel, and paper towels in the room—this will facilitate hand hygiene when entering and leaving the room
- A supply of the patient's own toiletries—this promotes personal hygiene and will also allow the patient to maintain his or her own identity
- Necessary clinical equipment including thermometer, sphygmomanometer, and stethoscope. This equipment should be used exclusively by the patient and will allow you to provide nursing care without increasing the risk of infection spread to others
- Dishes and cutlery; these will be for the patient's personal use and should not be removed from the room
- A door sign to indicate to patients, visitors, and staff members that the patient is being nursed in source isolation. This will ensure that everyone is informed

and will allow all concerned to take appropriate precautions
- An area immediately outside the room to allow visitors and staff the opportunity to don appropriate protective clothing
- Waste disposal equipment for sharps, linen, clinical, and domestic waste should be placed in the room; this will promote safe disposal while minimizing the chances of contaminating the wider environment, adhering to local policies and guidelines

Key point: Patients with a mental health problem, young children, or those with a learning disability may not be permitted to have sharps containers or waste disposal bags in their room as they may pose a risk. Seek further local guidance when caring for these individuals.

Developing your skills

It is essential that the nurse becomes familiar with each patient and the rationale for initiating either protective or source isolation. This knowledge can contribute to reducing the risk of transmission of infection and will help to ensure that appropriate nursing care is initiated.

Other factors to consider

Communication is important when caring for the patient in isolation. The patient may become bored and frustrated from the lack of companionship; there is also the risk of anger and anxiety. When providing care, the nurse should make sure that the patient is fully informed about each task performed, is encouraged to ask questions (this can sometimes alleviate anxiety) and also knows how to call for assistance if necessary.

Family members must be fully informed regarding the correct procedures when visiting a relative being cared for in isolation and, as such, the nurse must provide families with relevant information and guidance at

Protective and source isolation

Step	Rationale
1 A plastic apron should be put on before entering the room.	Your uniform will be protected.
2 Depending on the patient's diagnosis, it may be necessary to wear additional protective clothing.	Supplementary precautions may be necessary to protect staff, other patients, or the patient in isolation. This will either be necessary for your protection (source isolation) or for the protection of the patient (protective isolation).
3 Any breaks in your own skin should be securely covered by a waterproof dressing.	This will help to prevent transmission of organisms to or from the patient.
4 Undertake hand hygiene immediately on entering the room.	This will reduce the risk of transmission of new microorganisms.
5 Communication and provision of information.	The use of protective clothing can make the patient anxious and apprehensive; ensure that the patient understands why this is necessary.
6 Patient assessment; this should be carried out immediately on entering the room. It may be a simple visible assessment or it may include measurement of temperature, pulse, respiration, and blood pressure, as deemed necessary.	This will allow you to establish baseline parameters and should be recorded in the patient notes. The patient's condition may have altered since your last contact.
7 Specimen collection: protective clothing must be worn at all times when collecting body fluids for laboratory analysis. These may be labelled HIGH RISK and double-bagged, depending on the microorganism.	The presence of body fluids increases the risk of transmission of microorganisms. The HIGH RISK label warns all staff of potential danger.
8 Cleaning of equipment, dishes and cutlery: wash with warm water and general purpose detergent, making sure to dry thoroughly.	This will help to remove any microorganisms and will reduce patient risk.
9 Disposal of waste: clinical and domestic waste bags should be placed in a second bag held by another staff member outside the room. They should be secured with a ward-specific identifiable tag and then disposed of.	This procedure (double-bagging) is only necessary when nursing a patient in source isolation. It prevents the spread of infection outside the room and reduces the risk to other patients and staff. The tag allows the waste to be traced back to the ward should a query arise.

continued

10 **Disposal of linen: dirty linen is stored in a dissolvable plastic bag in the room. This should then be passed to a second staff member outside the room for double-bagging (as for waste.)**

This is also only necessary when nursing a patient in source isolation and is a measure designed to reduce the transmission of infection to other patients and staff.

the outset. This may be a good opportunity to educate patients and families. This activity can contribute to achievement of placement-specific learning outcomes.

2.4.4 **Cleaning and decontamination**

Definition

This involves the maintenance of a safe environment to support and enhance the delivery of optimal patient care. It is a cluster of skills that will help to reduce the risk of spread of infection and will ultimately contribute to the safety of the environment for patients, visitors, and staff. The key elements are:

- Cleaning equipment
- Managing accidents and spillages safely
- Disposing of clinical waste and linen safely

These particular aspects of infection control are guided by government policy, on which local guidelines and standards for practice are based. As a result, on arrival in the clinical area, it is your responsibility to familiarize yourself with local policy documentation and thereafter to adhere to the guidelines therein. General guidance is provided here in relation to each aspect of cleaning and decontamination.

When to perform cleaning and decontamination

You will be required to use these skills during the day to day routine when caring for patients. Equipment has

to be cleaned regularly if it is used over a period of time.

Procedure: Cleaning equipment

The following guidance should be considered in conjunction with local policy. However, equipment is normally cleaned by using a clean cloth soaked in a solution of warm water and detergent. If the soiling is difficult to remove, a soft brush can be used. It is important to remember to wear protective clothing when undertaking this procedure and also to dry the equipment thoroughly, as a warm damp surface can promote the growth of microorganisms.

Equipment is also often labelled to indicate its potential use. When deciding whether or not to clean the equipment it may be useful to consider the following;

- **Single-use equipment** This should not need to be cleaned and is usually discarded after use or if soiled
- **Single-patient use equipment** This equipment is usually cleaned according to local policy guidelines. However, it should only be used by one patient and then discarded
- **Reusable medical devices** This can include items such as a blood pressure cuff. This requires a more complex assessment of risk in relation to cleaning: if the item is soiled, has been in contact with body fluids or has been used be a patient with a known infection, then specialized sterilization may be necessary. Alternatively, if the item is visibly clean and has not been in contact with any of the above, then it may be possible to decontaminate this in the clinical area

Needlestick injury

Step	Rationale
1 Should this occur, your first response should be to call for assistance if caring for a patient.	This will allow you to administer the treatment necessary as soon as possible.
2 Encourage the wound to bleed.	To promote any infection that may have entered the wound to come out with the blood flow.
3 At the same time, wash the area under warm running water with soap or antiseptic solution.	To cleanse the wound.
4 Dry the wound and apply a waterproof dressing.	To protect the area from further contamination.
5 Report the incident to your line manager.	To advise you of what further action is required and also of the necessary paperwork to complete.

Procedure: Management of accidents and spillages

The unexpected can often occur when caring for patients and it is important to be as prepared as possible for this eventuality. Again, local policies and guidelines will dictate local procedure. However, some general principles apply in these situations, see p. 60.

Procedure: Safe disposal of clinical waste and linen

Clinical waste and dirty linen are generated when caring for patients and must be disposed of appropriately in relation to risk posed for the patients, staff, and the general public. Consider local policy, however, the following international guidelines provided in **Table 2.6** should apply to all areas, see p. 60.

Family members must be fully informed should an accident or spillage occur; this will reduce the risk for all concerned.

Developing your skills

All members of the healthcare team must communicate effectively to reduce the risk of contracting infection. This communication not only incorporates discussion, but also involves adhering to local policy guidelines and standards for safe and effective practice.

Scenario

Consider what you should do in the following situation, then turn to the end of the section to check your answers.

You have been asked to dispose of equipment used for a **subcutaneous** injection. Whilst doing this, you accidentally pierce your finger with the needle.

What action must you take?

Further scenarios are available at ☻ **www.oxford textbooks.co.uk/orc/docherty/**

Website

☻ **www.oxfordtextbooks.co.uk/orc/docherty/**
You may find it helpful to work through our short online quiz and interactive scenarios intended to help you to develop and apply the skills in this chapter.

Spillages

Key point: Once again, it is important to adhere to local policy guidelines. These should specify what is deemed appropriate to decontaminate the area. However, consider the following basic principles for guidance.

Step	Rationale
1 Cordon off the area where the spillage has occurred. Make sure that patients, visitors, and staff are in no immediate danger.	To prevent any danger to staff, patients, and visitors, and to stop any further spread of the contamination to footwear and the wider environment.
2 Assess the extent of the spillage and put on the necessary protective clothing and gloves.	To protect yourself from any contamination.
3 Mop up the spillage using disposable towel – discard this according to local waste disposal policy guidance.	To clear the area of the spillage.
4 Clean the area with warm water and detergent. If blood formed part of the spillage, then it may be necessary to use a chlorine-based disinfectant (refer to local policy for further guidance).	To clean the area.
5 Leave the area clean and dry.	To reduce the risk of injury and to prevent any further risk to staff, patients, and visitors.

Table 2.6 Disposal of clinical waste and linen

Type of waste	Method of disposal
High-risk waste This is usually generated from clinical activity and may include soiled dressings or infected material. This waste is usually incinerated.	Yellow bag
Domestic waste This may comprise foodstuffs and other normal household items. This waste is normally disposed of at landfill sites.	Black bag
Sharps Usually needles and syringes. This waste is also usually incinerated.	Yellow sharps container
Linen Used linen and visibly soiled linen are separated and disposed of differently. Protective clothing should be worn to reduce the risk of spreading infection. In particular, linen should be gathered or rolled up for disposal, as this will generate fewer bacteria-containing dust particles than dragging. Linen bags should also be positioned nearby to reduce the carrying distance. This will also reduce the transmission of infection.	Used linen: white cloth linen bag Soiled linen: red plastic bag inside red linen bag.

References

Department of Health (2006). *Code of Practice for the Prevention and Control of Healthcare Associated Infections*. Department of Health, London.

Department of Health (2007). *Uniforms and Workwear: An Evidence Base for Developing Local Policy*. Department of Health, London.

Gould D, Gammon J, Donnelly M, *et al.* (2000). Improving hand hygiene in community healthcare settings: the impact of research and clinical collaboration. *Journal of Clinical Nursing*, **9**, 95–102.

Health Protection Scotland (2008). *Personal Protective Equipment Policy and Procedures*. www.documents. hps.scot.nhs.uk/hai/infection-control/sicp/ppe/mic-p-ppe-2008-02.pdf.

Jenkinson H, Wright D, Jones M, *et al.* (2006). Prevention and control of infection in nonacute healthcare settings. *Nursing Standard*. **20**(20), 56–63.

ICNA (2005). *Audit Tools for Monitoring Infection Control Guidelines Within the Community Setting 2005*. Infection Control Nurses Association; Meridian, Huntingdonshire. www.ips.uk.net/icna/Admin/uploads/AuditTools2005.pdf.

Leggett NKJ and Watterson L (2005). Provision and decontamination of uniforms in the NHS. *Nursing Standard,* **19**(33), 41–5.

NMC (2005a). *An NMC Guide for Students of Nursing and Midwifery.* Nursing and Midwifery Council, London.

NMC (2005b). *Guidelines for Records and Record Keeping.* Nursing and Midwifery Council, London:

NMC (2008). *The Code: Standards of Conduct, Performance and Ethics for Nurses and Midwives.* Nursing and Midwifery Council, London.

Storr J and Clayton-Kent S (2004). Hand hygiene. *Nursing Standard*, **18**(40), 45–51.

Storr J, Topley K, and Privett S (2005). The ward nurse's role in infection control. *Nursing Standard*, **19**(41), 56–64.

Useful further reading and websites

Chalmers C and Straub M (2006). Infection control of undergraduate nurses. *Nursing Standard*, **20**(37), 35–41.

This explains the implementation of the Cleanliness Champion Programme to undergraduate nurses.

Department of Health (2005). *Saving Lives: A Delivery Programme to Reduce Healthcare-associated Infection (HCAI) Including MRSA*. The Stationery Office, London.

Hill D and Hadfield J (2005). The role of the modern matron in infection control. *Nursing Standard*, **19**(23), 42–4.

This article explains how the modern matron can help with the control and spread of infection.

Jeanes A (2005). Keeping hospitals clean: how nurses can reduce healthcare-associated infection. *Professional Nurse*, **20**(6), 35–7.

This article is acute-care based, and looks specifically at how to prevent the spread of infection.

King D (2005). Development of core competencies for infection prevention and control. *Nursing Standard*, **19**(41), 50–4.

This article explores competencies required for infection prevention and control for infection-control specialist nurses.

Murdoch S (2007). Infection prevention and control: principles of. In Jamieson EM, Whyte LA, and McCall JM, eds, *Clinical Nursing Practices*, 5th edn, Chapter 19, pp. 151–63, Churchill Livingstone, Edinburgh.

This chapter looks at safe practices, safe environment, and procedures for coping with the unexpected.

Wiseman S (2006). Prevention and control of healthcare-associated infection. *Nursing Standard*, **20**(38), 41–5.

This article explores auditing of the prevalence of healthcare-associated infections.

Check 🌐 **www.oxfordtextbooks.co.uk/orc/docherty/** for changes and new developments. Updated research, guidelines, or equipment will be added every four months.

Answers to scenario

- Call for immediate assistance from another staff member; they can take over the task freeing you to care for your injury
- Go to the nearest sink and turn the warm water tap on
- Encourage your finger to bleed by squeezing it below the injury point
- At the same time, hold your finger under the warm water—this will also help to encourage bleeding
- After this procedure, dry the injury thoroughly and apply a waterproof dressing
- Let the ward manager know about your injury and complete the necessary paperwork to ensure that a log of the incident is recorded
- It may be necessary to seek further medical attention—discuss this with the ward manager and take appropriate action thereafter

2.5 **Resuscitation**

Introduction

The aim of this chapter is to provide you with primary knowledge of the skills involved in basic life support and cardiopulmonary resuscitation (CPR) for adults, children, and infants. The main focus is dealing with the casualty as a healthcare provider both inside and outside the hospital environment. This is appropriate to you as a first-year student nurse, since the clinical skills involved in more advanced life support (ALS) are built on this solid foundation in the remaining years of your programme. The initial focus will be the adult patient, followed by the infant and child, and will be based on the resuscitation guidelines of the Resuscitation Council UK (Biarent *et al.* 2005; Handley *et al.* 2005; Nolan *et al.* 2005). Following on from the CPR sections, this chapter will also describe the steps to be taken for all age groups in the event of choking.

Learning outcomes

These outcomes relate to numbers 1, 3, 7, 9, 10, 13, 14, 17, and 22 of the NMC's Essential Skill Clusters and specifically to Care Domains 2 and 3 of the NMC's Standards of Proficiency for Pre-registration Nursing (outcomes to be achieved for entry to branch).

On reading the chapter and associated web pages and undertaking supervised activities, you will be able to:

- Define the term cardiac arrest
- Identify potential causes of cardiac arrest in adults and children
- Recognize signs of cardiac arrest
- Initially manage patients who require cardiopulmonary resuscitation

Prior knowledge

To use the skills in this chapter, it is important that you have a good understanding of the relevant anatomy and physiology. This can be found in a large range of textbooks.

Specifically you should be familiar with:

- The cardiovascular system
- The respiratory system
- The anatomical structures that comprise the chest and mediastinum

Background

Normal cardiac function

To maintain adequate performance of the vital organs, it is essential that we have:

1 An open **A**irway,
2 The capability to **B**reathe in oxygen and achieve adequate gas exchange in the lungs,
3 A functioning heart that will act as a pump to **C**irculate this oxygen to the organs of the body sustaining life.

Disruption to this 'ABC' process at any point will, within minutes, result in reduced oxygen delivery, organ failure, and death. When the amount of circulating oxygen in the arterial blood is diminished, this is referred to as hypoxaemia and when the oxygen level in the tissues falls, we refer to this as **hypoxia**.

Cardiac arrest is the abrupt cessation of cardiac function and is the ultimate clinical emergency. Cardiopulmonary resuscitation is a dramatic emergency exercise that aims to restore effective circulation and breathing following cardiac arrest. In adults the most common cause of sudden cardiac arrest, out of hospital, is acute coronary syndrome (heart attack). However, in children and infants this is unlikely, unless there is a piedisposing congenital cardiac condition. Cardiac arrest in children and infants tends to be the result of a primary respiratory problem. However, in all cases, other causes may exist, including:

- Drowning
- Choking
- Bleeding
- Drug overdose
- Hypoxia
- Trauma

(Resuscitation Council 2006)

2.5.1 **Cardiopulmonary resuscitation for adults**

Definition

Cardiopulmonary resuscitation is the act of artificially maintaining respiratory and cardiac function. It involves maintaining a clear airway, artificial breathing, and compressing the chest to circulate blood.

When to perform cardiopulmonary resuscitation

The skill should be performed in any casualty who has suddenly collapsed and is unresponsive with absence of signs of circulation. Basic life support measures, as shown in **Fig. 2.20**, may be commenced in any environment, however in hospital, where expertise is at hand, these will quickly be supplemented by more advanced interventions. There may be situations where it has been agreed that an individual patient should not be resuscitated (e.g. terminal illness). As part of the healthcare team you should be made aware of such decisions and it should be clearly recorded in the patient's notes. If you have not been made aware of this, and if there is no one around to guide you, then you should not hesitate in commencing resuscitation.

The diagnosis of cardiac arrest is confirmed by:

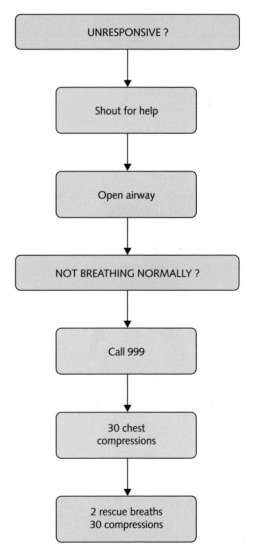

Adult Basic Life Support

UNRESPONSIVE ?

Shout for help

Open airway

NOT BREATHING NORMALLY ?

Call 999

30 chest compressions

2 rescue breaths 30 compressions

Figure 2.20 Basic life support for an adult. Courtesy of the Resuscitation Council UK.

- A sudden loss of consciousness
- Absent or abnormal breathing (for example, slow, laboured breathing, gasping, or an absence of breathing)
- The absence of signs of circulation

Procedure: confirming cardiac arrest in adults

The sequence of steps used to confirm a diagnosis of cardiac arrest can be remembered using the mnemonic 'Dr's ABC'. These initials represent:

- **D**anger—check for obvious signs—your own safety is paramount!
- **R**esponse—of the casualty
- **S**hout—for assistance
- **A**irway—check and open
- **B**reathing—check for breathing
- **C**irculation—check for signs

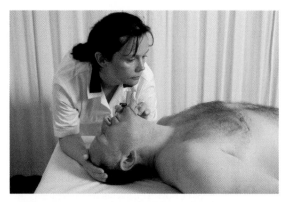

Figure 2.22 Performing look, listen, and feel (adult)

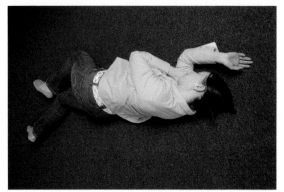

Figure 2.23 The recovery position

Key point: Agonal breathing (infrequent, occasional gasps) will be evident in 40% of victims; DO NOT confuse this with normal respiration (ILCOR 2005). The emergency medical services (EMS) must be alerted prior to commencing CPR in adults; therefore, if you are alone you should leave the casualty and call them. However, if you have a second rescuer one should call the emergency medical services while the other begins CPR.

Aftercare

Once expert help arrives, a safe handover should be given and the casualty removed from the scene and transferred to the nearest Accident and Emergency Department. You may be asked to continue with CPR by the ambulance personnel while they attend to more advanced life support measures. If you are too exhausted to continue, you should make this known.

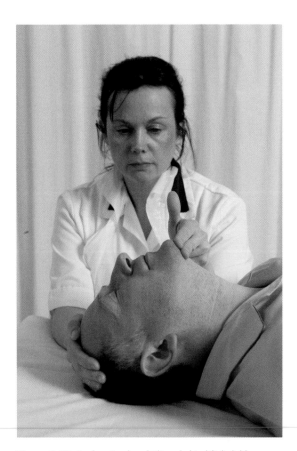

Figure 2.21 Performing head tilt and chin lift (adult)

Responding to cardiopulmonary resuscitation in adults

▶ Step   Rationale

Danger

1 Remove any obvious danger to the rescuer.

To prevent causing harm to the rescuer and prevent harm to the victim and rescuer.

Response

2 Check response of the casualty by shaking and asking, 'Are you alright?'

Confirm the conscious level of the casualty and assist in diagnosis.

3 If the casualty responds, leave in position in which found and alert help if you need it.

To check the casualty's condition, and allow an opportunity to reassess.

4 If the casualty does not respond, shout, 'HELP!'

To obtain assistance if you should need it.

Airway

5 Check the airway for obvious signs of obstruction. If a solid obstruction is detected, remove this with a hooked finger and sweeping motion. Well-fitting dentures should remain in place, as this helps to create a good seal during assisted ventilation. Loose or broken dentures should be removed.

To clear airway and optimize the casualty's airway.

6 Open the airway, using the head tilt and chin lift manoeuvre (see Fig. 2.21).

To prevent the tongue blocking the airway and allow for accurate assessment.

Breathing

7 While maintaining an open airway, position your ear over the mouth and nose and direct your eyes towards the chest. Look, listen, and feel (see Fig. 2.22) for expired air for no more than ten seconds.

To confirm or refute diagnosis.

8 If the casualty is breathing, place in the recovery position (see Fig. 2.23) and call for help, continually assessing condition.

To maintain a patent airway and identify signs of deteriorating condition.

continued

9 If after ten seconds, the breathing appears absent or abnormal (occasional, noisy, laboured gasps) and there are no obvious signs of circulation (movement, swallowing, etc.), alert the emergency medical services and begin CPR.

To summon expert help and access essential advanced resuscitation equipment.
To minimize delay in resuscitation and act as holding mechanism to keep the vital organs alive.

Circulation

10 Place the casualty in a supine position on a firm flat surface.

To permit easy access to the patient's chest and airway.

11 Place one hand on top of the other, on the centre of the chest, at the lower half of the sternum.

To safely locate the correct landmarks.

12 The arms should be straight and the elbows locked, lean over the casualty with the shoulder positioned in line with the heel of the hand, keeping the fingers off the ribs.

To use minimal exertion of the rescuer and prevent unnecessary harm to the casualty.

13 Press the chest by 4–5 cm, aiming for a rate of 100 compressions per min. Give 30 compressions, followed by two ventilations (see Fig. 2.24).

To maintain a cardiac output.

14 To deliver mouth-to-mouth ventilation: place the palm of one hand on the hairline while using the thumb and forefinger to occlude the nose.

To occlude the casualty's nose.

15 Allow the casualty's mouth to remain open, while placing the fingers of the opposite hand on the chin and lifting up.

To open the airway.

16 Ventilation is then achieved by placing your lips around the casualty's open mouth and blowing steadily to raise the chest.

To create a good seal.

17 Take about one second, allow the chest to fall fully between the first and second breath.

To prevent hyperinflation of the casualty and early exhaustion of the rescuer.

18 After the second breath do not delay before returning to the chest for 30 compressions and continue this pattern.

To deliver optimal resuscitation to the casualty.

19 This procedure should continue at a ratio of 30 compressions: 2 ventilations and should continue until expert help arrives, the casualty displays signs of life, or the rescuer becomes exhausted (Handley *et al.* 2005).

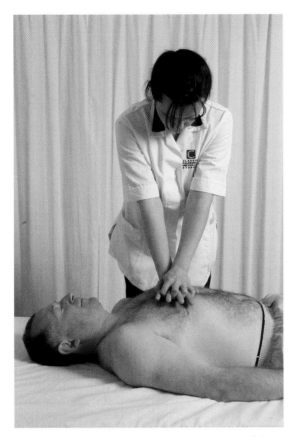

Figure 2.24 Performing chest compressions on an adult.

Alternative interventions

Compression-only CPR

Compression-only CPR can be used when attempts at mouth-to-mouth resuscitation have been unsuccessfull or you are unable or unwilling to do this. Occasions where you may be unwilling to perform mouth-to-mouth may include situations which can compromise your personal safety (e.g. exposure to blood). This involves following the steps for life support as described previously without stopping to ventilate. Compressions should be delivered continuously at a rate of 100 compressions per minute (ILCOR 2005).

In a hospital environment

As soon as the diagnosis of cardiac arrest is confirmed, ensure that appropriately experienced clinicians are alerted, and the emergency equipment is gathered; in hospital this will be the cardiac arrest team or equivalent. Begin chest compressions with minimal delay. This could be achieved by sending a second person for help, to make best use of the elapsing time and gain support from skilled personnel.

You may see airway adjuncts being used to help maintain an open airway. These include oral and nasal airways, and should only be used by personnel experienced and trained in their use.

Mouth-to-mouth ventilation should be discouraged within the hospital environment, unless it is absolutely necessary and if there is no alternative available. This will be in extreme circumstances only. Therefore, within the hospital setting, devices such as a pocket mask or bag-valve-mask device, as shown in **Fig. 2.25** will be used with supplementary oxygen (if available).

A single rescuer may find it necessary to combine mouth-to-mask ventilation and over-the-head chest compressions to minimize the disruption to compressions (Handley and Handley 2004).

If more than one healthcare provider is available, a two- person technique for ventilation and compressions should be used. Swap every 2 minutes. When the nurse tires during chest compressions, roles may be changed. Again, this should be with minimal disruption to chest compressions (Resuscitation Council UK 2006).

Once an airway is secured with an endotracheal tube, chest compressions should continue uninterrupted at a rate of 100 per minute and the patient should be ventilated at a rate of 10 breaths per minute (Resuscitation Council UK 2006).

Out-of-hospital environment

The situation in a community setting is individual to that particular area (for example, a patient's or client's own

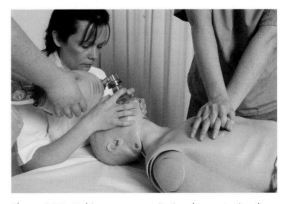

Figure 2.25 Multi-rescuer resuscitation demonstrating three roles: maintaining the airway, bag-breathing, and chest compression.

home; a GP practice; or supported accommodation). As a student nurse you should ensure that when on placement in community settings you are aware of the procedure specific to that clinical environment. In the absence of any clinical emergency team, calling for help will involve contacting the ambulance service on 999 or 112. Individuals should be aware of the information required when calling these services and that it can take a few moments to relay the necessary information. This may include: who you are; where you are; what you're dealing with; who the casualty is, and the age of the casualty.

Defibrillation

The use of automated external defibrillators (AEDs) is becoming more common in the community. These should only ever be used by personnel trained in their use. Once the defibrillator is switched on, the operator is guided by the voice prompt to the defibrillator and will attach the monitoring pads to the bare chest. This should be done with minimal disruption to chest compressions. The operator will instruct rescuers to stand clear while the defibrillator assesses the cardiac rhythm and to remain clear while the shock is delivered.

Developing your skills

You will be given the opportunity to learn this skill by using mannequins and simulated patients. However, you should recognize that the real situation will be very different and you may feel nervous or anxious when faced with this. There is no way of determining how you will react, and for this reason it is vital that you continue to take any opportunity to practice these skills in a controlled environment to prepare you for the real situation.

Other factors to consider

This clinical emergency is stressful for all involved and for those witnessing events as they unfold. For this reason, appropriate care of fellow patients and clients must be considered, since often these individuals require emotional support. This is of particular importance when dealing with potentially emotionally labile individuals (for example, those patients encountered in mental-health and learning-disabilities specialties).

Further consideration may be required of the relatives of patients who, if they are present at the time of the incident, may request to stay and observe. Relatives can find this useful. However, one staff member should be allocated to care for them during this time and explain procedures in language they will understand (Kidby 2003; Rattrie 2000). If the resuscitation attempt is unsuccessful, allowing the relatives to witness the event may help in the grieving process. However, this should not be forced on them, if it is not their desire. (Further information is available in Chapter 12.)

It is good practice to follow clinical emergencies with debriefing sessions, and often this will happen within the hospital environment. As a student nurse, you may wish to reflect on the experience and record those aspects that require clarification so you make the most of this learning opportunity. You can then discuss your queries with your mentor and academic staff (McGuinness 2008).

Do not attempt resuscitation

Recommendations for this sensitive topic have been compiled in a joint statement by the Resuscitation Council UK; British Medical Association, and Royal College of Nursing. Ultimately, this statement of best practice suggests that this very complex decision should only be made by an experienced, qualified practitioner and should be clearly documented. The information documented should include the date of the decision, the rationale for the decision, and a clear indication of the name and job title of the individual responsible for making it (Resuscitation Council UK 2007). Once this decision is made, it should be communicated to staff and respected.

Living will

It is the prerogative of an adult, with the appropriate intellectual capacity, to request that resuscitation is not attempted in the event of a cardiac arrest. In this situation, this should be clearly documented according to local policy and all members of the healthcare team should be made aware of the situation. The onus is on the patient to ensure that staff are made aware of the existence and content of any advance directive (Resuscitation Council UK 2007).

2.5.2 **Paediatric healthcare provider basic life support**

Definition

This section is aimed *only* at those student nurses who will have a professional responsibility or duty to care for children. It will describe the key points of basic life support for children and review some of the adaptations made in the in hospital environment. For the purpose of this chapter, the age definitions used by the Resuscitation Council UK (Biarent *et al.* 2005) will be used:

- Infant: child under 1 year
- Child: between 1 year and puberty.

Alternative intervention

For those who do not normally have a professional duty to care for children and are not familiar with the different requirements that children have, the preceding procedure for adults may be used with the following adaptations in the event of a paediatric emergency, where the child is unresponsive and not breathing normally it is recommended that:

- Five initial breaths are given before starting chest compression
- If alone, carry out CPR for approximately 1 minute before going for help
- The chest should be depressed by around one-third of its depth:
  - Use two fingers if the casualty is an infant under 1 year,
  - Use one hand if the casualty is over 1 year and **prepubescent**.

When to perform paediatric cardiopulmonary resuscitation

The most common primary cause of paediatric cardiorespiratory arrests tend to be the result of **hypoxia**, and it is unusual for children to have a sudden cardiac event. For this reason, swift oxygenation is the most pressing requirement. This can be achieved by delivering good basic life support (BLS), as shown in **Fig. 2.26**. For a lone rescuer, the priority is initiating BLS for approximately one minute

before summoning the emergency medical services (EMS). If more than one rescuer is available, one rescuer should initiate BLS while the other activates the EMS.

Procedure: Basic life support sequence for an infant

The sequence of steps used to confirm a diagnosis of cardiac arrest in adults can also be applied to children using the mnemonic 'Dr's ABC'. These initials represent:

- Danger—check for obvious signs - your own safety is paramount!
- Response—of the casualty,
- Shout—for assistance
- Airway—check and open
- Breathing—check for breathing
- Circulation—check for signs

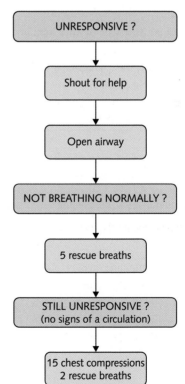

Paediatric Basic Life Support (Healthcare professionals with a duty to respond)

UNRESPONSIVE ?

↓

Shout for help

↓

Open airway

↓

NOT BREATHING NORMALLY ?

↓

5 rescue breaths

↓

STILL UNRESPONSIVE ? (no signs of a circulation)

↓

15 chest compressions 2 rescue breaths

After 1 minute call resuscitation team then continue CPR

Figure 2.26 Paediatric basic life support. Courtesy of the Resuscitation Council UK.

Paediatric basic life support sequence for an infant

Key point: This procedure should only be performed by student nurses who will have a professional responsibility or duty to care for children.

▶ Step	Rationale
Danger	
1 Remove any obvious danger to the rescuer.	To prevent causing harm to the rescuer and prevent harm to the infant.
Response	
2 Check the response of the infant by stimulating and asking loudly 'are you alright?'.	To confirm the conscious level of the infant and assist in diagnosis.
3 Avoid unnecessary vigorous shaking and take care not to exacerbate any potential injury sustained in the events leading to the collapse.	To prevent further injury.
4 If the infant does not respond, shout 'HELP!'	To obtain assistance if you should need it.
Airway	
5 Check the airway for obvious signs of obstruction. If a solid obstruction is detected, remove this with care by using a hooked little finger to gently sweep the obstruction.	To clear airway and optimize the casualty's airway.
6 DO NOT attempt blind finger sweeps.	To prevent unnecessary damage.
7 Open the airway using a head tilt and chin lift and position the head in the neutral position.	To clear airway and optimize the infant's airway.
8 Be careful not to press on the soft tissues of the neck.	To prevent damage. Pressing on the neck tissues may block the airway.
Breathing	
9 While maintaining an open airway, position your ear over the mouth and nose and direct your eyes towards the chest. Look, listen and feel for expired air for no more than 10 seconds.	To confirm or refute the presence of adequate breathing.

10	If the infant is breathing normally, place in the recovery position.	To maintain a patent airway and identify signs of deteriorating condition.
11	If the breathing is absent or inadequate (occasional noisy laboured gasps) proceed to deliver five initial rescue breaths.	To optimize oxygen uptake and potentially reverse any hypoxic event.
12	Place head in neutral position with chin lift applied. Take a breath and cover the mouth and nose with your mouth.	To create a good seal.
13	If it is too difficult to ventilate both the mouth and nose of the infant, attempt to ventilate through either the nose or mouth, while occluding the other.	
14	Inflate steadily for 1–1.5 seconds, watching for the chest rising, maintain head tilt and chin lift while you remove your mouth and watch the chest fall.	Prevent hyperinflation of the chest and allow for observation of any response from the infant.
15	Repeat until five attempts have been made.	
16	If there is no chest movement during the procedure; check the mouth for signs of obstruction and remove any obvious blockage carefully.	Ensure airway insufficiency is not the result of poor technique or foreign body airway obstruction.
17	If there is no obstruction; reposition the head each time until a rise and fall of the chest wall has been observed	
18	**Circulation** Check the circulation by looking for obvious signs of life (movement, swallowing, and so on). If you are experienced in clinical assessment, you may wish to perform a brachial artery pulse check.	To confirm the diagnosis.
19	If you are certain you can detect signs of circulation within ten seconds, continue rescue breathing, continuously observing the response.	To maintain oxygenation and early detection of deterioration.
20	If you are uncertain of the signs of circulation and either there is no pulse or it is below 60 beats per minute, with poor perfusion – commence chest compressions.	To create a blood flow to the vital organs.
21	Place the casualty in a supine position on a firm flat surface.	To optimize delivery of chest compressions.

continued

22	Place two fingers on the lower half of the sternum, one finger's breadth up from the xiphisternum (see Fig. 2.27).	To avoid damage to abdominal organs.
23	Press the chest by approximately one third of its depth, aiming for a rate of 100 compressions per min. Deliver a series of 15 compressions combined with 2 ventilations and continue with a ratio of 15:2.	To achieve optimal perfusion.
24	If there are two rescuers available, the encircling method may be used to deliver compressions and ventilation, see Fig. 2.29.	Make best use of space and a more effective method of achieving adequate compressions.
25	After 1 minute, briefly stop to reassess ABC and ensure that the emergency medical services have been called.	To confirm the diagnosis.
26	This procedure should continue at a ratio of 15 compressions: 2 ventilations until expert help arrives.	

Key point: Exert caution when opening the airway, particularly in an infant. Be careful not to press on the soft tissues of the neck, as this can cause damage and may occlude the airway.

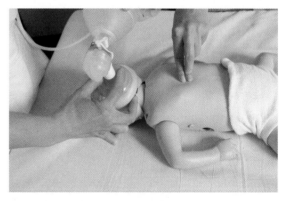

Figure 2.28 Single rescuer performing chest compressions on an infant while maintaining the airway.

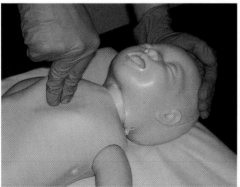

Figure 2.27 Placing fingers for chest compression.

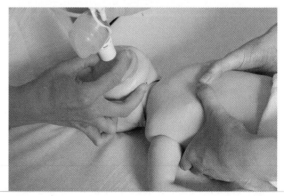

Figure 2.29 Alternative method for chest compression using thumbs and both hands. Requires second rescuer to maintain airway.

Paediatric basic life support sequence for a child

Key point: This procedure should only be performed by student nurses who will have a professional responsibility or duty to care for children.

▶ Step   Rationale

	Step	Rationale
	Danger	
1	Remove any obvious danger to the rescuer.	To prevent causing harm to the rescuer and prevent harm to the child.
	Response	
2	Check response of the child by stimulating them and loudly asking 'are you alright?'.	To confirm the conscious level of the infant and assist in diagnosis.
3	Take care not to exacerbate any potential injury sustained in the events leading to the collapse.	To prevent further injury.
4	If the child does not respond, shout 'HELP!'	To obtain assistance if you should need it.
	Airway	
5	Check the airway for obvious signs of obstruction. If a solid obstruction is detected, remove this with care.	To clear airway and optimize the casualty's airway.
6	DO NOT attempt blind finger sweeps.	To prevent unnecessary damage.
7	Open the airway using a head tilt – chin lift.	To clear airway and optimize the child's airway.
8	Be careful not to press on the soft tissues of the neck.	To prevent damage and blocking of the airway.
	Breathing	
9	While maintaining an open airway, position your ear over the mouth and nose and direct your eyes towards the chest. Look, listen and feel for expired air for no more than 10 seconds.	To confirm or refute the presence of adequate breathing.
10	If the child is breathing normally, place in the recovery position.	To maintain a patent airway and identify signs of deteriorating condition.

continued

11	If the breathing is inadequate (absent, or occasional, noisy, laboured gasps) proceed to delivering five initial rescue breaths.	To optimize oxygen uptake and potentially reverse any hypoxic event.
12	Position the child: head tilt, chin lift.	To allow delivery of mouth to mouth ventilation.
13	Pinch the soft part of the nose the between the thumb and forefinger of the hand which is positioned on the forehead.	To prevent air escaping from the nose.
14	Allow the child's mouth to remain open, while placing the fingers of the opposite hand on the chin and lifting it up. Ventilation is then achieved by placing your lips around the child's open mouth and blowing steadily to raise the chest.	To create a good seal.
15	While delivering the rescue breaths, observe the child for signs of gag or swallowing reflex.	This may indicate the presence of a circulation.
16	Inflate steadily for 1–1.5 seconds, watching for the chest rising, maintain head tilt and chin lift while you remove your mouth and watch the chest fall.	
17	Repeat until five attempts have been made.	Prevent hyperinflation of the chest and allow for observation of any response from the infant.
18	If there is no chest movement during the procedure; check the mouth for signs of obstruction and remove any obvious blockage carefully.	Ensure airway insufficiency is not the result of poor technique or foreign body airway obstruction.
19	If there is no obstruction; reposition the head each time until a rise and fall of the chest wall has been observed.	
	Circulation	
20	Check the circulation by looking for obvious signs of life (e.g. movement, swallowing, and so on) and if you are experienced in clinical assessment, you may wish to perform a carotid artery pulse check, see Fig. 2.30.	To confirm the diagnosis.
21	If you are certain that you can detect signs of circulation within ten seconds, continue rescue breathing, continuously observing the response.	To maintain oxygenation and early detection of deterioration.

22	If you are uncertain of the signs of circulation and either there is no pulse or it is below 60 beats per minute, with poor perfusion, prepare to commence chest compressions.	To create a blood flow to the vital organs.
23	Place the casualty in a supine position on a firm flat surface.	To optimize delivery of chest compressions.
24	Place the heel of one hand on the lower half of the sternum, one finger's breadth up from the xiphisternum.	To avoid damage to abdominal organs.
25	Press the chest by approximately one third of its depth, aiming for a rate of 100 compressions per min. Deliver a series of 15 compressions combined with 2 ventilations and continue with a ratio of 15:2.	To achieve optimal perfusion.
26	If it is difficult to achieve a compression depth of one third of the chest, two hands and a compression ratio of 30:2 should be used.	
27	If there are two rescuers available, one should take control of the airway while the other performs compressions, see Fig. 2.31.	Makes best use of resources and is an effective method.
28	After 1 minute, briefly stop to reassess ABC and ensure that the emergency medical services have been called.	To confirm the diagnosis
29	This procedure should continue at a ratio of 15 compressions: 2 ventilations until expert help arrives.	

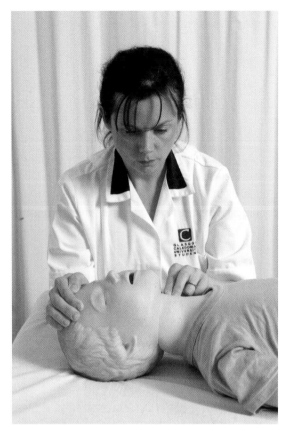

Figure 2.30 Maintaining the airway while finding the carotid pulse on a child

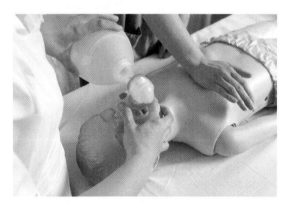

Figure 2.31 Two-rescuer method, showing chest compression

Key points Only attempt to remove airway obstruction if it is clearly visible and easily reached with the little finger.

Aftercare

Once expert help arrives, a safe handover should be given and the casualty removed from the scene and transferred to the nearest Accident and Emergency Department with paediatric specialty.

Developing your skills

Within most universities you will be given the opportunity to learn this skill. However, you should be advised that this sequence might only be taught to those students who will have a responsibility to care for paediatric patients. The opportunity to develop this skill will be achieved by using manikins and simulated patients. As with adult resuscitation, however, you should recognize that the real situation will be very different and you may be anxious when faced with this situation. There is no way of determining how you will react, and for this reason it is vital that you continue to take any opportunity to practice these skills in a controlled environment to prepare for the real situation.

Alternative interventions

In-hospital environment

As soon as a critical problem with a child or infant has been identified, local policy and procedure should be followed. The clinical emergency team (or equivalent) should be alerted and emergency equipment must be gathered.

Mouth-to-mouth ventilation should be discouraged within the hospital environment unless it is absolutely necessary and there is no alternative available; this will be in extreme circumstances. Therefore, within the hospital setting, devices such as a pocket mask or bag-valve-mask device (see **Figs 2.29** and **2.31**) will be used with supplementary oxygen (if available). If more than one healthcare provider is available, the two-person technique for ventilation and compressions should be adopted.

Once an airway is secured with an endotracheal tube, chest compressions should continue uninterrupted at a rate of 100 compressions per minute and the patient should be ventilated at a rate of 10 breaths per minute (Biarent *et al.* 2005).

Defibrillation

The use of automated external defibrillators (AEDs) is becoming more common in the community. These should only ever be used by personnel trained in their use. Once the defibrillator is switched on, the operator is guided by the voice prompt of the defibrillator and will attach the monitoring pads to the bare chest. This should be done with minimal disruption to chest compressions. The operator will instruct rescuers to stand clear while the defibrillator assesses the cardiac rhythm and remain clear while the shock is delivered.

Defibrillation is not frequently required in paediatrics; however, if a child does require defibrillation, this should be done with minimum delay. A standard automated external defibrillator can be used in children over eight years old. However, children younger than eight require either a manual defibrillator or an automatic external defibrillator that has purpose-made paediatric pads and a device that alters the current delivered to suit the size of the child. If no such system is available, an adult defibrillator may be used, since the evidence to support or oppose this is insufficient at present (Biarent *et al.* 2005).

Alternative mnemonics

You may encounter alternative mnemonics to Dr's ABC. Two other mnemonics used in paediatrics are SSSABC(R) and the SAFE approach to resuscitation. Respectively, these translate as:

Safety; **S**hout; **S**timulate; **A**irway; **B**reathing; **C**irculation; **R**eassess, and

Shout help; **A**pproach with care; **F**ree from danger; **E**valuate ABC.

Other factors to consider

This clinical emergency is stressful in all cases, and could be considered even more so in the case of children and infants. The emotional needs of staff, relatives, and other patients or clients must be considered, identified, and supported. With this age group, additional support will be required for the parents or carers of the child, particularly if they have witnessed the event. Often they will request to stay and observe, indeed this opportunity should be made available to parents, but under no circumstances should this be forced on them if it is not their desire.

Facilitating this will involve ensuring that a suitably qualified staff member is available to remain with the parents or carers and to explain all procedures to them, and appropriately answer any questions which may arise. Ultimately, this may ease the grieving process should the resuscitation be unsuccessful (Kidby 2003; Rattrie 2000). (Further information is available in Chapter 12).

It is good practice to follow clinical emergencies with debriefing sessions, and often this will happen within the hospital environment. As a student nurse, you may wish to reflect on the experience and record those aspects that require clarification so that you can make the most of this learning opportunity. You can then discuss your queries with your mentor and academic staff (McGuinness 2008).

2.5.3 **The choking casualty**

Definition

Early detection of a choking casualty, regardless of age, is paramount for the rescue attempt to be successful. Choking is sometimes referred to as a foreign body airway obstruction (FBAO) and can cause a mild or severe blockage in the casualty's airway.

Background

Signs of choking include sudden onset of an attack while eating or grasping the neck. The recognition and removal of any airway obstruction should be performed swiftly and safely, as soon as the diagnosis has been confirmed. Onset is usually sudden in the absence of other illness.

There may be signs to which the rescuer should be sensitive (for example, the casualty has been eating; children may have been playing with small toys) prior to the symptoms. Without exception, you must always consider your own safety first before attempting to respond to the needs of any casualty. Flow diagrams to illustrate the procedures for adults and children are given in **Figs. 2.32** and **2.33**, respectively.

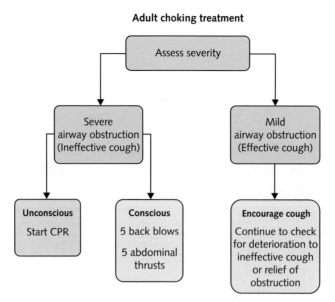

Figure 2.32 Adult choking treatment. Courtesy of the Resuscitation Council UK

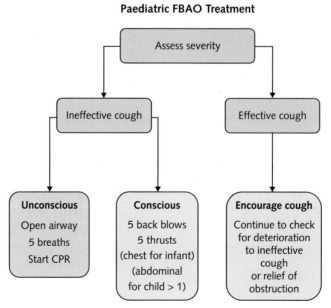

Figure 2.33 Paediatric choking treatment. Courtesy of the Resuscitation Council UK

The choking adult

Key point: It is essential that the student nurse acknowledges his or her own clinical limitations and acts always in the best interests of the casualty (NMC 2008).

Step	Rationale
1 Confirm the severity of the attack: is it mild or severe? Ask the casualty, 'Are you choking?'	To avoid asking open questions that the casualty will be unable to answer and to establish the immediate action required.
2 If the casualty replies and is coughing, encourage the coughing.	To reduce stress and prevent inflicting unnecessary procedures on the casualty.
3 If the casualty is unable to speak, has a silent cough, noisy breathing, or can only reply by nodding, there may be a severe obstruction.	If the airway is partially obstructed, attempts at breathing will be noisy. If the obstruction is complete, attempts at breathing will be silent.
4 Deliver up to five back blows. Stand at the side, lean the casualty forwards, support the chest, and deliver five firm blows between the shoulder blades, checking after each blow for signs of dislodgement.	To attempt to dislodge the obstruction.
5 If after five back blows the obstruction is not cleared, progress to abdominal thrusts. Stand behind the casualty, leaning the casualty forwards. Position your fist between the navel and breastbone, grab this with the opposite hand and with apply a sharp upwards and inwards motion.	To try an alternative method and create changes in abdominal pressure.
6 If after five attempts, the obstruction is not dislodged, alternate between back blows and abdominal thrusts until the obstruction is dislodged or the casualty becomes unconscious.	To try an alternative method and create changes in abdominal pressure.
7 If the casualty becomes unconscious, call the EMS and begin CPR.	This is now a hypoxic event and advanced life support measures are required.

The choking infant or child

Step		Rationale
1	Confirm the severity of the attack, is it mild or severe? Are attempts at coughing effective or ineffective?	To establish the immediate action required.
2	If the coughing is effective, crying or verbal response can be given; the casualty can manage a loud cough, with a breath before each and is fully responsive. Encourage coughing and observe for signs of improvement or deterioration.	To help the casualty to dislodge the obstruction without further help.
3	If the coughing is ineffective: the patient is quiet or silent; unable to vocalize; has a silent cough, noisy breathing or is unable to breathe; if there is cyanosis, or a decreasing conscious level, there may be a severe obstruction.	If the airway is partially obstructed, attempts at breathing will be noisy, if the obstruction is complete, attempts at breathing will be silent.
4	Deliver up to five back blows. **For an infant:** Support the infant in a head down, prone position supporting the infant safely. Place the thumb at the angle of the jaw and the forefinger at the opposite side; gently apply a chin lift, avoiding the soft tissues, while supporting the head. Check after each blow for signs of dislodgement. **For a child:** Ideally the child will be positioned head down with support similar to the infant position. However, if this is not possible, lean the child forwards, supporting the chest and deliver the blows from the side. Check after each blow for signs of dislodgement.	This allows gravity to help and maintains the safety of the infant.
5	Deliver up to five sharp back blows with the heel of the opposite hand.	To create an artificial cough and attempt to dislodge the obstruction.
6	If after five blows, the obstruction is not cleared, progress to the next step.	To try an alternative method and create changes in abdominal pressure.

Infant: Carefully turn the infant over into the head down, supine position. Place your free arm down the infants back and hold the occiput as you rotate the infant round. Identify the landmarks for chest compressions, and deliver five slow deliberate sharp chest thrusts.	To reduce harm and protect the organs of the abdominal cavity.
Child: Deliver abdominal thrusts. Stand behind the child, leaning the child forwards. Position your fist between the navel and breastbone, grab this with the opposite hand and apply a sharp upwards and inwards motion.	To create an artificial cough.
7 If after five attempts, the obstruction is not dislodged, alternate between back blows and abdominal thrusts until the obstruction is dislodged or the casualty becomes unconscious.	To try an alternative method and create changes in abdominal pressure.
8 If the casualty becomes unconscious, call the EMS and begin CPR.	This is now a hypoxic event and advanced life support measures are required.

Aftercare

Depending on the severity of the obstruction, it may be necessary for the casualty to attend the local accident and emergency department for review by experienced medical personnel.

Developing your skills

Take the opportunity to use the relevant manikins to practice positioning and the technique required when dealing with a choking victim. This technique can be difficult to master, and because of the nature of the clinical situation, opportunities to practice will be nonexistent.

Patient scenarios

Consider what you should do in the following situations, then turn to the end of the section to check your answers.

Further scenarios are available at 🌐 **www. oxfordtextbooks.co.uk/orc/docherty/**

 Scenario 1

You are standing in the checkout queue in the supermarket when a middle-aged lady collapses in front of you. What action do you take?

 Scenario 2

You are in a restaurant having lunch, when you hear a baby sitting in a high chair at the next table, begin to cough noisily. The loud coughing rapidly deteriorates to a quieter cough and the baby is turning blue. The mother and father are obviously distressed and are not coping with the situation. Consider your immediate response and action to address the situation.

Website

🌐 **www.oxfordtextbooks.co.uk/orc/docherty/**

You may find it helpful to work through our short online quiz and interactive scenarios intended to help you to develop and apply the skills in this chapter.

References

Biarent D, Bingham R, Richmond S, *et al.* (2005). European Resuscitation Council guidelines for resuscitation 2005: Section 6 Paediatric life support. *Resuscitation*, **67**(suppl. 1), S97–S133.

Handley AJ and Handley JA (2004). Performing chest compressions in a confined space. *Resuscitation*, **61**(1), 55–61.

Handley AJ, Koster R, Monsieurs K, Perkins GD, Davies S, and Bossaert L (2005). European Resuscitation Council Guidelines for Resuscitation 2005: Section 2 Adult basic life support and use of automated external defibrillators. *Resuscitation*, **67**(suppl. 1), S7–S23.

ILCOR (International Liaison Committee on Resuscitation) (2005) Part 2 Adult basic life support. *Resuscitation* **67**(2–3), 187–201.

Kidby J (2003). Family-witnessed cardiopulmonary resuscitation. *Nursing Standard*, **17**(51), 33–6.

McGuinness C (2008). *Nursing Diary and Reflective Journal 2008–9*. Elsevier, London.

NMC (2008). *The Code: Standards of Conduct, Performance and Ethics for Nurses and Midwives*. Nursing and Midwifery Council, London.

Nolan JP, Deakin CD, Soar J, Böttiger BW, and Smith G (2005). European Resuscitation Council guidelines for resuscitation 2005: Section 4 Adult advanced life support. *Resuscitation*, **67**(suppl. 1), S39–S86.

Rattrie E (2000). Witnessed resuscitation: good practice or not? *Nursing Standard*, **14**(24), 32–5.

Resuscitation Council UK (2006). Lay rescuer basic life support. In *Immediate Life Support Course Manual*, 2nd edn, Resuscitation Council UK, London.

Resuscitation Council UK (2007). *Decisions relating to Cardiopulmonary Resuscitation – A Joint Statement from the British Medical Association, the Resuscitation Council UK, and the Royal College of Nursing*. Resuscitation Council UK, London.

Useful further reading and websites

www.resus.org.uk/pages/bls.pdf
Basic life support for adults.

www.resus.org.uk/pages/pbls.pdf
Basic life support for paediatrics.

www.resus.org.uk/pages/dnar.pdf
Information on 'do not attempt resuscitation' decisions.

www.resus.org.uk/pages/pals.pdf
Paediatric advanced life support skills.

Check **www.oxfordtextbooks.co.uk/orc/docherty/** for changes and new developments. Updated research, guidelines, or equipment will be added every four months.

Answers to scenarios

Scenario 1

- Assess for signs of danger.
- Shake and shout and ask the casualty if she is alright.
- Shout for help.
- Check and open the airway.
- Assess for signs of breathing and circulation for no more than ten seconds.
- Confirm cardiac arrest.
- Instruct help to summon the emergency medical services and to come back.
- Placing interlocked hands one on top of the other on the lower half of the sternum, begin chest compressions:
  - Rate 100 compressions per min,
  - Depth 4–5 cm.
- Give 30 compressions.
- Then give two ventilations:
  - Pinch nose,
  - Tilt head,
  - Lift chin,
  - Cover mouth with your lips,
  - Inflate for about one second,
  - Allow to deflate and repeat.
- Continue at ratio of 30 compressions to two ventilations until expert help arrives, you become exhausted, or the casualty responds.

Scenario 2

- Ensure personal safety.
- Diagnose severe foreign body airway obstruction with ineffective coughing.

- Summon help.
- Determine whether conscious level is deteriorating.
- Hold infant's jaw with the thumb at the angle of the jaw on one side and the forefinger at the other, taking care with the soft tissues, and lift chin.
- Hold infant in head down prone position and deliver up to five firm back blows, checking the effectiveness of each blow.
- After five unsuccessful back blows, cup occiput with hand, lie arm down the infant's back and rotate infant into the supine head down position – deliver five chest thrusts locating landmarks for chest compressions, deliver slow, deliberate, sharp thrusts up to a maximum of five thrusts.
- Repeat until obstruction clears or becomes unconscious, and then follow infant basic life support.

2.6 **Administration of medicines**

Introduction

The administration of medicine is an essential component of nursing. The term 'medicine' literally means any substance used therapeutically in the treatment of disease. An understanding of medicines and their effects on patients is, therefore, a crucial part of nursing knowledge. The supply, storage, prescription, and administration of medicines are governed by legislation, and drug errors can cause devastating effects. It is, therefore, vital that nurses are aware of the correct procedures, to maintain safe and accurate administration of medicines to patients.

Learning outcomes

These outcomes relate to numbers 33 to 41 of the NMC's Essential Skill Clusters and specifically to Care Domains 1 to 3 of the NMC's Standards of Proficiency for Pre-registration Nursing (outcomes to be achieved for entry to branch).

On reading the chapter and associated web pages and undertaking supervised activities, you will be able to:

- Demonstrate knowledge of the professional, legal, and ethical issues surrounding the administration of medicines.
- Recognize what constitutes a valid prescription.
- Administer medicines to patients safely and accurately, based on a comprehensive assessment.
- Understand the different routes in which medications can be administered and the appropriateness of each.
- Understand the importance of following policy in relation to covert medicines and drug errors.

Prior knowledge

When administering medication, nurses must ensure that they have appropriate knowledge and understanding of the professional, legal, ethical, pharmacological, and calculation issues associated with this skill.

Professional and ethical responsibilities

You should be familiar with the appropriate legal and professional guidelines in relation to administering medicine. This can be obtained by reading:

- The *Standards for Medicines Management* (NMC 2008a). These replace the *Guidelines for the Administration of Medicine*. These guidelines have been updated to reflect changes in nursing and midwifery practice. They are broad principles and should act as the standard to which practice is conducted.
- *Guidelines for Records and Record Keeping* (NMC 2005a). These address communication, documentation, and the dissemination of information.
- *An NMC Guide for Students of Nursing and Midwifery* (NMC 2005b). This document provides guidance for students in the clinical area and addresses aspects that

may relate to administration of medication including client confidentiality and student accountability.

- *The Code: Standards of Conduct, Performance and Ethics* (NMC 2008b). It is important to recognize and understand the nursing professions' expectations in relation to conduct and performance. As such, all nurses proposing to administer medication must ensure that they have read and understood this professional guidance.

Legal and Health Authority requirements

You are also legally accountable for your actions when administering medicines and should, therefore, be familiar with:

- The Medicines Act (1968),
- The Misuse of Drugs Act (1971/1985),
- The Consumer Protection Act (1987),
- The Medicinal Products: Prescription by Nurses Act (1992).

Pharmacology and drug calculation

Nurses also require a comprehensive knowledge of prescribed medication including the indications for its use, normal dosage range, permitted routes of administration, possible side effects, interactions with other drugs, and **contraindications**. This information has to be combined with information about the patient's condition and treatment.

The ability to carry out accurate drug calculations is also essential to maintain patient safety. There are many books and websites available that facilitate the practice of this skill.

- *The British National Formulary 55* (British Medical Association 2008a)

- *The British National Formulary for Children* (British Medical Association 2008b)
- *The Nurse Prescribers' Formulary* (British Medical Association 2007)

2.6.1 **Patient assessment**

Definition

Before administering any medication it is essential that the nurse is knowledgeable about the patient; therefore, individual patient assessment is one of the first stages in medicine administration.

Procedure

Some of this information will be contained on the prescription so that the patient can be identified; however, knowledge of the many other important factors influencing this patient's care is essential. These can be divided into physical, psychological, sociocultural, environmental and politico-economic, as shown in **Table 2.7**.

Aftercare

Following a full patient assessment, the nurse can then conclude whether the prescription is appropriate. For example, is the medication, the dose, the timing, and the route appropriate for this particular patient?

Depending on the age of a child the drug of choice and drug dosage will vary. It is important to ensure that there are no contraindications prohibiting administration of prescribed medication to the patient. For example, premature or newborn infants should be assessed individually, as their liver and renal function is immature and certain drugs are not suitable for this age group. Aspirin should not be prescribed or administered to any child under the age of 16 years.

Table 2.7 Influencing factors to include in a patient assessment

Physical	• Patient's weight, **body mass index** or surface area. This is particularly relevant when caring for children, as body weight is always used when calculating drug dosage. • Pregnancy, • Past medical history, for example, gastrointestinal ulcers, asthma, • Other medications (including over-the-counter and alternative medicines), • Allergies or sensitivities to medications or other substances, for example, some depot injections contain nut oil, • Ability to swallow, • Previously used injection sites, • Age.
Psychological	• Knowledge and understanding of the medication, • Ability to consent, capacity (see section on covert medication), or dependence, • Compliance, • Fears (needles, or previous experiences),
Sociocultural	• Ingredients of the drug (for example, pig insulin), • Alcohol. smoking, illegal drugs, other lifestyle factors, • Experiences or opinions of friends or family.
Politico-economic	• Most appropriate drug (costs).
Environmental	• Hospital patients: fasting for surgery, drug round timings, • Normal routine, for example, diuretics before bedtime.

2.6.2 **Basic principles of medicine administration**

Prescriptions

There are many rules in relation to prescriptions. Prescriptions must be written in indelible ink (so that they cannot be erased) and only standardized abbreviations are acceptable. Before issuing a drug, the nurse must check that the information listed in **Box 2.4** is provided. Figure 2.34 shows a common prescription chart.

Patient group directions (PGDs)

As well as prescriptions, you may also see patient group directions (PGDs). These are written agreements between

Box 2.4 Information needed before issuing a drug	
Patient details	Name and address (if appropriate), hospital or other identification number, Age (if under 12 years old), Any known allergies, Weight. This is good practice and especially important in children as body weight and, increasingly, surface area are used to calculate drug dose.
Medication details	Name, dose, route and frequency or timing
Prescriber information	Signature of the prescriber

PATIENT DETAILS		DRUG SENSITIVITIES		OTHER CHARTS IN USE	
Hospital Name:				**PRESCRIPTION FORM (5 WEEK)**	
Name:				Insulin	☐
Hospital Number:				PCA and other infusions	☐
DOB:				Anticoagulants: Heparin	☐
				Oral	☐
Date of Admission:		Consultant Name:		Topical:	☐
Ward:	Height:	DVT Risk on Admission (SIGN Guideline) High ☐ Moderate ☐ Low ☐		TPN: Enteral Nutrition:	☐ ☐
Weight:	Surface area:	Assessed by: Date: ___/___/___		Other:	
Date of writing discharge prescription: ____ / ____ / ____		Prescription sheet number: _____		Date and time form re-written: ____ / ____ / ____ Time:_____	

ONCE ONLY AND PREMEDICATION DRUGS

DATE	DRUG	DOSE	ROUTE	TIME	SIGNATURE OF DOCTOR	GIVEN BY	TIME GIVEN

Figure 2.34 Prescription chart. Reproduced with permission from Greater Glasgow and Clyde Health Board.

medical staff and pharmacists to allow nurses to supply or administer certain drugs to patients using their own assessment and without having to refer to a doctor for an individual prescription. They will have been agreed by the relevant NHS healthcare body. Some employers require their staff to have completed additional training before being allowed to use them.

This is different from nurse prescribing where certain nurses are allowed to prescribe drugs within their competence. The NMC (2006) has published standards and proficiencies for the programme of preparation for nurses, midwives, and specialist community public health nurses to prescribe either as a community practitioner nurse prescriber or as an independent nurse or supplementary prescriber. These nurses are experienced practitioners who have completed an approved programme of preparation and training for independent nurse prescribing and have sufficient knowledge and competence to prescribe medications to patients.

Storage of medicines

All medications and prescription pads need to be stored according to law and local policy. Medications may be stored is in a cupboard trolley (see **Fig. 2.35**) or fridge and these should be locked up at all times.

Controlled drugs should be stored in a locked cupboard within a locked cupboard. The two keys for these cupboards should be kept separately and a red light should automatically light up when the inner cupboard is opened. Keys to these cupboards should be kept by a registered nurse at all times – you, as a student, should NEVER hold these keys.

Medications should remain below 25 °C, as some drugs can be damaged above this temperature. If medications must be stored in a fridge, then the fridge should have a maximum and minimum thermometer, which should be monitored daily. Please note that some of these medications need to be brought to room temperature prior to administration.

Repeated handling of some drugs can cause contact **dermatitis**. Examples are cytotoxics, **antibiotics**, local **anaesthetics**, **topical** preparations). Gloves should be worn when handling drugs that can be absorbed through the skin. These include cytotoxics, hormone preparations, and iodine preparations.

Pregnant staff should not handle **cytotoxic** agents and should be advised against other teratogenic substances, such as anaesthetic gases and radiopharmaceuticals that can harm the unborn child.

Drug calculations

Nurses need to be able to perform drug calculations accurately and confidently if they are to administer the correct dose of medication to patients. Failure to do so will

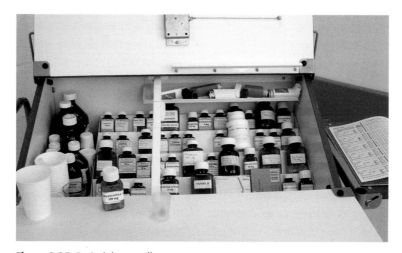

Figure 2.35 Typical drugs trolley

compromise patient safety. Calculating drug doses is often an area of concern for nurses, perhaps because of poor preparation, or pressures of time in the clinical area. Drug errors are still common and are often caused by errors in calculation. Two different approaches to drug calculation can be used. The first method is based on using the information you have about the prescription and drug strength. The second method is based on the use of a formula. Examples of suitable formulas are

number of tablets = amount prescribed (what you want)
÷ amount in each tablet (what you've got)

volume to be given = (amount prescribed × unit volume)
÷ amount per unit volume

Good practice recommends that the calculation should first be made mentally or in writing and then checked with a calculator (if appropriate) (Downie *et al.* 2006). Most doses are small numbers or volumes, so if your answer is large check it and then ask a more experienced nurse or refer to the *British National Formulary*. Most students find it very useful to practice drug calculations throughout their training and once qualified. We have included some useful resources in the reference list at the end of this chapter.

If your answer looks wrong, double-check it!

Surface area

In children and in certain specialized forms of therapy (for example, chemotherapy), drug dosage is often calculated using weight or, more frequently, by calculating the patient's surface area. The reasons that surface area is now the preferred measurement are:

- Drugs are absorbed in different ways and surface area may impact on the dosage required,
- Children with more body fat may have a different rate of absorption. This should be taken into account when calculating the dose required.

To calculate surface area you need to use a table called a nomogram. These can be found in the *British National Formulary for Children*. You find the patient's height on one side of the scale and the patient's weight on the other side of the scale and draw a line (with a ruler) between these two points to find the patient's surface area.

Administration routes

There are numerous routes by which medications can be administered. For the majority of clients, the most appropriate method of receiving medication is by mouth and swallowed, that is, oral medication. Other oral routes can be **sublingual** (dissolves under the tongue) and **buccal** (held against the mucous membrane of the gum and the inside of the cheek). The route of administration should be clearly stated on the prescription and must be followed. A dose of drug prescribed for one route may be lethal or ineffective if given through another route.

There are many types of medicinal preparations of drugs: tablets, **capsules**, lozenges, **elixirs**, **linctuses**, syrups, and mixtures. Tablets can also come in different shapes, sizes, colours, and types; for example, they may be **enteric-coated** (this prevents the drug irritating the gastric lining or prevents it from being broken down by gastric acid) or slow-release (this controls the rate of release of drug from the tablet as it passes through the **alimentary** canal). Capsules are beneficial when the drug is difficult to make into a tablet or is particularly unpalatable.

If the oral route is not appropriate, then medicines can be administered by injection. These can be administered subcutaneously (into the fatty connective tissue beneath the skin), **intramuscularly** (into skeletal muscle), or **intravenously** (into a vein). Other, less common, routes of injection can be used to deliver a drug to a particular tissue or organ. These include **intra-arterial** (into the artery supplying the organ), **intra-articular** (into the joint), **intradermal** or **intracutaneous** (into the lower layers of the skin), and **intrathecal** (within the subarachnoid space).

- **Subcutaneous injections** tend to be used for administering small doses of nonirritating, water-soluble substances, such as insulin, heparin, hyosine, and vaccines.
- **Intramuscular injections** tend to be used for administering irritating drugs and those in an oily solution or aqueous suspension, such as **analgesics**, **anti-emetics** and corticosteroids.

- The **intravenous** route is used to administer a drug directly into the vein and, therefore, can result in an effective blood level of the drug in seconds. This is very useful in emergency situations, but is also a useful way of administering larger volumes or of administering drugs where other injection routes would be too painful.

There are many other routes that can be used when oral and injection methods are inappropriate. One such route is through the **mucosa**; this includes rectal, vaginal, **aural** (ears), nasal (nose), sublingual, and buccal. This route is effective if the drugs cannot be swallowed, cause severe irritation to the upper gastrointestinal tract, require a prolonged reaction, need rapid absorption due to the **systemic** blood supply or need to be delivered close to the site of the lesion or directly to the source of an infection.

Other commonly used routes are inhalation, that is, using **inhalers** and **nebulizers** to allow rapid relief from respiratory symptoms and topically, that is, directly on to the skin.

2.6.3 **Procedure for the administration of any medicine**

Definition

This section discusses the safe and legal administration of a prescribed medicine.

The following principles apply to the administration of any medicine. However; it is essential to remember that each client is an individual and, as such, may require a tailored assessment prior to administration. The five RIGHTS will also be explained individually. These are:

1. The right point
2. The right route
3. The right time
4. The right drug
5. The right dose

Student nurses should always be directly supervised when administering medications and a registered nurse must countersign all student signatures (NMC 2008a).

When to administer medicine

Issues of consent must be considered when administering any medicine. The guidance in relation to consent in childhood is complex and can vary depending on local guidelines and laws in different countries. For example, the guidance for consent in childhood in England differs from that operating in Scotland. It is, therefore, important that you clarify that the consent process adopted in the clinical area accurately reflects the appropriate guidance. References to support further reading around this issue have been provided.

Key point: In many clinical areas, when administering medicines to children, it is common practice that all medications are checked and administered in the presence of two nurses; one of whom must be a registered practitioner. Both must sign the drug kardex to verify that the medicine has been administered as prescribed. This differs from adult practice, where medications are often administered by only one registered nurse.

Administration of any medicine

Key point: There are safety checks that should always be made when administering medication. However, these checks should be carried out before approaching the patient:

- **Case notes and prescription chart**: check these documents for any known patient allergies.
- **Prescribed dose**: ensure the dose prescribed is within the correct range for the patient.
- **Prescribed date and time**: confirm this information.
- **Prescription**: the writing must be legible – make sure that the prescription has not been discontinued.
- **Administration**: make sure that the medicine has not already been given.

continued

Administration of any medicine

Step		Rationale
1	Assess patient's knowledge of medicine and verify any allergies.	To allow informed consent and to prevent a reaction to the medicine.
2	Discuss what you propose and ensure that the patient is aware of his or her rights regarding consent.	The patient has a right to informed consent.
3	Wash your hands.	To reduce the risk of spreading infection.
4	Identify a suitable working area; this should be clean and provide space to prepare the medicine.	To prevent infection and to facilitate administration.
5	Check that you have the **RIGHT PATIENT**. You can ask for the patient's name, however, other safeguards are necessary depending on the environment: **If in a hospital:** check the patient's name-band. This information should match the prescription chart. The patient's details should match the prescription chart (full name and hospital number). **If in the community:** verbal confirmation of the patient's name should be received from either the patient or the patient's carer if they are unable to communicate. It is also now common practice to have a photo board with the patient's name on it.	To ensure it is the correct prescription for this patient.
6	Check that you have the **RIGHT ROUTE**.	To safeguard against errors.
7	Check that it is the **RIGHT TIME** to give the medicine and that the medicine has not already been given.	To safeguard against errors.
8	Also check that there are no other special requirements in relation to the administration of this medicine, for example, after food, depending on blood pressure.	
9	Check that it is the **RIGHT DRUG** and check the drug's expiry date	To ensure that the patient is given the correct drug and that it is not out of date.
10	Check that it is the **RIGHT DOSE**.	To ensure patient receives the prescribed amount.

Administration of any medicine

11	Administer the medicine as prescribed. Do not leave the medicine unattended at any time.	To ensure that the medicine is received by the correct patient.
12	Remember to talk to the patient whilst carrying out the procedure.	To allay any fears and to allow the patient to ask questions or express concerns.
13	Observe the patient for any adverse reactions or signs of discomfort. Refer to local policy documentation for guidance regarding how long you should remain with the client afterwards; this will be of particular importance when administering medicines in the community setting.	Adhering to this procedure will also allow you to react promptly should the patient experience any adverse reaction to the medicine.
14	If you suspect that an adverse reaction is related to a drug or a combination of drugs (adverse drug reaction [ADR]) then a Yellow Card should be completed. These are available in the BNF, the MIMS Companion, and from the MHRA, and are then sent to the MHRA (Medicines Healthcare products and Regulatory Authority. They can also be accessed from http://yellowcard.mhra.gov.uk.	To detect and report reactions to certain drugs.
15	Record that the medicine has been given. Your signature must be legible and both the date and time of administration should be clear for others to read.	This process provides a permanent record of the procedure and will safeguard both the nurse and the patient.
16	If the patient experienced any adverse reactions to the medicine this must be recorded and reported thereafter to medical staff.	To meet legal and hospital requirements.
17	Dispose of any soiled equipment. Refer to local policy guidelines for disposal of waste and infection control.	To prevent transmission of infection.

Aftercare

On administration of the prescribed drug, the date, time, and dose should be recorded in the patient's medicine kardex. This information should be accompanied by a signature from both members of staff. This provides both a permanent record of the drug administered and also ensures that other staff can access this information as necessary.

After administration and documentation, the patient should be advised to report any adverse reaction or response. Should this situation arise, the nurse should both advise medical staff and document what has occurred in the patient's notes, again ensuring that a permanent record is maintained.

Other factors to consider

Sometimes it is not possible to administer the drug prescribed. In these situations, the nurse must document that the drug has not been given and should also record the reason. Medical staff should also be advised, as the drug prescription chart may have to be reviewed.

Anaphylaxis

When administering a medication, nurses must be aware of the possibility of **anaphylaxis**. This is a sudden severe allergic reaction. It is sometimes referred to as *anaphylactic shock* and can be triggered by a severe allergy to, amongst other things, medication. If this situation arises, the client may experience all, or a selection, of the following symptoms:

- Increased anxiety
- Tingling or increased warmth
- Itching
- A metallic taste in the mouth
- Swelling of lips and tongue
- Skin rash
- Breathlessness or wheezing
- Vomiting or diarrhoea
- Dizziness or chest pain

If you suspect anaphylaxis, it is imperative that you act quickly. Consider the following guidelines for practice:

- Raise the alarm and make sure that a qualified practitioner or member of medical staff is aware of what's happening as medical intervention is essential. In the community, this will mean dialling 999
- Follow the anaphylaxis protocol (Resuscitation Council 2005). Be ready to provide an update to qualified practitioners and medical staff when they arrive

Covert or hidden administration of medicine

Another way of administering medication, which you may see when you are on clinical placements, is the covert or hidden administration of medicine. This often means that the medication needs to be crushed or capsules opened.

In most instances this is bad practice and has both legal and ethical implications, as it removes the patient's fundamental right to *consent to treatment* (NMC 2008a). However, there are circumstances when it may be justifiable if it is in the patient's best interests. Further advice can be found on the NMC website.

It is sometimes used when it is impossible to administer oral medicine to certain clients as they may:

- Have **dysphagia** (have difficulty swallowing)
- Frequently spit out their medication
- Chew medication when immediate swallowing is indicated
- Hide their medication, leading to missed or reduced doses with the possibility of a future overdose if drugs are accumulated over time

It may also be suitable when patients are unable to consent to treatment. This may present with certain clients:

- People with a learning disability
- People with mental health problems
- Elderly
- Neonates, infants, and children
- The critically ill.

Therefore, covert administration of a medication can *only* be carried out if the nurse is able to demonstrate that:

- The action is in the best interest of the client,
- The medication is necessary to preserve life,
- The method of administration has been discussed and agreed on by the pharmacist, medical team, and nursing staff, and
- The method chosen is safe and will not alter the absorption of the drug and, therefore, its mode of action

Crushing tablets or opening capsules

Crushing tablets or opening capsules and adding it to food may seem pragmatic but is classed as unlicensed drug administration. It can be dangerous as it can change the site and rate of absorption and the strength of the medication. It can also cause irritation to the gastrointestinal lining, for example, in the case of enteric-coated medicines, Dingwall 2007). Before this unlicensed method is chosen, the following advice should be considered:

- All other possible methods of administration have been reviewed and discussed with nursing, medical and pharmacy staff before choosing this approach
- Attempts have been made to obtain a licensed liquid formulation of the medicine

Administration of a controlled drug

Keypoint: This table summarizes the requirements of the Act as applied to nurses.

Action	Rationale
Follow the procedure for administration of any drug, but with these additions:	
Two nurses or a registered nurse and another approved professional must be involved in the procedure at all times.	To comply with legislation and hospital regulations.
Take the drug from the controlled drug store.	
Check stock number with the number in the controlled drug book.	To ensure that the numbers of drugs matches the number in the register.
Check date, time, method, route, dose, and patient.	To ensure that the correct patient receives the correct prescription.
Record stock number of the remaining medicine.	To comply with legal and hospital regulations.
Administer the drug.	

If an unlicensed method is chosen, it must be agreed on and authorized by the prescriber. A written record of this authorization should be recorded in both the prescription chart and the clients' notes. In addition to discussion with the pharmacist, it may also be useful to speak to the medicine manufacturer or the local medicines information centre for advice on alternative medicines or formulations.

These situations often arise in nursing homes. Each nursing home should have a protocol which they follow when faced with residents who have swallowing difficulties or have medicines administered via PEG tubes.

2.6.4 **Administration of controlled drugs**

Definition

This section explains the administration of controlled drugs in accordance with existing legislation. Controlled drugs are drugs that are dangerous and have stricter legal controls to prevent them from being obtained illegally. They are also associated with a potential for abuse and dependency.

Background

Under the current regulations, controlled drugs are classified into five schedules, each representing a different level of control. Level 1 is the strictest level, while level 5 has the most lenient controls.

- Schedule 1 drugs have no approved medicinal use. An example is lysergic acid (LSD). These are not used in nursing practice
- Schedule 2 is the next highest level of control and includes drugs such as diamorphine, morphine, and pethidine
- Schedule 3 includes most of the barbiturate dugs and a few minor stimulants
- Schedule 4 is divided into two parts. The first includes the benzodiazepines and the second includes the anabolic and androgenic steroids

- Schedule 5 includes preparations that contain a drug with a potential for abuse, but in a low dose form, where the risk of abuse is very small. For example codeine phosphate has a very small dose of codeine, which is a schedule 2 drug

Aftercare

The administration details should be documented in the controlled drug book (date, time, patient's name, dose, and the signature of both staff). This ensures that a permanent record is kept.

If the prescription does not involve the full dose of drug in the **ampoule**, then any unused drug should be discarded. This needs to be witnessed by the second nurse and documented in the controlled drug book (**Fig. 2.36**).

Other factors to consider

In a community setting, the patient or carer may be able to administer the controlled drug if it is in oral form. In this instance, the controlled medicine belongs to the patient or carer and a controlled medicine record sheet and prescription sheet for this medicine (signed by the GP or consultant) will be in the patient's home.

If patients bring in their own controlled drugs, which they have been prescribed, to hospital, then the pharmacist (but not the nurse) can lawfully accept these drugs for destruction. If the drugs are brought in illegally, then the police need to be contacted.

2.6.5 **Self-administration of medication**

Definition

Patients administer their own prescribed medications to themselves. This can be in any form, for example, tablets or capsules, ointments, or injections.

When self-administration is appropriate

Self-administration of medicines (SAM) programmes are becoming increasingly popular, as they improve patient compliance and independence. They can also reduce potential drug errors in drug rounds, which can be caused by the trolley being full of different medications and nurses being interrupted. As these programmes involve individual patient histories, they improve patient assessment and allow patients to receive their

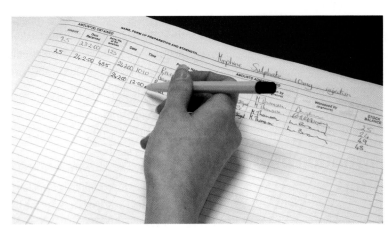

Figure 2.36 Controlled drug book

Self-administration of medicines

Key points: The system must have been fully documented and agreed by all parties. There must be full patient information and patient consent. A detailed protocol, including patient assessment, stages of the process (prescription sheet, record of administration, checks, and actions) and clear guidelines on the role of the healthcare professionals, must be provided.

Step	Rationale
1 Assess the patient and document findings in the nursing notes.	Knowledge, compliance, and any special needs can be identified.
2 Review proposed prescription with pharmacist.	If drugs are to be changed regularly, then self-prescription may not be suitable.
3 If successful, patient is given access to bedside medicine cabinet under nurse's supervision.	To allow continued assessment and evaluate any compliance aids used.
4 If successful, patient is given the key to the cabinet and allowed to self-administer with only limited supervision checks.	Patient can be given further information and education at this point as confidence improves.
5 Check that the drugs are being taken, records are being kept, and discuss progress with the patient.	To ensure that treatment is received and to promote patient involvement.
6 If successful, patient is allowed to self-administer with reduced level of checks on compliance.	To allow the patient to prepare for discharge.

medication at the most appropriate times. Self-administration programmes also encourage patient-centred care, empower patients and increase the opportunities for patient learning with the expectation that enhanced patient knowledge will lead to improved compliance on discharge from hospital (McGraw and Drennan 2001).

Aids to compliance

- Daily dose reminder (DDR) devices are divided into days of the week (see **Fig. 2.37**). On the reverse is a label listing the contents of the device and instructions for administration. The box is loaded by the pharma-

cist, carer, patient, or nurse and opened at the instructed times.

- Monitored dosage (MD) systems differ in that the medication is usually provided in heat-sealed foil blister packing and must be dispensed in a pharmacy.

Aftercare

If the patient is to be discharged home then the nurse should check the drugs in the locked cabinet against the discharge prescription. If they are prescribed, then the remaining drugs can be given to the patient to take home along with any others supplied by the hospital pharmacy. The keys to the locker will be given back to the nurse on discharge.

Developing your skills

It is important to evaluate the effectiveness of the SAM programme and record any difficulties and actions taken. This will then identify further teaching and learning needs and allow the plan to be changed accordingly.

Other factors to consider

The patient must be able to keep the key to the locked cabinet safe and must tell staff if any visitor or other patient tries to access the medication.

With children it may be possible to have a locked medicine cabinet at their bedside over which the nurse has complete control but which remains individualized to the patient.

2.6.6 **Administration of medicine through other common routes (except injection)**

Definition

There are many routes that can be used to administer a medication. This section covers the skills involved in administering:

When to administer medicine through different routes

These routes are effective for a variety of reasons. For example, eye drops and ointments are administered to patients for various eye conditions, such as infections, red eye, tear **deficiency**, or inflammatory conditions, often to allow absorption at the direct site of infection or inflammation.

Rectal preparations can take the form of **suppositories** (in a solid form that melts at body temperature) or **enemas** (as a solution, suspension, or foam) and are used when other methods are unsuitable, when a prolonged affect is desired, or to allow the medication to act directly on the lower bowel. It should go without saying that the patient must be fully informed of the procedure and that dignity and privacy must be maintained at all times.

Vaginal preparations that contain drugs should be prescribed, administered, and recorded according to local

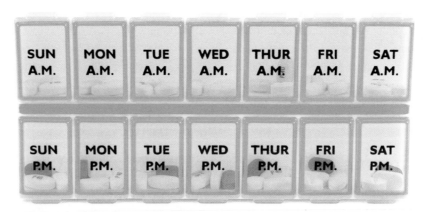

Fig. 2.37 Daily dose reminder (DDR) device. Jurie Maree/istock.com

Administration of an oral medicine (in any form)

Step	Rationale
Follow the guidelines for the administration of any medicine.	
1 Calculate how much drug is to be given. Do not break tablets unless there is a score on them: use a file or tablet cutter.	To ensure that the prescribed amount is given to the patient.
2 **Tablet or capsule:** empty into a medicine container or pot without touching the medicine (use a blister pack or tip into the lid of the bottle and then transfer to the pot). **Liquid:** the liquid should be drawn up using a syringe for accuracy. If a larger volume is required, then pour into a measuring cup and check the level against the measuring line at eye level. For other forms of oral medication, for example, soluble, buccal, sublingual, see individual drug instructions.	To prevent cross-infection and to reduce harm to the nurse. To ensure accuracy.
3 Take the medicine and the prescription chart to the patient and check the patient's identity.	To ensure that the medicine is administered to the right patient.
4 Administer with food or between meals if required.	To prevent gastric upset or problems with drug absorption.
5 Administer the drug. Do not leave the medicine at the bedside.	To ensure that the patient takes the medication.
6 Give the patient a glass of water if allowed.	To aid swallowing.

policy. Where possible, the patient should apply the preparation herself. Privacy, tact, patience, and gentleness are essential at all times, as this can be very embarrassing for patients.

In babies and young children, oral medications are usually given in liquid form. Dosage can be measured more accurately using a syringe rather than a spoon or medicine cup. The use of the syringe also makes it much easier to administer the medicine if the child is uncooperative. The tip of the syringe should be placed towards the side of the mouth and the contents should be slowly discharged into the cheek.

Administration of eye drops or ointment

Step	Rationale
Follow the guidelines for the administration of any medicine.	
1 **Assess the eye for any negative changes, such as inflammation, discharge, or alterations in vision.**	To prevent further damage.
Record any negative changes and seek appropriate advice if required.	The eye is a very delicate and vital structure which has many ways of protecting itself, for example, the blink reflex, tears, eyelashes.
2 **Clean eyes ONLY if the lids are sticky.**	Eyes have effective self-cleaning mechanisms: tears and lid closure.
3 **Clean hands**	To prevent cross-infection.
4 **Instil one drop into the lower fornix (see Fig. 2.38).**	Eyes cannot cope with any more fluid. Overflow can be absorbed into the systemic system.
If the bottle or dropper comes into contact with the patient's eye then the bottle or dropper should be discarded as appropriate and a new bottle received from the pharmacy.	To prevent the spread of infection.
The bottle or tube should be labelled 'left' or 'right' specifically for the affected eye. If both eyes are to receive medication then often two bottles or tubes will be provided, and should be labelled 'left' and 'right'.	To prevent cross-infection from one eye to another.
5 **Ask the client to close the eyes gently and count to 60. Ask the client to close the eyes gently and count to 60.**	Prevents the drop from being moved into the systemic system. Allows it be absorbed correctly.
6 **Leave for 3–5 minutes before applying a second drop to the same eye if prescribed.**	Otherwise, the previous drop will be washed away and not absorbed.
7 **If eye ointment is prescribed, then it should be applied now.**	Ointment 'waterproofs' the eye and so drops would not be absorbed if administered afterwards (Marsden and Shaw 2003).

Administration of ear drops

Key point: When administering ear drops in children over three years old, the pinna should be pulled straight back. In a child younger than three years old, the pinna should be pulled down and back. It may be necessary to use distraction techniques to keep the child still for several minutes.

Step	Rationale
Follow the guidelines for the administration of any medicine.	
1 Ear drops should be used at the temperature between room temperature and body temperature.	If eardrops are too cold they can cause a mild vertigo.
2 If instructed, clean external auditory meatus gently with cotton bud.	To allow better penetration of the medication.
3 Position patient either sitting with head tilted to one side or lying on side with ear to be treated uppermost.	To minimize discomfort and ensure penetration of the medication to the intended part.
4 Clean hands.	To prevent cross-infection.
5 Shake bottle if it contains a suspension.	To mix the active ingredients.
6 Draw required amount into dropper.	
7 Pull up and back the cartilaginous part of the pinna (a child's pinna should be pulled back or down and back).	To allow the medication to reach the intended part.
8 Instil drops in external canal without allowing dropper to come into contact with ear.	To prevent cross-infection.
Bottles should be labelled 'left' or 'right', as appropriate.	To prevent cross-infection from one ear to another.
9 Apply gentle massage over tragus.	To help work in the drops.
10 Encourage patient to maintain position for several minutes.	To allow the drops to reach the eardrum.

continued

| 11 | Lightly place a cotton wool ball in external meatus, if necessary. | To ensure that the drops remain in contact with the epithelium. |
| 12 | Wipe any excess medication away. | To ensure patient comfort. |

Administration of nasal drops

Step		Rationale
	Follow the guidelines for the administration of any medicine.	
1	Nasal drops should be at room temperature prior to installation.	The membrane structures are delicate.
2	Patient should be positioned in the supine position with the head hyperextended, for example, head over edge of bed or pillow under shoulders.	To minimize discomfort and ensure penetration of the medication to the intended part.
3	Clean hands.	To prevent cross-infection.
4	Ask patient (or assist if required) to close off one nostril and insert drop or drops into the other nostril without touching any part of the nose with the dropper.	To allow the drops to reach the intended part.
5	Encourage patient to sniff liquid into the back of the nose or, if unable, maintain position for about one minute.	To ensure that the drops remain in the intended place.
6	Instruct patient not to blow nose.	To ensure that the drops remain in the intended place.
7	If the patient sneezes immediately after receiving nasal drops then you should not repeat the dose.	You cannot determine how much medication has been absorbed.
8	Offer patient a tissue into which excess drops can be collected or spat out.	To ensure patient comfort.

Administration of topical preparations

Step	Rationale

Follow the guidelines for the administration of any medicine.

1 Before applying, the skin should be cleansed. — Removes previous applications to prevent accumulation.

2 Wear polythene gloves (use aseptic technique if the skin is broken). — To minimize risk of cross-infection and protect the nurse from absorption.

3 Apply preparation gently and sparingly. — To ensure patient comfort and prevent over-absorption of medication.

4 Keep dressing to a minimum size, if necessary.

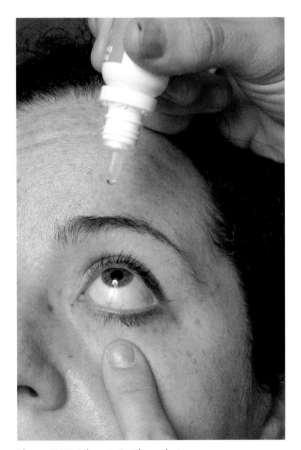

Figure 2.38 Where to instil eye drops

Aftercare

If you are not sure that the patient has swallowed the medication then you should check. Look in the mouth, under the tongue, and between the cheek and the gum. This is important in certain patients with mental health problems who may be trying to store medication.

If the patient vomits immediately after taking the medication, then you should assess the vomit for any signs of the medication. If a whole pill can be seen and identified, then the doctor may wish to administer the medication again or by a different route.

As with the administration of all medications, it is a legal requirement to document that the drug has been administered in the patient's drug record. As with any medication, ongoing assessment is important to detect any adverse reactions and to evaluate the effect of the medication.

Where a rectal or vaginal preparation has been administered, it is very important to ensure that the patient is comfortable and has been allowed the opportunity to wash.

Administration of rectal preparations

Step	Rationale
Follow the guidelines for the administration of any medicine.	
1 Assess bowel tone.	Some patients, for example, older adults, may find it difficult to retain a rectal suppository owing to decreased muscle tone or loss of sphincter control.
2 Position patient correctly. Use incontinence pad and have commode at the bedside if appropriate.	To facilitate the correct insertion of the medication and allow ease of passage.
3 Clean hands and wear disposable gloves.	To minimize the risk of cross-infection.
Suppositories: **4** Lubricate the suppository using lubricant jelly or soften tip in hot water, according to directions on packet.	To reduce **friction** and so ease insertion.
5 Locate anus and insert suppository gently and slowly. Insert the tapered end first if used to evacuate rectum and the blunt end first when the suppository is to be retained. Withdraw finger smoothly.	
6 If the patient expels the suppository before it is absorbed then you should put on gloves and apply further lubricant to the suppository and reinsert it past the internal sphincter.	The suppository will not have been inserted long enough for the drug to be absorbed and so the patient won't receive the therapeutic dose.
If the suppository is too soft to reinsert then you should discard it and notify the doctor.	The doctor may prescribe an additional dose.
Enemas: **4** Warm the enema, expel the air, and lubricate the nozzle.	To prevent damage to the intestinal mucosa and for patient comfort.
5 Locate the anus and insert nozzle for 4–6 cm and slowly roll up the enema pack to introduce contents into the anus.	To ensure tube is in the rectum.

6 Withdraw nozzle slowly.	To prevent pressure being exerted on the intestinal wall.
7 Wipe clean the anal region.	To ensure patient comfort.
8 For evacuant medications the patient should be encouraged to delay first urges to defecate. Elevation of the foot of the bed may help the medication to be retained.	To allow the medication to have the desired effect.

Developing your skills

It is essential, as a student nurse, that you become accustomed to administering medication and know the legal, professional, ethical, and pharmacological aspects surrounding its administration. Observing drug rounds when you are on placement and working with your mentor will help you become familiar with this skill.

2.6.7 **The administration of injections**

Definition

Injections are given using a needle and syringe and should only be given if this is the most appropriate route for the patient or the drug. There are various routes for injection but the subcutaneous (SC) and intramuscular (IM) are the two most common and so will be discussed first.

When to administer an injection

Whether an injection should be administered subcutaneously or intramuscularly depends on the individual drug.

Subcutaneous injections

These are used when the medication needs to be absorbed slowly and over a longer period of time and when only a small volume is to be injected (that is, less than 2 ml). These injections are less painful and so are suitable for frequent injections, such as insulin.

Subcutaneous injections are given under the epidermis into the fat and connective tissue of the subcutaneous layer. Suitable sites are shown in **Fig. 2.39**.

Intramuscular injections

These injections are chosen as more appropriate when rapid, systemic absorption is required (through well-perfused muscle, see **Fig. 2.40**) or when the drug is likely to irritate the subcutaneous tissues, or if a larger volume is required (for example, 5 ml).

Intramuscular injections are given into the skeletal muscle. Needles should be long enough to reach

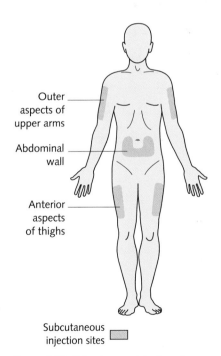

Outer aspects of upper arms

Abdominal wall

Anterior aspects of thighs

Subcutaneous injection sites

Figure 2.39 Subcutaneous injection sites

Administering a vaginal pessary

Step	Rationale

Follow the guidelines for the administration of any medicine.

Step	Rationale
1 The patient should be positioned correctly, preferably in the supine position with knees flexed and thighs abducted or in the left lateral position with buttocks at the edge of the bed.	For ease of insertion and patient comfort.
2 Clean hands and apply gloves.	To protect the patient and nurse from acquiring infection or the nurse from absorbing any of the medication.
3 Apply lubricant to the pessary.	For ease of insertion and patient comfort.
4 Insert pessary as high as possible along the posterior vaginal wall in an upwards and backwards direction for the full length of the vagina, using the applicator.	To allow the medication to be absorbed at the correct site.
5 Wipe dry the vulval area, make the patient comfortable, and apply sanitary pad.	Prevent staining of the clothes. Tampons should not be used in the presence of an infection.

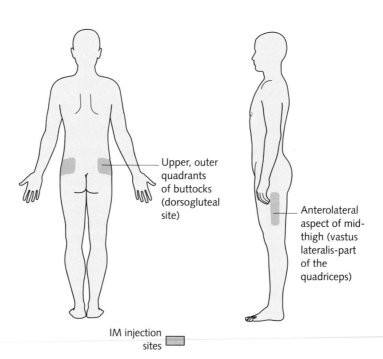

Upper, outer quadrants of buttocks (dorsogluteal site)

Anterolateral aspect of mid-thigh (vastus lateralis-part of the quadriceps)

IM injection sites

Figure 2.40 Intramuscular injection sites

the muscle and still allow a third of the needle to remain outside the skin. In selecting the most appropriate needle the nurse needs to assess the patient's muscle mass, subcutaneous fat, and weight. The volume of the injection should also be considered and, if greater than 3 ml, two separate sites may have to be used.

Aftercare

After administering an injection, you should never re-sheathe the needle: this will help prevent needle-stick injuries. The correct documentation should be completed and sharps and nonsharp waste should be disposed of appropriately according to local hospital or health board policy. Care must be taken to ensure that sharps are not carelessly disposed of with linen, or in plastic bags, as this then creates a serious hazard for others.

Ongoing assessment of the patient is very important to evaluate the patient's response to the medication and to detect any adverse effects.

Developing your skills

Giving injections is a skill that many student nurses are apprehensive of. Observing this skill on placement and carrying it out in a supportive environment should help ease this anxiety. It is important that you do not exhibit and transmit your fear and anxiety to the patient.

Other factors to consider

Fear of needles or fear of injections

Some patients are afraid of needles and it is important to determine the reason. It may be that a previous injection was very painful. There are ways to reduce the pain, for example, preparing the patient better, freezing the skin with ice or a local anaesthetic, selecting a different site, technique, patient position relaxation and distraction techniques. It is particularly important for intramuscular injections that the muscle is relaxed: should the muscle be tense through anxiety or fear, the injection will require

more force and be more painful as a result. If none of these techniques are appropriate, then it may be necessary to use a different route.

Interruption in injection

If the patient pulls away from the injection before you have fully delivered the medication, you should remove and discard the needle and attach a new one and administer the remaining medication at a different site. This should all be documented.

2.6.8 **Managing drug errors**

Definition

Drug therapy is becoming more and more advanced and, therefore, the potential for errors is increasing. These errors can be made by medical staff in prescribing, by pharmacists in dispensing, or by nurses in administering the drugs. The errors can be caused by lack of basic mathematical skills, staff becoming deskilled as a result of using pre-measured drugs, lack of knowledge regarding medicines (for example, overdosing, underdosing, wrong route), complacency, overconfidence, and lack of resources, time pressures, or distractions. An error can lead to anything from no ill effects to death.

Background

Previously, drug errors were seen as a cause for punitive measures to be taken against the person making the error; this led to under-reporting. The NMC (2008a) now encourage an open culture in relation to reporting errors and recommends that ward managers, in their investigation of the error, consider the reasons behind the error (environment, influencing factors), the drug and its effect, whether the incident was disclosed, whether policy was followed, and the nurse's experience and previous involvement in any drug errors.

The following guidelines should be followed so that the patient's best interests are acted on.

The administration of any injection

The administration of any injection

Action	Rationale

Follow the guidelines for the administration of any medicine.

1 Put on gloves.

Protect against infection and prevent contamination by the medicine.

Single-dose ampoule solution

2 Check the solution for cloudiness or matter and if present discard according to hospital policy.

Prevents the patient from receiving a contaminated drug.

3 Break the neck of the ampoule using a gauze swab.

To prevent the nurse from receiving lacerations from glass splinters.

4 Inspect the solution for fragments of glass.

Prevents glass splinter contamination.

5 Withdraw the prescribed amount of solution.

Ensures that the patient receives the prescribed amount.

6 Tap the side of the syringe to dislodge air bubbles.

To prevent air from entering the patient.

Single-dose vial solution

2 Remove the cap and clean the rubber top with an alcohol swab.

To prevent cross-infection.

3 Insert a needle into the vial.

To release the vacuum.

4 Draw air (equal to the amount of solution to be withdrawn) into a syringe and attach it to a second needle. Insert this needle and syringe into the vial and insert the air.

To allow easier withdrawal of the solution from the vial.

5 Draw up the required dose and expel air bubbles.

Prevents the solution spraying into the air on withdrawal.

Single dose vial powder

2 Inject the correct diluents slowly into the vial.

To dissolve the drug.

3 Shake the vial to mix the powder with the diluents.

To dissolve the drug.

4	When the solution is clear, withdraw the prescribed amount (can tilt the ampoule if helpful).	To ensure that the drug is dissolved and to avoid drawing in air.
5	Change the needle to a new needle of the appropriate size.	To make sure that a sharp needle point is used. The needle point can be blunted by insertion into the ampoule.
6	Expose the selected area.	
7	Cleanse the patient's skin with an alcohol swab (if appropriate) and allow to dry.	Cleansing the skin prior to injecting is unnecessary unless the skin is contaminated or the patient is immunocompromised. In these cases this will prevent infection. Allowing the skin to dry will prevent stinging caused by the alcohol entering the skin along the needle track (Downie *et al.* 2008).

The administration of a subcutaneous injection

Action	Rationale

Follow the guidelines for the administration of any medicine.

1	Select an appropriate site such as those shown in Fig. 2.39: • The middle outer aspect of the upper arm, • The middle anterior aspect of the thigh, • The anterior abdominal wall below the umbilicus, • The back and lower loin. If the patient receives many injections, the site should be rotated.	To reduce subcutaneous tissue irritation and maintain drug's absorption rate.
2	Pinch the skin up into a fold, as shown in Fig. 2.41.	
3	Insert the needle into the skin at a 45° angle and release the skin (except insulin).	To elevate the subcutaneous tissue. Some pre-filled syringe medications, such as low molecular weight heparin, have shorter needles, and insulin needles are also shorter, therefore a 90° angle is more appropriate.
4	Inject the drug slowly: there is no need to draw back.	To prevent pain. No blood vessels will be reached, owing to pinch and needle size.
5	Withdraw the needle gently and apply pressure to any bleeding	To prevent a haematoma forming

The administration of an intramuscular injection

Key points: In older patients, it is important to assess the patient's muscle mass (muscle mass reduces in older adults) and select an appropriate needle length and gauge accordingly.

In children, the anterior lateral aspect of the thigh is the preferred site for intramuscular injections.

Step	Rationale
Follow the guidelines for the administration of any medicine.	
1 Assist the patient into the appropriate position and remove necessary garments.	To make the patient more comfortable and the site accessible.
2 Select an appropriate site such as those shown in Fig. 2.40: • Upper outer quadrant of the buttock (dorsogluteal), • Anterior lateral aspect of the mid-third of the thigh (vastus lateralis), • Deltoid region of the arm, • Ventrogluteal.	
3 Clean the site with alcohol swab (if appropriate) and allow to dry.	To prevent infection and prevent stinging from the alcohol entering the skin along the needle track (Downie *et al.* 2008).
4 Stretch the skin around the injection site (with nondominant hand).	To displace the subcutaneous tissue.
5 Hold the needle at a 90° angle and inject the needle two-thirds of the way into the skin quickly.	To ensure that the needle reaches the muscle.
6 Withdraw the syringe plunger and, if no blood is aspirated, inject the drug slowly at a rate of 1 ml in 10 seconds If blood appears, withdraw the needle completely, replace it, and begin again.	To confirm that the needle is not in a vein. To prevent pain and ensure that the muscle has absorbed the drug.
7 Wait ten seconds, withdraw the needle rapidly, and apply pressure to any bleeding.	To allow the drug to diffuse into the muscle. To prevent a haematoma forming.

Managing a drug error

Action	Rationale
Immediately inform medical staff, ward manager, patient and patient's relatives, pharmacist.	To alert the incident to their attention and instigate necessary treatment. To allow investigation to prevent further errors occurring. To maintain open and honest culture.
Implement any intervention as directed by medical staff.	To maintain patient safety by counteracting the effect or reducing further risk or complications.
Complete a critical incident form (a student nurse should also inform the university).	To follow hospital or health board policy and report the incident. To record personal account for use in future investigation.
Document the incident in the patient's record.	To follow legal requirements.

Aftercare

It is important to monitor the patient and report any changes in the patient's condition, to maintain patient safety and comfort.

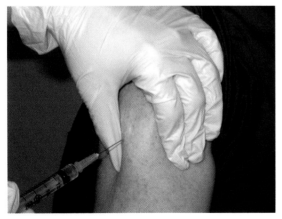

Figure 2.41 Pinching the skin to administer a subcutaneous injection. With permission of Vicki Shawyer and her patient.

Other factors to consider

Errors can never be totally prevented. However, there are many strategies that can be used to reduce the number or errors. These include:

- Having two nurses administer medicines,
- The promotion of self-administration,
- Minimized interruptions during the administration of medicines,
- The adoption of an honest, open culture in reporting errors,
- Nurses keeping their knowledge and skills up-to-date (Preston 2004).

Increasingly, technological systems are being introduced into clinical environments to improve patient safety. These include the use of barcoded patient, drug, and prescription identification, to ensure that identification and calculation errors are minimized.

In the community, devices now exist to encourage compliance with medicines; for example, smart medicine bottles exist that detect whether the bottle has been opened at the appropriate time. If not, a text message is sent either to the client or carer as a reminder that the drug has yet to be taken.

Scenario

Consider what you should do in the following situation, then turn to the end of the section to check your answers.

You have been asked to administer oral medication to one of your patients, Mr Jones. He is having difficulty swallowing the tablet. What options do you have?

Further scenarios are available at 🌐 **www.oxford textbooks.co.uk/orc/docherty/**

Website

🌐 **www.oxfordtextbooks.co.uk/orc/docherty/**

You may find it helpful to work through our short online quiz and interactive scenarios intended to help you to develop and apply the skills in this chapter.

References

British Medical Association and The Royal Pharmaceutical Society of Great Britain (2008a). *The British National Formulary 55*, 55th edn. Pharmaceutical Press, London.

British Medical Association and The Royal Pharmaceutical Society of Great Britain (2007). *Nurse Prescribers' Formulary for Community Practitioners 2007–2009*. BMJ Group and RPS Publishing, London.

British Medical Association, The Royal Pharmaceutical Society of Great Britain, Royal College of Paediatrics and Child Health, Neonatal and Paediatric Pharmacists Group (2008b). *The British National Formulary for Children*. Pharmaceutical Press, London.

Dingwall L (2007). Medication issues for nursing older people (part 2). *Nursing Older People*, **19**(2), 32–6.

Downie G, Mackenzie J, and Williams A (2006). *Calculating Drug Doses Safely: A Handbook for Nurses and Midwives*. Elsevier, Edinburgh.

Downie G, Mackenzie J, and Williams A (2008). *Pharmacology and Medicines Management for Nurses*, 4th edn. Elsevier, Edinburgh.

Marsden J and Shaw M (2003). Correct administration of topical eye treatment. *Nursing Standard,* **17**(30), 42–4.

McGraw C and Drennan V (2001). Self administration of medicine and older people. *Nursing Standard*, **15**(18), 33–6.

NMC (2005a) *Guidelines for Records and Record Keeping*. Nursing and Midwifery Council, London.

NMC (2005b). *An NMC Guide for Students of Nursing and Midwifery*. Nursing and Midwifery Council, London.

NMC (2006). *Standards of Proficiency for Nurse and Midwife Prescribers*. Nursing and Midwifery Council, London.

NMC (2008a). *Standards for Medicines Management* Nursing and Midwifery Council, London.

NMC (2008b). *The Code. Standards of Conduct, Performance and Ethics for Nurses and Midwives*. Nursing and Midwifery Council, London.

Preston RM (2004). Drug errors and patient safety: the need for a change in practice. *British Journal of Nursing*, **13**(2), 72–8.

Resuscitation Council UK (2005). *The Emergency Medical Treatment of Anaphylactic Reactions for First Medical Responders and for Community Nurses*. Resuscitation Council UK, London. The Resuscitation Council UK anaphylaxis algorithm is available from www.resus.org.uk/pages/anaalgo.pdf.

Useful further reading and websites

British Medical Association (2006). *Parental Responsibility*. www.bma.org.uk/ap.nsf/content/parental. This site provides advice from the BMA ethics department in relation to some consent issues in children and the responsibilites of parents.

Finney A and Rushton C (2007). Recognition and management of patients with anaphylaxis. *Nursing Standard*, **21**(37), 50–7. This is a useful article that discusses the nurse's role in identifying and managing patients with anaphylaxis.

Gatford JD, Phillips N (2006). *Nursing Calculations*, 7th en. Churchill Livingstone, Edinburgh. This is a useful book which should enable you to calculate drug doses accurately.

Griffith R, Griffiths H, and Jordan S (2003). Administration of medicines part 1: the law and nursing. *Nursing Standard*, **24**(18), 47–53. This is a useful article that discusses the legal implications of medicine administration.

Houghton J (2006). Understanding the biological differences between adults and children. *Nurse Prescribing*, **4**(2), 54–9. This article describes the differences between children and adults in relation to pharmacokinetics and suggests strategies for ensuring that these are considered when prescribing for children.

James A (2004). The legal and clinical implications of crushing tablet medication. *Nursing Times*, **100**(50), 28–9.
This articles discusses the legal implications of crushing medications and concealing them in patient's food.

Jordan S, Griffiths H, and Griffith R (2003). Administration of medicines: pharmacology. *Nursing Standard*, **18**(3), 45–54.
This articles discusses pharmacology and practice implications, including the consequences for patients of changes, nonadherence, and failure to accommodate drug–food interactions.

Lambert J and Adams E (2006). Anaphylaxis: how to respond with confidence. *Practice Nursing*, **17**(5), 236–41.
This article discusses how to respond to a patient suffering an anaphylactic reaction in the general practice setting.

Pentin J and Smith J (2006). Drug administration. Drug calculations: are they safer without a calculator? *British Journal of Nursing*, **15**(14), 778–81.
This paper discusses medication administration in relation to drug calculation errors and how competence in practice can be maintained.

Royal Pharmaceutical Society (2003). *The Administration and Control of Medicines in Care Homes and Children's Services*.
www.hcsu.org.uk/index.php?option=com_docman&task=doc_download&Itemid=99999999&gid=192.
This document discusses how owners or managers of care homes (residential, nursing homes, and children's homes) can safely handle medicines to meet the standards regulating private care.

Scottish Executive (2006a). *Consent: A Guide for Children and Young People Under 16 (Version 1)*. Scottish Executive, Edinburgh.
www.nhs24.com/content/mediaassets/doc/Consent%20your%20righrts%20(under%2016s).pdf.

Scottish Executive (2006b) *Consent: It's Your Decision (Version 1)*. Scottish Executive, Edinburgh. www.scottishhealthcouncil.org/shcp/files/Consent.pdf.
These are easy to read leaflets that discuss healthcare consent issues in Scotland. The first leaflet is for those under 16 years old and the second is for people of all ages.

Watt S (2003a). Safe administration of medicines in children (part 1). *Paediatric Nursing*, **15**(4), 40–3.

Watt S (2003b). Safe administration of medicines in children (part 2). *Paediatric Nursing*, **15**(5), 40–4.
These are two useful articles on the preparation and administration of medicines to children and the role and responsibility of the nurse.

Wright D (2002a). Swallowing difficulties protocol: medication administration. *Nursing Standard*, **17**(14–15), 43–5.
This article describes an evidence-based protocol used in practice when administering medication to patients who have swallowing difficulties.

Wright D (2002b) Medication administration in nursing homes. *Nursing Standard*, **16**(42), 33–8.
This study looks at the difficulties faced when administering oral medication to patients with swallowing difficulties in nursing homes and how these can be overcome.

Medicines Healthcare products and Regulatory Authority (MHRA). www.mhra.gov.uk/index.htm.
This is an agency of the Department of Health that safeguards the public by ensuring that medicines and medical devices are safe.

http://yellowcard.mhra.gov.uk/.
This site can be used to report suspected side effects to any medication.

Brush up on Your Drug Calculation Skills. www.nursesaregreat.com/articles/drugcal.htm.
This is a useful site in relation to drug calculations and gives some calculations and exercises to complete to practice your skills.

www.mathemagic.org/nursing/#Intro-Intro.
This is the numeracy course for the Department of Health Sciences at the University of York

Test and Calculate. www.testandcalc.com/.
This is a very useful website that contains examples of calculations.

Quick Reference Guide – Numeracy Skills. www.nursing-standard.co.uk/archives/ns/residentpdfs/quickrefPDFfiles/Quickref1.pdf.

Quick Reference Guide – Calculating Drug Dosage. www.nursing-standard.co.uk/archives/ns/residentpdfs/quickrefPDFfiles/Quickref2.pdf.

The *Nursing Standard* has published two quick reference guides in relation to drug calculations. Check **www.oxfordtextbooks.co.uk/orc/docherty/** for changes and new developments. Updated research, guidelines, or equipment will be added every four months.

A Answers to scenario

You should firstly assess Mr Jones's swallowing reflex. It may be that a swallowing assessment needs to be carried out.

If Mr Jones has a swallowing reflex, you could investigate whether there is a liquid form of the medication available. You could consult the pharmacy to establish whether it is possible to crush the tablet. Not all medications can be altered, for example, long-acting or slow-release drugs. You could combine the medication with some soft food to facilitate administration (this should **not** be hidden from the patient).

If Mr Jones does not have a swallowing reflex, look at other routes of administering the medication, for example, injections or suppositories.

3 Maintaining a safe environment

JAYNE DONALDSON AND VALERIE NESS

Introduction

By 'maintaining a safe environment', we mean the safety of the patient taking into account the patient's surroundings. Recognizing and preventing risks to patients' safety is an essential element of the nurse's role. It is important that once a risk has been identified, it is managed effectively to prevent harm. Where actual problems arise, the appropriate action must be taken by the nurse to prevent further deterioration in the patient's condition. This chapter introduces the fundamental skills of maintaining a safe environment and will help you develop your knowledge and underlying skills base to assess patients, and to recognize anyone who is at risk.

There are many potential risks to an individual's safety from the environment. Many of the reasons why a patient needs treatment or support involve some form of harm from the environment, ranging from infections, accidents, and pollution, all of which have obvious physical consequences, and can cause mental health problems created by a stressful environment. The level of risk in the environment often depends on the patient's ability to withstand and avoid these risks. The same environment may be 'safe' for one person but 'dangerous' for another. For example, patients with mental health problems, such as those with severe depression, may not exercise their social and interpersonal skills to communicate health issues and important clinical features may go unreported. Children, those with learning disability, or those with a confusional state may also be unable to report, comment on or even ask questions relating to aspects of their care. Some patients may be unable to make decisions for themselves, or be engaged in any

patient-centred decisions that other patients may be involved in. In these cases, it is essential that nurses have fully developed skills so that the patient is fully and holistically assessed.

This chapter focuses specifically on the physiological systems that help protect healthy individuals against external hazards, and the nursing role of assessing and maintaining their function. The areas that will be addressed within this chapter include:

1 Assessing the patient's **skin**,
2 Assessing the patient's level of **pain**,
3 Assessing the patient's **neurological status**.
4 Assessing and recognizing signs of **acute** and **critical illness** and the immediate actions to take to maintain life.
5 Assessing the patient's risk of **falls**.

The patient's skin is essentially an interface between the internal and external environments. It has an important function in being a barrier to potential infection. It also helps maintain **homeostasis**. For these reasons, the skin should be regularly assessed for signs of damage (further care of the skin is covered in Chapter 8). There are measures that could be taken to prevent damage to the skin surface. For example, using a structured assessment tool will help to identify those at risk of developing **pressure ulcers** and also help to indicate a cause, such as immobility. Implementing an effective intervention thus becomes more logical: the next stage may well be to provide a pressure-relieving mattress for the patient. As a student nurse, you will be placed in a number of different care environments and you will encounter many patients whose skin will be at risk.

Pain

Pain is an experience that everyone encounters in life. As a healthcare professional, you will come to appreciate that pain in others is an everyday event. Pain in health is an unpleasant experience that, consciously and subconsciously, persuades us to adopt healthy behaviours and protects us from harming ourselves. For example, if we touch a hot object we immediately react to the potential tissue damage by subconsciously removing our hand from danger in a **reflex** action. Similarly, if an individual accidentally bites his or her tongue, the pain incurred is sufficient to make the person more wary when chewing their food. A lesson to be learned here is that for pain to be an effective protective mechanism, an intact nervous system and full consciousness is essential. However in ill health, and for some medical interventions, such as surgery, pain serves no useful protective purpose, and can be damaging to health if allowed to continue unchecked. For example, if someone has bruised ribs and lungs, they will experience pain on breathing. This pain will discourage deep breathing, and a chest infection becomes more likely, complicating recovery from injury. Similarly, a child with painful mouth ulcers will be disinclined to eat and may suffer from hunger as a consequence.

Pain can be acute (short-lived) or chronic (long term) and can cause physiological and psychological stress if uncontrolled, affecting the patient's lifestyle, social functioning, and quality of life. It is important that nurses are able fully to assess patients who are in pain and effectively help them take some control in any part of their pain-management regime It is, thus, essential that nurses have the skills and knowledge to recognize symptoms of pain, to understand the underpinning pathophysiology, and to be able to manage pain in any patient across the lifespan.

The protective functions of the nervous system are severely compromised when consciousness is lost. Conscious level must be monitored in those most at risk, as an unconscious patient will need an extra level of care. When assessing a patient's neurological status, the most commonly used validated scale is the 'Glasgow Coma Scale'. This chapter will introduce you to its use within assessment and help you identify signs of stability, improvement, or deterioration in a patient's condition. In addition to the Glasgow Coma Scale, for consciousness, the overall assessment of a critically ill patient will be facilitated by using the systematic ABCDE approach, which assists in identifying appropriate treatment.

A functioning sense of balance and control over our movements allow us to navigate safely through our environment without falling or bumping into objects. If this is compromised, there is an increased risk of falling and causing injury. The section on the assessment of falls will highlight those patients most at risk, describe how to conduct an individualized assessment and outline the preventative measures that could be taken.

Learning outcomes

These outcomes relate to numbers 2, 4, 9, 10, and 18 of the NMC's Essential Skill Clusters and specifically to Care Domains 2 and 3 of the NMC's Standards of Proficiency for Pre-registration Nursing (outcomes to be achieved for entry to branch).

On reading the chapter and associated web pages and undertaking supervised activities, the student will be able to:

- Describe and explain the assessment of patient's skin,
- Discuss the preventative measures that could be implemented to prevent initial, and any further breakdown of the skin
- Describe and explain the assessment of a patient's level of pain, demonstrating an awareness of underlying pathophysiology of pain
- Describe and explain the assessment of a patient's neurological status using the Glasgow Coma Scale and other vital signs
- Discuss what factors may indicate improvement or deterioration within the Glasgow Coma Scale and other 'vital signs', such as pulse
- Discuss the signs of critical illness and identify patients at risk of cardiorespiratory arrest
- Discuss the immediate assessment of critically ill patients using the ABCDE approach

Prior knowledge

To perform the clinical skills in this chapter it is important that you know and understand the following, which can be obtained from a range of reference books:

- The anatomy and physiology of the skin (also refer to Chapter 8 for the skills associated with skin care)
- Basic life support (refer to Chapter 2.5)
- The cardiovascular system
- The respiratory system, including oxygen and carbon dioxide transport and utilization (refer to Chapter 5)

Since each of these topics differs, the relevant background information that underpins each skill can be found in the section immediately following the skill's definition.

3.1 **Skin assessment**

Definition

Skin assessment is an essential skill that is required of all nurses caring for clients, across the lifespan. Often skin assessment is carried out at the same time as other procedures. However, a careful, structured assessment will allow a wide-ranging assessment reflecting the function and performance of other organs, such as the heart, liver, and lungs. Careful observation of the skin and its characteristics can provide useful clues in the assessment of the patient's body temperature, level of hydration, and circulation. Skin can become infected, inflamed, and even damaged by mites, infection and pressure (further information on wound assessment is given in Chapter 8). In addition, the patient's psychological status and general well-being can also be ascertained by examining how well the skin is cared for.

Patients with skin conditions can have symptoms such as pain, scratching, and breaks in the skin, and this can often affect social and psychological functioning (such as where the patient is embarrassed by the skin condition). It is important that the psychological and social aspects of the assessment are considered in any assessment.

Background

The skin

To assess the skin it is useful to have an understanding of the underlying anatomy and physiology, as it will help to explain the problems that may occur within the skin.

The skin has a number of purposes as an organ:

1. The skin provides a natural defence to infection, being the interface between our internal and external environments.
2. The skin is an essential organ in the control of body temperature through promoting or reducing heat loss by vasodilation and vasoconstriction of the blood vessels and producing sweat.
3. The skin is a source of **sensory** input through the nerve endings within it. This is particularly well-developed in the fingertips and provides the sensation of touch. Nerve endings and reflex actions also help to prevent the patient from harm (such as from touching hot substances) and to provide the patient with the sensation of pain.

The structure of the skin is divided into three layers: the epidermis, the dermis, and the **subcutaneous** layer, as shown in **Fig. 3.1**.

- The epidermis is renewed every 50–70 days and can renew and repair itself against the damage it receives from external factors
- The dermis lies below the epidermis and contains connective tissue, collagen, elastic fibres, and specialized cells. The dermis also contains nerve endings, sweat glands, hairs, and blood and lymph vessels
- The subcutaneous layer consists mainly of fat (adipose tissue) and can vary between individuals. This layer provides insulation to organs below and provides a long-term energy resource

The skin contains **commensal** microorganisms, which live on the skin without causing any harm. A baby is born from a sterile world into a world rich in microbial diversity. Very soon the baby's skin becomes colonized by these microorganisms, which are acquired through contact with its parents, brothers, and sisters. These harmless microbes serve the useful purpose of keeping harmful, **pathogenic** microorganisms at bay.

Pressure ulcers

Extrinsic factors, such as pressure, friction, and **shearing** can damage the skin (see **Fig. 3.2**).

Pressure is the force applied on the skin: usually it arises from the weight of the body on a surface such as a bed or chair. Blood supply to the area is reduced as the blood

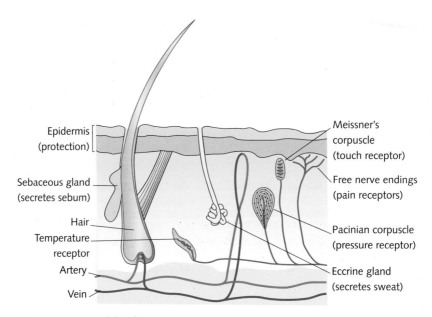

Figure 3.1 Layers of the skin

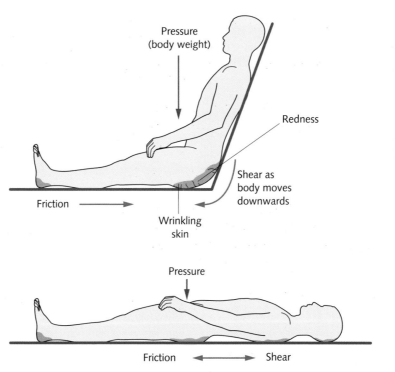

Figure 3.2 Pressure, shear, and friction (a) Sliding in a chair (b) Lying on a bed or trolley

vessels become compressed. As a result, body cells are starved of oxygen and can die (necrose).

Friction occurs when the skin moves against a static surface. For example, the patient may slide down in bed, or be repositioned inappropriately.

Shearing occurs when the skin is static against a surface, but the subcutaneous structures, such as bone and muscle, are relatively mobile, placing the tissues under tension. This creates localized tissue and blood vessel damage, eventually reducing blood supply to the surrounding area.

The result of pressure, friction, and shearing, singly or in combination, is referred to variously as a pressure ulcer, decubitis ulcer, or pressure sore.

Since pressure, shearing and friction are extrinsic factors that increase the patient's risk of pressure ulcer development, these should be reduced or removed by using appropriate pressure-relieving devices, careful repositioning, and appropriate moving and handling techniques.

A survey by EPUAP in 2002 suggested that as many as 22% of hospitalized patients develop some degree of pressure ulceration. The survey also revealed that the incidence of pressure ulcers occurs across all age groups, nursing and medical specialties, and care settings. In terms of patient outcome, they are a significant contributor to **morbidity** and **mortality**, and patients, carers, and families often state that pressure ulcers are a deep source of distress for them.

Classification of pressure ulcers

Within the EPUAP (1999) review, four grades of pressure ulcers were identified, as shown in **Box 3.1**. These are now internationally recognized and referred to in the literature. See **Fig. 3.3** for photographs of graded pressure ulcers.

Patients most at risk of developing pressure ulcers include those with:

- Reduced mobility or immobility
- Sensory impairment
- Acute illness
- Compromised consciousness/sensory loss
- Increasing age
- Vascular disease
- Severe chronic or terminal illness

- Previous history of pressure damage
- **Malnutrition** and **dehydration**
- Extremes of weight, both underweight and overweight
- Communication difficulty preventing the reporting of discomfort or pain, for example, patients with **dementia**

When to asses the patient's skin condition

As a nurse you should be able to identify patients at risk from developing pressure ulcers and employ preventative measures to reduce that risk. It is essential that initial assessment begins immediately. NICE (2003) and NHS Quality Improvement Scotland (2005a) guidelines recommend that these should be carried out and documented within the patient's case notes within six hours of admission in keeping with NMC guidance on good record keeping (NMC 2005; NMC 2007). Reassess for pressure ulcer risk when there has been any change in the patient's condition, and be observant as an ongoing component of care, for example, whenever you reposition the patient you should examine their skin for any signs of tissue damage.

Often this assessment is carried out when performing other tasks, such as the administration of sanitary dressings, or even just spending time in the patient's company. The skin may also be assessed during observation of the patient's vital signs or during skin cleansing (refer to Chapter 8).

Box 3.1 Classification of pressure ulcers	
Grade 1	Nonblanchable hyperaemia of intact skin. Discolouration of the skin, warmth, oedema, induration, or hardness may also be indicators, particularly on individuals with darker skin.
Grade 2	Partial thickness skin loss involving epidermis, dermis, or both. The ulcer is superficial and presents clinically as an abrasion or blister.
Grade 3	Full thickness skin loss involving damage or necrosis of subcutaneous tissue that may extend down to, but not through, underlying fascia.
Grade 4	Extensive destruction, tissue necrosis, or damage to muscle, bone, or supporting structures with or without full thickness skin loss.

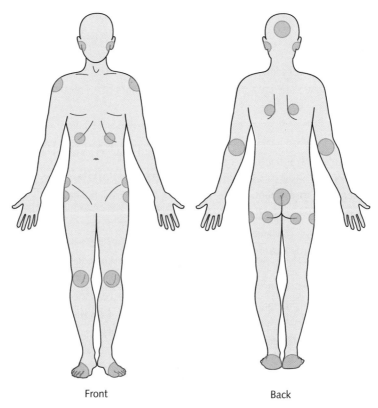

Front   Back

Figure 3.3 Areas susceptible to pressure ulcers

Procedure

Assessment of areas of skin normally covered by clothes can take place while helping the patient bathe or dress. Normally, skin is warm to the touch, dry on the surface, intact, and of a colour consistent with the patient's racial origins. Skin should be assessed for signs of redness, clamminess, rashes, signs of scratching or breaks in the skin's integrity (including signs of parasitic infection such as scabies).

The nurse should either perform the skin inspection regularly or teach the patient to inspect his or her own skin for signs of tissue damage. Particular attention should be paid to those areas most susceptible to pressure ulcers, as shown in **Fig. 3.3**.

Aftercare

Repositioning schedules are usually worked out with the nursing staff, patient, and family, or carer and should be clearly documented in the patient's care plan or pathway. These schedules are also based on clinical judgement and

the risk identified with the scoring tool employed, and should be individualized to each patient. Position itself is important. Even the pressure of top sheets on toes while in bed can damage the tips of the toes in susceptible patients. Every carer and family member who is willing and able to reposition the patient should be taught how to do this in a safe and effective manner.

Best practice states that we should reposition using a 30° tilt where the patient is positioned on areas of large muscle, such as the buttocks. If the patient lies in a **prone** position (face down) this provides the most pressure relief by distributing weight over a large surface area. However, deciding on the best position for the patient should take into account the patient's wishes, medical condition, and comfort, and the overall plan of care.

Refer to Chapter 10 for manual handling devices and techniques that could be employed to minimize friction and shear on the patient, while being safe for practitioner, families, carers, and the patient. Ensure that slings, sleeves, or other equipment are not left underneath the patient.

Skin assessment

Key point: The signs of pressure ulcer development include persistent **erythema, nonblanching or blanching hyperaemia**, blisters, discolouration, localized heat, localized oedema, and induration. For patients with pigmented skin, observe for a purplish or bluish localized area with heat, oedema, and induration. Once tissues have been compressed and the blood vessels seriously damaged, localized heat is replaced by coolness.

Step

Rationale

Step		Rationale
1	Cleanse hands prior to the assessment.	To prevent cross-infection.
2	Explain the assessment to the patient.	To facilitate informed **consent**.
3	Gain patient consent.	To gain cooperation.
4	Ensure privacy.	To prevent embarrassment and maintain dignity.
5	Observe the condition of the skin.	To check skin integrity.
6	Note and document any signs of inflammation, bruising, discolouration, or rash.	To provide continuity of care. To manage any problems that are noted.
7	Note and document the integrity and hydration of the skin (for example, dry, clammy, sweaty). Look for signs of infection: pus, swelling, warm, smelly, and so on. If infection found, swab, and send for microscopy, culture, and sensitivity testing (MC&S).	To provide continuity of care. To manage or evaluate any problems that are noted.
8	Assist patient with clothes and ensure that patient is in a comfortable position.	To prevent further damage to skin. To promote comfort and compassion.
9	Explain your findings to the patient, senior, and other staff where appropriate.	To provide continuity of care. To liaise with other staff's expertise in preventing and managing any problems. To promote patient involvement.

Other factors to consider

Pressure ulcer risk assessment tools

There are a number of tools that are available to identify those at risk of pressure ulcers forming. These should be used to supplement your developing clinical judgement. These tools are based on known risk factors, which are allocated a numerical score. Adding the scores for the different factors provides a total score, which helps define the level of risk, for example, low, medium or high.

An example of such a score is the Braden scale (Braden and Bergstrom 1988), where a low score indicates high risk. In contrast, when using the **Waterlow scale** (Waterlow 2005), a high score indicates high risk. Training is required to use these, and any other scales that are used within practice areas. You should practice using the scores under your mentor's supervision to ensure that you use them properly. It is recommended that all patients requiring nursing care should have their levels of risk assessed (NHS Quality Improvement Scotland 2005a; 2005b).

Pressure-redistributing equipment

This includes any equipment that enables patients to maintain their independence (such as bed frames) and encompasses a wide range of pressure area care mattresses, cushions, and seating. Each patient should be assessed and the appropriate piece of equipment chosen by experienced members of the multidisciplinary team. The decision to use pieces of equipment should be based on identified levels of risk, skin assessment, comfort, lifestyle and abilities, critical care needs, and acceptability of the piece of equipment to the patient, family, or carer.

Where seating is required (for example, for wheelchair users) this assessment is usually carried out by the occupational therapist or physiotherapist. Generally, patients in a sitting position should not be in that position for longer than two hours without movement.

On occasions, the need for pressure-relieving devices may change quickly, for example, during surgery, during a hospital transfer, or immediately following surgery. At these stages the patient's condition can fluctuate dramatically over a short period of time and it is necessary to assess the skin and review the use of pressure-relieving devices at short intervals.

Referral to multidisciplinary team

Referral to the multidisciplinary team is essential for managing pressure ulcer prevention. The Tissue Viability Nurse can be accessed for specific advice and education on all aspects of pressure ulcer management and prevention. It may also be worth considering specialist advice from the specialist nutrition nurse or dietician, the physiotherapist, to improve mobility, and an occupational therapist, for providing aids to increase mobility (for example, moulded specialist wheelchairs and seats). Advice can also be sought from the moving and handling coordinator about correct positioning and handling of the patient to prevent pressure, friction, and shear forces. The specialist continence nurse may also be employed if there are issues with incontinence that put the patient at greater risk. Medical and nonmedical prescribing staff and pharmacists may be able to provide guidance on medication.

3.2 **Pain assessment**

Definition

So that nurses can adequately manage pain, it is important that the patient's pain is assessed and methods employed to alleviate pain are evaluated. Most patients within hospital will experience some degree of pain and everyone has experienced pain of some kind in their lives (for example, toothache, childbirth, headache, illness, or trauma).

This section introduces you to the nature and characteristics of pain and provides an overview of underlying pain theory. Secondly, you will be introduced to a variety of methods that could be employed to assess the patient's pain.

Pain can have a dramatic effect on all aspects of a person's life, and nurses have an important role to play in its assessment and management. Nurses can contribute uniquely by viewing the patient holistically, by conveying a sense of compassion, and by maintaining a therapeutic relationship with the patient.

People react differently to pain and experience it in different ways. Nurses, too, carry misconceptions about pain, which can lead to the extent of the patient's suffering being underestimated (White 2004). This highlights the importance of nurses being aware of the complexity of pain and its perception, in order to individualize the assessment and management of pain. By working with the patient, the best possible outcome for pain management can be achieved. Most importantly, nurses must remember that pain is 'what the patient says it is' (McCaffery 1972, p. 8).

Background

The purpose of pain

Pain, although not a pleasant sensation, has a protective function: it means that the patient will, for example, withdraw a body limb from danger and prevent the repetition of behaviours that are injurious to the body. For example, children learn quickly that behaviours that cause pain, for example, through falling, should be avoided. In this way, pain can help to maintain the child's safety by encouraging the children to avoid hazards that cause them to fall.

However, some patients will not experience pain and this will endanger their safe environment. For example, a patient who has had a spinal injury may not have pain sensation and the skin may be more susceptible to pressure damage, as there is no sensation of pain to encourage the patient to change position.

Repetitive strain injury (that is, pain usually experienced by repeating the same manoeuvre over and over again) can involve the patient experiencing pain, for example, by operating a piece of machinery at work over and over again. Pain is experienced and can often highlight to the patient that the muscle is being injured by repeating the same manoeuvre again and again. If the manoeuvre is reduced or changed in some way, this can often minimize the pain experienced and help to maintain a safe environment for the patient.

Theory of pain

As we learn more about the transmission of pain, the evolving pain theories enable our understanding of pain to develop. The gate-control theory of pain (Melzack and Wall 1965) proposes that pain is transmitted at the level of the spinal cord by a gate-like process (see **Fig. 3.4**). The 'gates' are thought to be in the dorsal horn of the spinal cord. The gate is open or closed depending on the combination of the sensory impulses from the **peripheral** nerves and the descending impulses from the brain. This has

helped to explain the influence of anxiety and depression: pain increases when the patient is more anxious or depressed (that is, the gate is open). Interestingly, we can help to reduce pain (that is, close the gate) when we can distract or relax the patient using the descending fibres from the brain. We can also reduce pain by using techniques, such as cold, heat, or massage, using the ascending messages from the peripheral fibres.

This theory has helped health professionals understand the nature and complexity of pain and the need to assess the patient holistically. As the theory suggests, there are psychological, physiological, behavioural, emotional, and social elements to the assessment of pain.

Assessment of pain

To manage pain effectively, McCaffery and Pasero (1999) advocate that precise assessment, appropriate intervention, and regular evaluation are necessary. Assessing pain is a nursing skill that is complex in nature, but so important that it is considered to be the fifth 'vital sign' after blood pressure, temperature, pulse, and respiration (Schofield and Dunham, 2003). It can be inferred from this that pain should be assessed on all patients and as frequently as the other vital signs.

Pain assessment that is carried out well can lead to substantial improvements in patient care (Schofield and Dunham 2003), while poor pain assessment can lead to inadequate pain relief, affecting the quality of care and recovery (Wood 2004). Nurses have a professional responsibility to provide adequate pain assessment. To do this effectively, there must be a trusting, therapeutic nurse–patient relationship where patients feel that they are being listened to. However, Middleton (2004a, 2004b) states that although pain assessment is simple, it is not performed frequently enough.

The physiological response to pain

This is an important aspect to assess. In a sudden, acute episode of pain, the body responds by using the 'flight or fight' mechanism of the sympathetic nervous system. Adrenaline (epinephrine) and noradrenaline (norepinephrine) are released, causing an increase in blood pressure, pulse, respiration rate, and perspiration, and dilation of the pupils. However, these physiological

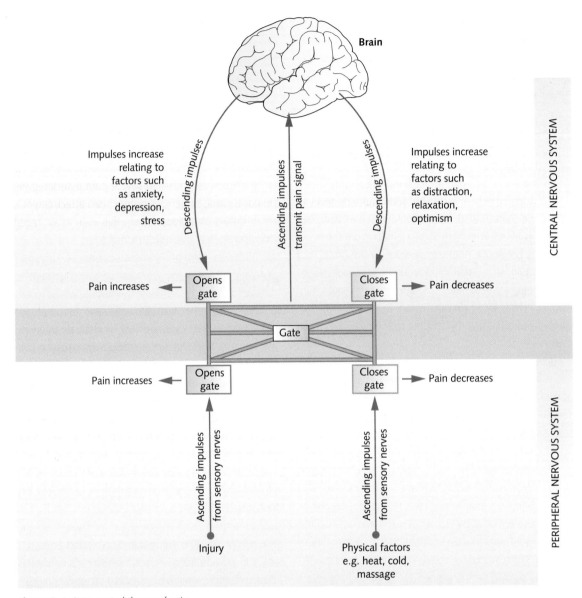

Figure 3.4 Gate-control theory of pain

responses will not be seen in patients with chronic pain. It is also important to realize that these initial responses may also be indicators of stress and anxiety.

There are numerous causes of pain and also numerous ways in which a patient can react to painful stimuli. There is research evidence to suggest that we remember our experiences of pain from an early age. The **threshold** (the level of stimulation at which pain is experienced) varies between individuals and can vary within the same person at different times. The tolerance of pain relates to its intensity and duration. Both **pain threshold** and tolerance vary and can be affected by external factors, such as cultural and spiritual beliefs, sex, previous experience, emotion, and stress, as well as the individual's coping mechanisms and locus of control.

The psychosocial response to pain

It is essential to take account of this when assessing pain, particularly for those with long-standing, chronic pain, as relationships, employment, and career prospects can suffer, causing psychological distress. Research into the relationship with pain, fear, and anxiety have undoubtedly shown that fear and anxiety can increase the perception of pain. Therefore, it is essential that you assess these factors when considering pain assessment. Box 3.2 summarizes the detrimental effects of pain.

Pain is, therefore, a complex phenomenon which is difficult to define. It is recognized that the experience of pain is a **subjective** one for each individual. This should be considered when assessing your patient's level of pain. The seminal work often quoted is that of McCaffery (1972, p. 8), which described pain as 'whatever the experiencing person says it is, existing whenever he says it does.' The International Association for the Study of Pain (IASP) endorsed the more complete definition proposed by Merskey *et al.* (1979): 'Pain is described as a sensory and emotional experience associated with actual and potential tissue damage or described in terms of such damage.'

Historically, pain assessment, especially of children, has been ignored (Carter 1994; Twycross *et al.* 1998). However with the advent of hospital 'pain teams', nurse specialists, and clinical guidelines, the assessment of pain has received more attention both in the literature and in clinical practice. You will be required to develop your knowledge and skills in assessing pain so that you can provide detailed, relevant information to the pain team, evaluate any interventions that may be made and also document that you have thoroughly assessed the patient.

Types of pain

Pain can be described and classified, although any patient may suffer from more than one type of pain. The classification includes: acute, chronic, neuropathic, malignant, and idiopathic pain.

Acute pain has a recent onset and limited time duration (usually less than six weeks) and is commonly associated with surgery or injury. Acute pain is associated with actual tissue damage causing damage to the nerve endings, known as nociceptors. This is a very common type of pain and can range in intensity from a minor injury, such as a small bruise, to severe pain associated with major trauma, surgery, or even a heart attack (**myocardial infarction**). Sometimes, this pain may require medical intervention; at other times it can be managed at home with simple analgesia. It is only through a thorough assessment that this clinical judgement can be made.

There are occasions where acute pain may be 'referred', which means that pain arises in the internal organs (viscera) but is then experienced in another region of the body. An example of referred pain could emanate from an acute myocardial infarction (heart attack). This varies, but there could be central chest pain with referred pain occurring down the left arm, or through to the back, or into the jaw. In its mildest form, a heart attack may even be mistaken for indigestion. The roots of this can be found in embryology but, simply put, the sensory impulses from the left arm and the heart enter the same level of the spinal cord.

Chronic pain may be defined as persistent, either continuous or intermittent, pain that lasts for three months or more. Chronic pain affects around 18% of people in Scotland (NHS Quality Improvement Scotland 2006), and is widespread amongst the elderly population (Gagliese and Melzack 2003), a group within which pain is badly controlled (Proctor and Hirdes 2001). Chronic pain can have serious effects, such as mobility problems, disrupted sleep patterns, and poor appetite, and can cause problems at work or with close relationships or families. Children can have problems with education and play activities, while adults experience feelings of isolation, may not be able to continue working, and generally have to make major changes to their lifestyles (Wilson 2002; McHugh and Thoms 2001). For all groups, pain can have a detrimental effect on mental health. Chronic pain syndrome, a psychosocial disorder, can also develop, where pain

---

Box 3.2 The detrimental effects of pain

- Cardiovascular effects
- Gastrointestinal effects
- Nervous system and hormones
- Poor or reduced mobility
- Psychological effects
- Respiratory effects
- Social effects

becomes the main focus of the sufferer's life (Middleton 2004a).

Neuropathic pain is a condition resulting from injury, such as nerve damage or irritation, to the nervous system. Receptors on the skin, which may only be sensitive to touch or pressure, can become hypersensitive to stimuli that would not normally produce a response (for example, patients report a burning or shooting pain). Examples of this type of pain include phantom limb pain following an amputation, or post-herpetic neuralgia following shingles. This type of pain is notoriously difficult to manage.

Malignant pain is pain resulting from malignant disease (cancer) where progression and spread of the disease leads to pain. Often patients initially present with acute pain associated with treatments and surgery; this pain can then become chronic and more complex to manage as the disease progresses and spreads. This type of pain is often described by patients as 'total pain' as it often affects the patient's whole life, including physical, psychological, social, and spiritual aspects.

Idiopathic pain is pain for which there is no known cause.

Pain transmission

In simple terms, the pain transmission process occurs from the site of the pain, to the spinal cord, and then to the brain. Pain fibres or nociceptors are specific neurons located throughout the body, particularly within the skin (see **Fig. 3.1**). When tissue damage occurs chemical substances are released, and nociceptors recognize the damage exciting peripheral nerve fibres to carry impulses to the spinal cord. Here they enter the dorsal horn of the grey matter and are then carried to the thalamus and on to the cortex of the brain producing our perception of pain.

When to assess pain

An initial assessment is essential on any admission to hospital. Similarly, an assessment is required when a new patient is adopted in the community, or there is in any change in the patient's condition, or if you suspect that a patient has pain. The assessment of pain is normally incorporated into any nursing documentation and should be part of your normal record-keeping procedures (NMC 2005, 2007).

Procedure: Selecting a pain assessment tool

Perhaps the most challenging part of pain assessment is measuring the intensity of the pain objectively. Since pain is a subjective experience this is difficult, but it is not impossible. There are a number of tools that can help measure pain intensity: these often work by asking the patient to rate the pain on a chart. **Figure 3.5** shows examples of different types of scale. The patient is asked to identify which part of the rating scale best describes the intensity of the pain.

Bird (2005) notes that assessment tools can be spilt into two categories: unidimensional and the more complex multidimensional. An example of a unidimensional tool that is easy to use is provided in **Fig. 3.5**.

Procedure: Performing an initial pain assessment

Communication skills are absolutely essential for effective pain assessment. The patient needs to feel comfortable to report the pain to you and to feel that you will listen. The table on p. 127 is an overview of the initial questions that you could ask the patient, carers, and families about the patient's pain.

Before beginning any assessment process, you should always ensure that you have followed appropriate infection control measures that are in place (for example, hand washing), and that you have explained to the patient what you are about to do and given the reasons why. Ensure that you protect the patient's privacy and dignity during the assessment.

Selecting a pain assessment tool

Pain assessment tool	Description and rationale
Unidimensional	Measures pain using a single dimension or aspect.
Visual analogue scale	This is normally a 10 cm line with 'no pain' at one end and 'worst pain ever' at the other end. The patient marks on the line where the pain is judged to be. This scale can also be used for children or patients with a learning disability.
Intensity rating scale	These can have numbers, such as 0 to 10, with zero being no pain at all and 10 the worst pain ever, or they may use verbal ratings, such as 'no pain' to 'worst pain'. These can be read out if the patient has visual impairment, or for a child or other person who cannot read, but the adjectives used can be open to varying interpretations (Bird 2005).
Verbal rating scale **Specific child pain rating scale (Fig. 3.6)** **Neonatal pain rating scale (Fig. 3.7)**	
Multidimensional	Chronic pain, in particular, needs a more detailed assessment because of its multidimensional nature (Schofield and Dunham 2003), and because of this a holistic, multidimensional approach is usually required (Wood 2004).
McGill Pain Questionnaire (MPQ) (Melzack 1975).	The MPQ takes about ten minutes to complete, and is used to obtain information about three qualities of the pain: sensory, affective, and evaluative (Schofield and Dunham 2003). There are long and short versions. The long version takes the form of a patient self-report designed to assess the intensity and quality of the pain. There are three parts to this; a pain rating index, a present pain intensity scale, and a body chart (Wood 2004). The shorter version has 15 adjectives that describe pain: the patient rates these to achieve an overall score (White 2004).
	The MPQ has a number of advantages: firstly, it is an excellent tool for assessing chronic pain, and is quick and easy to use (White 2004); secondly, the questions help with diagnosis and planning of treatment, and can be used to evaluate the effectiveness of interventions as part of a nursing model (Wood 2004). However, the MPQ has been criticized for being more oriented towards research than clinical practice, on account of its length. It has been described as difficult to complete and time is needed for patient education for it to reach its full potential.

continued

The Brief Pain Inventory (BPI) (Fig. 3.10) (Daut *et al.* 1983)	Assesses pain on a scale of one to ten over a week, and records how the pain has interfered with the patient's daily activities. It is easy to use and parts of the questionnaire may be used to assess the management and treatment of the pain (White 2004). The BPI takes around 15 minutes to complete and focuses on the last 24 hours.
Chronic Pain Assessment Tool (Simon and McTier 1996)	For use with patients who have unresolved or poorly managed chronic pain. This tool provides a true multidimensional assessment of patients' chronic pain experiences. It comprises six sections and is a comprehensive, easy-to-use tool suitable for use in inpatient settings. However, it would need to be adapted for use in the community (White 2004). It also takes between 45 and 90 minutes to carry out, making it less suitable for patients who may become fatigued.
Pain diary	In some community areas, a pain diary can be used to record the patient's pain over the course of a number of days or weeks. This allows the patient and nurse to analyse changes in pain and potential triggers and aggravating or relieving factors, knowledge of which may help to manage the pain. The patient, however, needs to be motivated and have the cognitive ability and manual dexterity to write the diary.
The Liverpool Infant Distress Score (LIDS) (Horgan *et al.* 1996).	Many of the tools used in adult areas cannot be used by patients with learning disabilities, who are unable to communicate verbally, or by young children. There are a number of tools that have been developed specifically for this client group, including the Liverpool Infant Distress Score (LIDS) (Horgan *et al.* 1996). Within these client groups, it is imperative that families and carers are involved in care for the assessment of the individual's pain and for the comfort that they can provide.

Performing an initial pain assessment

Questions to ask   Rationale

Questions about the pain	
When did the pain occur?	To identify whether this is acute or chronic pain.
Is there a link to surgery, illness, trauma, or an unknown cause?	To identify any likely cause of the pain.
What was the patient doing at the time of onset?	To identify any triggers or exacerbating events that could also lead to the pain.
How intense is the pain?	To highlight the seriousness and urgency of the situation for the patient.
Where is the pain?	To highlight the possible cause of the pain and to determine whether the pain location will interfere with function. For example, a pain in the throat will interfere with swallowing and possibly affect dietary intake.
How would the patient describe the pain? For example, burning, aching, stabbing, headache.	To highlight the possible cause of the pain, as different types of pain sensation can indicate which type of body structure is involved. For example, waves of spasmodic abdominal pain point to the intestine being a possible source of the problem.
How long have you been in pain?	To highlight whether this is acute or chronic pain.
Is it intermittent or continuous?	To highlight the possible cause of the pain as some conditions produce constant pain, whereas in others, the pain fluctuates.
Was it improved or made worse by, for example, medication, positioning, heat, cold?	To identify the nature of the pain and whether simple remedies have an effect in its relief.
Has this pain been previously experienced? What treatment was used then?	To highlight whether this is acute or chronic pain; to evaluate the success of previous interventions.
Any other medical history.	To highlight the possible cause of the pain. To highlight whether this is acute or chronic pain.

continued

Questions about coping mechanisms

How has the patient been coping with this pain (or not)?	To determine the effect on the patient's social and psychological functioning and to have an insight into the coping mechanisms that the patient has found useful.
Has any medication been taken? If so, when and what? Check that the patient has actually taken any prescribed regular analgesia.	To determine how reliant the patient has become on pharmacological measures. This is important in determining the dose of any **analgesic** prescription if it is to be effective. Generally, the longer a patient has been receiving strong painkillers then the higher the dose that is required in subsequent prescriptions to achieve the same effect.
Have any nonpharmacological interventions been used (for example, heat, cold)?	To evaluate the possible benefits of these measures and to assess the patient's coping mechanisms.
How has the pain affected the patient's lifestyle (for example, behavioural changes, such as not being able to socialize, or communicate)?	To assess the likely effect on the patient's mental health and psycho-social well-being.

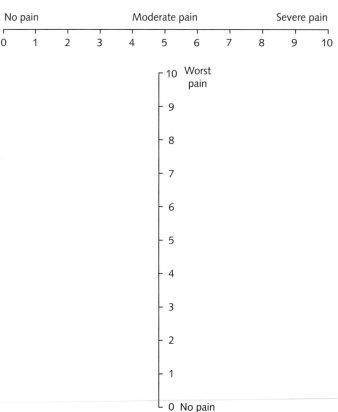

Numerical scale

No pain   Moderate pain   Severe pain

0   1   2   3   4   5   6   7   8   9   10

10 Worst
    pain

9

8

7

6

5

4

3

2

1

0 No pain

Figure 3.5 Pain rating scales. *PAIN, Clinical Manual,* 2nd edn, ISBN 9780815156093, 1999, Pasero, *et al.* 3 figures only 3.12, 3.8b, and 3.9b © Elseiver, 2008.

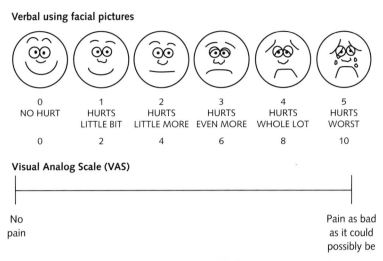

Figure 3.6 Child pain rating scale from Hockenberry MJ, Wilson D, Winkelstein ML, *Wong's Essentials of Paediatric Nursing*, 7th edn, St Louis, 2005, p. 1259. Used with permission, © Mosby.

Aftercare

It is important that you accurately record and document this assessment process and inform the patient of your conclusions. It may be necessary at this stage to inform more senior nursing staff if you feel that the patient is not in a comfortable state, so that pain control interventions can be initiated as soon as possible.

It may also be appropriate to take and record the patient's vital signs as these may indicate a physiological response to pain, such as raised pulse or respiratory rate. In touching the skin of a patient in severe pain, you will notice that it is cool and moist, indicating increased sympathetic nervous system activity. All of these factors are important to note particularly in unconscious or uncommunicative patients.

Other factors to consider

Children and other unique groups

Some patients will not have the verbal skills to give any, or a limited, account of their pain and you will need to rely on behavioural responses to pain alone. These include patients who are cognitively impaired (for example, because of dementia, mental illness, or physical or learning disabilities), patients with language and speech problems, unconscious patients, and neonates (see the neonatal pain scale, **Fig. 3.7**).

It is essential in these circumstances, as well as any time that you are assessing a patient in pain, to use observational skills to help in the assessment of pain. Look out for any nonverbal signs of pain, such as facial expression, mood, crying, screaming, wailing, and weeping (see the child pain rating scale, **Fig. 3.6**). The patient could also be reluctant to mobilize, have an unusual **gait** or posture, or be pressing or holding the painful areas. For other patients, the effect of pain may also cause symptoms such as nausea, vomiting, disrupted sleep pattern, and loss of appetite. Compare your findings to the pain assessment tools in **figures 3.6** and **3.7**.

Pain management

Both pharmacological (see Chapter 2.6 for more information on the administration of medicines) and nonpharmacological interventions (for example, alternative or complementary therapies) can be used in the treatment of pain, however, it is more appropriate to learn these interventions at a later stage. For now it is important for you to appreciate how effective these interventions are by repeating the assessment process at timely intervals. Where interventions have not had the desired effect, it may be appropriate to ask for further help, for example, from your mentor or other senior nurse.

Pain Assessment Tools

Neonatal/Infant Pain Scale (NIPS)

(Recommended for children less than 1 year old) - A score greater than 3 indicates pain

	Pain Assessment	Score
Facial Expression		
0 – Relaxed muscles	Restful face, neutral expression	
1 – Grimace	Tight facial muscles; furrowed brow, chin, jaw, (negative facial expression – nose, mouth and brow)	
Cry		
0 – No Cry	Quiet, not crying	
1 – Whimper	Mild moaning, intermittent	
2 – Vigorous Cry	Loud scream; rising, shrill, continuous (Note: Silent cry may be scored if baby is intubated as evidenced by obvious mouth and facial movement.)	
Breathing Patterns		
0 – Relaxed	Usual pattern for this infant	
1 – Change in Breathing	Indrawing, irregular, faster than usual; gagging; breath holding	
Arms		
0 – Relaxed/Restrained	No muscular rigidity; occasional random movements of arms	
1 – Flexed/Extended	Tense, straight legs; rigid and/or rapid extension, flexion	
Legs		
0 – Relaxed/Restrained	No muscular rigidity; occasional random leg movement	
1 – Flexed/Extended	Tense, straight legs; rigid and/or rapid extension, flexion	
State of Arousal		
0 – Sleeping/Awake	Quiet, peaceful sleeping or alert random leg movement	
1 – Fussy	Alert, restless, and thrashing	

Figure 3.7 Neonatal pain rating scale

3.3 **Early warning signs for critical illness**

Definition

Most patients who develop critical illness do so in a slow and progressive manner, often demonstrating a common pattern of clinical signs that, if not monitored or treated early enough, lead to significant deterioration (Kause *et al.* 2004). It is essential that you develop the knowledge and skills required to detect and report these signs of deterioration promptly in the patient's condition and be able to summon help from more senior colleagues. Patients whose deterioration is recognized early and treated appropriately are more likely to be stabilized, maximizing their chance of making a full recovery. One method commonly used to identify and treat problems in patients with critical illness is known as the ABCDE approach.

The Resuscitation Council (2006) suggests that all healthcare practitioners, irrespective or their training, experience, and expertise should be able to:

1 Carry out a systematic approach to assess and treat critically ill patients based on **A**irway, **B**reathing, **C**irculation, **D**isability, and **E**xposure (ABCDE),
2 Make an initial assessment and reassess regularly,
3 Always treat life-threatening problems first before proceeding to the next stage of an assessment,
4 Always evaluate the effects of their interventions,
5 Recognize when additional help is required and request it as early as possible,
6 Ensure that communication is effective.

This section will discuss the use of the ABCDE approach in assessing and treating critically ill patients. It is important to recognize that these patients may require **basic life support** (BLS) (refer to Chapter 2.5).

Background

To maintain function of the vital organs, we require:

1 An open **a**irway,
2 The ability to **b**reathe in oxygen and to obtain adequate gaseous exchange in the lungs,
3 A pump that can **c**irculate this oxygen to these organs to keep them perfused and alive.

Failure at any point in this process will result in reduced oxygen delivery; organ failure, and ultimately death. In hospital, the most common cause of cardiac arrest is hypoxaemia due to deteriorating respiratory, circulatory, and neurological systems (ILCOR 2005).

The Early Warning Scoring System can be used to document and record the patient's observations while alerting you to abnormal values within each observation. **Figure 3.8** provides an example of the early warning scoring system (**EWSS**), where for adults, white indicates normal, yellow indicates borderline, and red indicates danger. In this example, the patient has had three recordings:

- The first recording is normal; sews score = 0
- The second recording has most scores within the

yellow zones, indicating borderline results and signs of deterioration; sews score = 6
- The third recording has most scores within the red zones, indicating a definite deterioration in the patient's condition; sews score = 10

The score can then help you to identify that the patient needs help, for example, from the medical team.

When to use the Early Warning Scoring System

The use of the Early Warning Scoring System will help you to identify when you need to call the senior practitioner or other medical help when you assess a patient who has signs of clinical deterioration. Adam and Osborne (2005) state that when these signs are detected (**Box 3.3**) and treated early, this can often prevent cardiac arrest. The majority of cardiac arrests in hospital are not sudden or unexpected events. In the UK, as many as 80% of patients demonstrate warning signs of deterioration prior to the event. Close monitoring of the patient may allow early recognition, provide an opportunity for appropriate treatment, and, in some cases, may prevent cardiac arrest (Resuscitation Council UK 2006).

Box 3.3 Common clinical signs of critical illness

There are common clinical signs evident in the critically ill patient. These are:

Tachypnoea	A fast breathing rate in an attempt to breath in more oxygen,
Tachycardia	A fast pulse as the body attempts to circulate oxygen to the vital organs,
Hypotension	Low blood pressure,
Altered conscious level	As the perfusion of the brain is diminished (for example, lethargy, confusion, restlessness, or falling level of consciousness).

(Resuscitation Council UK 2006)

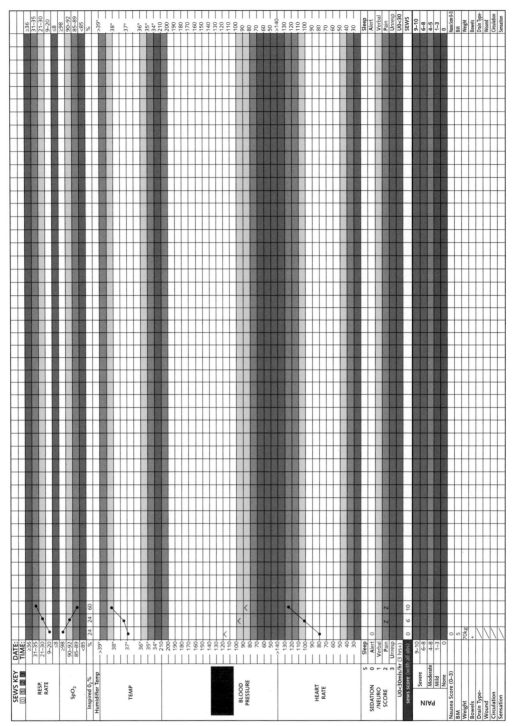

Figure 3.8 Early Warning Scoring System (EWSS). With permission of NHS Lothian.

Summarized ABCDE assessment

Key points:

- Problems *must* be dealt with as they arise.
- *Always* reassess after every action.
- If the patient's condition changes, go back to ABCDE.

Letter	Action	Follow-up
A = Airway	Check patency and maintain	See basic life support.
B = Breathing	Look Listen Feel Record rate, rhythm, and depth of breathing Record SaO$_2$ Work of breathing, use of accessory muscles	Monitor and record. See basic life support if inadequate. Refer to medical team for further assessment. Administer prescribed oxygen
C = Circulation	Pulse (carotid if collapsed) Record rate, regularity, volume of pulse Capillary refill time <2 seconds Blood pressure	Monitor and record. See basic life support if inadequate. Refer to medical team for further assessment.
D = Disability	Assess with Glasgow Coma Scale (GCS): Worrying if score drops by 2 points or more (refer to Section 3.4) E = 4 V = 5 M = 6 Record conscious level using AVPU scale: **A**lert Responds to **v**oice Responds to **p**ain **U**nresponsive An AVPU score of P or below indicates GCS of less than 8 and indicates that airway protection is required.	Monitor and record. See basic life support if inadequate. Refer to medical team for further assessment. Airway may be at risk.
E = Exposure	Exposure	Examine patient. Top-to-toe assessment.

Procedure: ABCDE assessment

This assessment has to be swift and efficient to be effective. Always check any change in the patient's condition with a senior member of nursing staff or medical team. The approach is summarized and then the procedures for each stage are outlined.

Throughout the ABCDE assessment, the nurse should also be sensitive to any change in the patient's condition. If any deterioration is suspected, the nurse should return to the beginning of the assessment and ensure that the airway, breathing, and circulation are being supported.

If you are in any doubt about whether the patient's condition is stable, do not hesitate to seek further guidance from more senior practitioners. If your mentor has called

Assessment of the patient's airway

Action	Rationale
Ask how the patient is feeling.	If a patient can give a verbal response, then the airway is patent. If the airway is completely obstructed, there will be no breath sounds at the mouth or nose. The look, listen, and feel approach can detect airway obstruction.
Look for 'see-saw' pattern of respiration, with a silent chest. See-saw respiratory pattern is confirmed by the abdomen moving in as the chest moves out and vice versa.	This is a sign of complete airway obstruction.
An anaesthetist should be contacted immediately according to local protocol and basic life support should be initiated (see Section 2.5).	This is an extreme clinical emergency and will require immediate, advanced airway management.
Listen for evidence of noise (for example, stridor or wheeze). Other noises associated with airway obstruction includes: gurgling, snoring, or crowing. In cases where these are found, apply basic life support (see Section 2.5).	This is a sign or partial airway obstruction. Stridor often indicates an upper airway obstruction and wheeze usually indicates a lower obstruction.
Feel: put your hand on the patient's chest and feel for any movement up and down with the patient's breathing.	These are signs of airway obstruction.

for another practitioner to review the patient's condition, you should take time to ask the mentor why this was done, and what made the practitioner act in this way.

The ABCDE approach is a systematic framework that allows the nurse to identify problems and to act on these without delay. The process is continuous and staff should reassess the casualty at each point that intervention takes place for signs of improvement or deterioration. Nurses should only work to their own level of clinical expertise and should be aware of their limitations. It is essential to call for help as soon as it is required and to acknowledge your limitations.

It is important to use all the information that is available to carry out as thorough an assessment as possible. Information about the patient's general condition and any previous recording of vital signs, such as blood pressure, temperature, pulse, respiration, and oxygen saturation, can help to provide insight into what is normal for this individual or any trends in deterioration of vital signs. Previous medical and other healthcare documentation can provide insight into aspects of the patient's previous medical history, current care provision, and results of any previous assessments.

Procedure: A = Assessment of the airway

The airway should be assessed to determine whether it is patent, partially obstructed, or completely obstructed. The airway can be obstructed by the tongue, vomit, blood, a foreign body, tissue swelling, and other numerous causes.

Procedure: B = Assessment of breathing

The rate, rhythm, and depth of respirations should be measured when assessing breathing. Normal breathing is quiet, but there could be rattling, stridor, or wheeze from the breathing effort. People actively inhale and passively exhale in normal breathing. During episodes of exercise, fever, fear, anxiety, or even pain, patients can experience higher respiratory rates than normal (tachypnoea). As a guide, it is suggested by early warning scoring systems that if the patient's respiratory rate is less than 5 breaths per minute or more than 36 breaths per minute, help should be called.

When assessing breathing, the respiratory rate should be observed and particular attention should be paid to the effort of breathing, tachypnoea, **bradypnoea**, the depth of breathing, equal movement on both sides, rhythm of breathing, and the use of accessory muscles of respiration should be noted and reported immediately. Note any presence of chest deformity. Chapter 5 provides an overview of the skill required in observing and documenting respiratory rate, rhythm, and depth.

The adequacy of breathing may also be assessed by heart rate, skin colour (that is, **cyanosis**), and mental state. However, these are late signs of deterioration and should not be relied on before any help is summoned. Cyanosis will only occur when the oxygen saturation has fallen to 80–85% (Giuliano and Higgins 2005). Pulse oximetry can be used to measure the percentage of arterial oxygenated haemoglobin in the patient's blood (see Chapter 5 for procedure). The normal value is >95%, but this may be lower, and still 'normal', for patients with existing conditions such as chronic obstructive pulmonary disease (COPD). Children can show signs of respiratory distress that are different from those in adults: grunting, nasal flaring, head bobbing, or drooling.

Other observations of breathing should include listening to the chest with a stethoscope and **percussion** of the chest by trained personnel.

If the patient is able to answer questions, or there is a family member or carer who is able to answer some questions, it is important that an initial assessment includes an overview of the physical, psychological, sociocultural, environmental, and any politico-economic factors that could be influencing the patient's breathing. Chapter 5 summarizes some of the questions that could be asked during the assessment of a patient's breathing.

In summary, respiratory rate is a very significant observation in the critically ill patient (Resuscitation Council UK 2006). As the body requires more oxygen, the respiratory rate will increase (tachypnoea). The rise may be subtle initially, but should be closely monitored. These patients should be administered prescribed high-flow oxygen as soon as possible, with due caution exercised for patients with pre-existing lung disease and help should be sought.

Procedure: C = Assessment of circulation

The nurse should observe the patient for signs of circulatory failure. An initial observation should include:

1 Monitoring pulse,
2 Capillary refill time,
3 Blood pressure,
4 General observation of the patient's colour and temperature.

Pulse

A pulse is produced when the pressure wave is created from each heartbeat following the expansion and recoil of arterioles. A pulse can be located and palpated in any artery that lies close to the surface of the body (**Fig. 3.9**). The most common site is the radial artery in adults and the brachial artery in children. The patient's pulse should be recorded, noting the rate, regularity, and volume (see Chapter 2.5 for carotid pulse check, which should be made if the patient is in a collapsed state).

The normal pulse rates for different client groups are demonstrated in **Box 3.4**. However, there may be variations within age ranges, which may be due to level of fitness, posture, recent activity, and amount of disease within the cardiovascular system. You may also find that different sources quote slightly different values.

The regularity and volume (or strength) of the pulse should also be noted. A pulse can be described as 'weak and thready' or 'full and bounding'. Normal pulses are regular and

Recording radial pulse

▶ Step   **Rationale**

	Step	Rationale
1	Explain the nursing practice to the patient.	To gain consent, understanding, and cooperation.
2	Ensure that the patient is in a position that is as comfortable and relaxed as possible.	To assist in obtaining a true baseline measurement.
3	Ensure limb is supported.	
4	Observe the patient throughout the activity for any signs of discomfort or distress.	To intervene immediately in the event of an adverse reaction.
5	Locate the radial artery, place the first and second fingers along it, and press gently.	So that the pulse of blood passing through the artery can be felt.
6	Sufficient pressure should be applied to allow the artery to be against an underlying bone.	Care must be taken not to press too hard or the artery may be occluded: it will then be impossible to feel the pulse.
7	Count the pulse for 60 seconds noting rate, rhythm, and volume.	To allow sufficient time to detect any irregularities or other defects. Rhythm is determined to identify any potential heart irregularities. Volume is indicative of the patient's fluid balance status.
8	Document the findings appropriately, compare past recordings, and identify any developing trends in this observation.	To enable early intervention to improve the situation.
9	Report this and any abnormal findings to a more senior member of staff and document in care notes.	

are in the sequence of beats of the heart. Any irregular pulse rate indicates a defect in the conduction system of the heart and should be reported to your senior colleagues. A note of the regularity of the pulse should also be documented.

It can also be important to assess the volume of the pulse, as this can reflect other problems, for example, blood loss.

Blood pressure and capillary refill time

Where there is a fall in cardiac output, the body will respond by further increasing the peripheral resistance in an attempt to maintain adequate blood pressure and organ perfusion. This will result in a fast but weak, thready pulse (tachycardia) and a delay in capillary refill time. Capillary refill time is measured by exerting pressure on the patient's finger tip for four or five seconds and releasing the pressure. Normal skin colour should return within two seconds. If this is delayed, it demonstrates that peripheral resistance has increased, thus limiting the blood supply to the peripheries while trying to maintain blood supply to the major organs. You should be aware that capillary refill time may be influenced by the patient's increasing age, environmental temperature, and is more difficult to observe in poor lighting. A delayed filling time should alert you to a circulatory problem for which you should immediately seek senior practitioner advice.

A blood pressure recording will determine the effectiveness of the cardiovascular system. Blood pressure is defined as the force exerted by blood against the walls of the vessels in which it is contained. Normal blood pressure ranges from 110/60 to 139/89 mmHg. **Box 3.5** summarizes the normal limits of blood pressure (Williams *et al.* 2004).

The compensation mechanisms to maintain blood pressure cannot be maintained indefinitely and ultimately perfusion of the organs will stop and subsequently they will fail. The organ that will be protected most is the brain. As the patient's conscious level begins to deteriorate, therefore, the brain is no longer being adequately perfused and the patient should be considered to be in severe difficulty. Urine output can also be used as a marker of end organ perfusion.

Procedure: D = Disability

Disability relates to the neurological assessment of the patient (see Section 3.4), which is used to identify signs of

central neurological failure. The neurological (**d**isability) assessment is performed after **a**irway, **b**reathing, and **ci**rculation have been assessed, and any problems with these must be dealt with first. Often problems with breathing and circulation can manifest as a neurological symptom (affecting consciousness, causing seizures). Similarly, some neurological problems can affect the breathing and circulation of a patient. The assessment of neurological function has three main components:

1 Conscious level,
2 Posture,
3 Pupils.

Conscious level

A quick and easy way to determine how well the brain is being perfused is to assess the patient using the AVPU score. This translates as:

- The patient is **a**lert
- The patient responds to **v**oice
- The patient responds to **p**ain
- The patient is **u**nresponsive

(Resuscitation Council UK 2006)

If a patient's condition deteriorates from one level to a lower one this is indicative of a significant change in neurological status and should not be overlooked. An AVPU recording of P or less indicates a Glasgow Coma Scale score of <8 and means that the patient's airway cannot be protected fully by the patient. Expert help is required immediately.

A potential indicator of altered conscious level that can be monitored at the bedside is the patient's blood glucose level. This is generally a skill that is taught in the branch programmes and, therefore, the procedure is not explained at this point.

Box 3.4 Normal pulse rates

Age	Normal range, beats per minute	Average, beats per minute
Newborn	120–160	140
1–12 months	80–140	120
12–2 years	80–130	110
2–6 years	75–120	100
6–12 years	75–110	95
Adolescent	60–100	80
Adult	60–100	80

Box 3.5 The normal limits of blood pressure

	Systolic pressure, mmHg	Diastolic pressure, mm Hg
Optimal	<120	<80
Normal	<130	<85
High normal	130–139	85–89
Hypertension	>140	>90

Measuring the patient's blood pressure

▶ Step   Rationale

	Step	Rationale
1	Explain the nursing practice to the patient.	To gain consent, understanding, and cooperation.
2	Wash your hands.	To reduce the risk of cross-infection.
3	Ensure the patient's privacy.	To reduce anxiety and maintain patient's dignity and respect.
4	Collect the equipment: an aneroid sphygmomanometer, correct size of cuff, and stethoscope.	To conduct the measurement effectively and efficiently.
5	Observe the patient throughout the activity.	To note any signs of distress: a little discomfort caused by the cuff is to be expected.
6	Apply the cuff 3–5 cm above the point at which the brachial artery can be palpated (Fig. 3.10). The cuff should be applied smoothly and firmly, covering 80% of the arm circumference, with the middle of the rubber bladder lying directly over the brachial artery.	To permit access to the brachial artery by the stethoscope and even pressure around the circumference of the limb. A bladder that is too large or too small will result in a respective under- or overestimation of the blood pressure.
7	Ask the patient to rest the arm on a suitable firm surface. The arm should be level with the heart.	To ensure patient comfort and prevent movement of the limb, which may lead to inaccurate results. If the arm is too high it can artificially lower the blood pressure reading, if the arm is too low it can artificially raise the blood pressure reading.
8	Palpate the radial pulse and inflate the cuff until the pulse has been obliterated. Inflate for a further 20 mmHg. Release the valve slowly, taking note of the reading on the dial when the radial pulse returns. Allow air to escape from the cuff.	To provide an initial assessment of the systolic pressure.
9	Palpate the brachial pulse, place the stethoscope over the site, and inflate the cuff to 20 mmHg above the previous reading. Release the valve of the inflation ball at a rate of 2–3 mmHg per second. When the first pulse is heard, the reading on the dial should be mentally noted – this is the systolic pressure.	To provide an accurate assessment of the systolic and diastolic pressure without excessive discomfort to the patient.

10 Continue to deflate the cuff: the pulse sounds changing to muffled sounds until it finally disappears. The reading on the dial at this point should also be mentally noted – this is the diastolic pressure.

11 Continue controlled deflation until a value of 20 mmHg below the diastolic pressure has been reached.

To eradicate the chance of a silent interval leading to a false recording.

12 Completely deflate the cuff, disconnect the tubing and remove the cuff from the patient's arm.

To prevent further compression of the limb.

13 Ensure that the patient is left feeling as comfortable as possible.

To ensure the quality of nursing practice.

14 If a communal stethoscope has been used, clean the earpieces and the diaphragm with an alcohol wipe.

To reduce cross-infection between staff or between patients.

15 Dispose of equipment safely.

To comply with health and safety criteria.

16 Wash your hands.

To reduce the risk of cross-infection.

17 Report this and any abnormal findings to a more senior member of staff (registered nurse or doctor) and record in care notes.

To allow remedial action to be taken immediately if necessary.

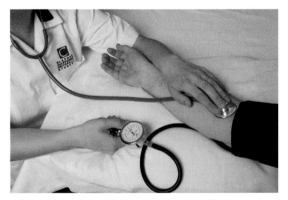

Figure 3.10 Location of cuff and stethoscope during blood pressure measurement

Posture

Serious problems with brain function will result in abnormal posturing. If a patient's posture changes to flexed arms and extended legs, this is a **decorticate** sign. If the patient's arms and legs become extended, this is a **decerebrate** sign. Both postures indicate severe damage to the brain and could be confused with the **tonic phase** of a seizure (Advanced Life Support Group 2005). Another change to posture to be aware of is **extension** or stiffness of the neck: this could be caused by irritation of the **meninges** and can be a sign of **meningitis**. In infants, you may also notice a bulging **fontanelle**.

Pupils

Pupils' size and reaction may be affected by **cerebral lesions**, therefore, this should be assessed using a pen torch and observing for equality of both (this procedure is explained in Section 3.4). The nurse should be aware that drug treatment can have an effect on pupils and may cause them to **dilate** or **contract**. It is useful to check the patient's prescription chart to establish any treatment the patient may have received. Further explanation of this can be found in Section 3.4.

Procedure: E = Exposure

This assessment is to identify signs of illness and is usually conducted by a member of medical staff. It has been included in this section for the purpose of completeness and to give some background information on what medical staff will be looking for. It is anticipated that this will help a student nurse to act as assistant in this assessment.

A top-to-toe examination of the patient should be performed; this helps to establish the potential cause of the change in the patient's condition. This should be conducted in such a way that the patient's dignity is not compromised. There should be no unnecessary exposure or heat loss suffered.

Any problems identified during this assessment should be dealt with immediately. For example, in an unconscious patient, clothes may be removed at this time to check for signs of obvious injury or illness (for example, fractures, bleeding open wounds, rashes). These can then be assessed and treated. Types of rash that may be seen include: **urticaria**, **purpura**, or erythema; these can indicate such problems as infection, allergy, and sepsis. Further assessment will include feeling the temperature of the skin. A formal temperature should be recorded to affirm the findings.

3.4 **Neurological assessment**

Definition

Neurological assessment is the assessment of the level of consciousness. Holistic neurological assessment will involve assessment of the neuromuscular, nervous, **motor**, and sensory systems. However, for the purposes of this chapter, and the functions you will be carrying out as a first-year student, we will concentrate on the assessment of consciousness. The word 'conscious' suggests that the patient is alert and aware of the environment, and can make deliberate and intentional decisions.

Assessment of conscious level can allow the nurse to observe the patient for signs of deterioration, stability, and improvement. The National Institute for Health and Clinical Excellence (NIHCE 2007) recommend that the minimum acceptable documented neurological observations are:

- Glasgow Coma Scale
- Pupil size and reactivity
- Limb movements
- Vital signs:
  - Respiratory rate (Chapter 5)
  - Heart rate (Section 3.3)
  - Blood pressure (Section 3.3)
  - Temperature (Chapter 9)
  - Blood oxygen saturation (Chapter 5)

This section will introduce you to assessing neurological status and will help you develop the knowledge and skills required to undertake this fairly complex procedure. The Glasgow Coma Scale, and measuring pupil size and reactivity and limb movements will be explained. The vital signs of respiratory rate, heart rate, blood pressure, temperature, and blood oxygen saturation are all covered elsewhere in this book (see list of procedures).

Background

Glasgow Coma Scale

The most commonly used tool to assist the nurse in carrying out part of a neurological assessment is the Glasgow Coma Scale (GCS), which relies on scores from the best eye response, the best verbal response, and the best motor response.

Developed by Teasdale and Jennet (1974), the Glasgow Coma Scale is the most common way to assess the patient's conscious level using eye opening, verbal response, and motor response to assess arousal, awareness, and activity level of the patient's behaviour. A score is associated with each aspect of the scale: the higher the score, the better the patient's condition. The highest score is 15, and indicates an alert and responsive patient. The lowest score achievable is three, which indicates unconsciousness. As well as the overall score, you should also report the separate score for each category, as this will provide a better overview of the patient's condition. **Figure 3.11** shows a typical chart for the GCS. There are many advantages to recording the Glasgow Coma Scale:

- It is a systematic approach to collecting and analysing data
- It is a means of communication between health professionals
- It aids diagnosis
- It provides a baseline of observations
- It helps determine subtle and rapid change in the patient's condition
- It helps monitor neurological status following neurological procedures
- It helps in the observation of deterioration and in establishing the extent of traumatic head injury
- It helps detect life-threatening situations
- It alerts nurses to seek urgent assistance when required

(Dawes *et al.* 2007)

When to perform a neurological assessment

Head injuries (such as those from sports, falls, and road traffic accidents, as well as illness, for example, stroke, head surgery, epileptic seizure), recent changes in mood or confusional states can require close neurological assessment and continuous observation of the patient. It is essential that when assessing neurological status, nurses understand the underlying pathophysiology and signs or symptoms of deterioration, stability, and improvement.

Procedure: Neurological assessment

It is essential that you wash your hands before and after the procedure. In some cases, neurological damage can cause the patient to become **aggressive** or violent. If this is the case it may be appropriate to seek help from more experienced practitioners before you approach the patient. If you do experience any aggressive behaviour, you must report this to more senior colleagues who will be able to assess the situation further in terms of the risk posed to staff and to the patient. **Figure 3.14** shows a chart for recording observations.

There is guidance on how often the Glasgow Coma Scale should be used: the NIHCE (2007) recommend:

- Perform and record observations on a half-hourly basis until GCS = 15
- When GCS = 15, minimum frequency of observations is:
  - Half-hourly for two hours
  - Then hourly for four hours
  - And at two-hourly intervals thereafter
- If the patient deteriorates to GCS < 15 after the initial two-hour period, revert to half-hourly observations and follow original schedule

In cases where the patient is unconscious, it is not unusual for observations to be carried out every 15 minutes and this should be reflected in local policies.

As with many scoring systems, in patients with learning disabilities that impair cognitive function, or with language difficulties or **dysphagia**, it can be very difficult to assess best verbal, best motor, or eye opening responses. Likewise, the intoxication by drugs or alcohol can make the neurological assessment of any patient particularly difficult, as these symptoms (such as slurred speech, confusion, drowsiness, cooperation to obey commands) can imitate decreased neurological function and mask 'true' neurological status.

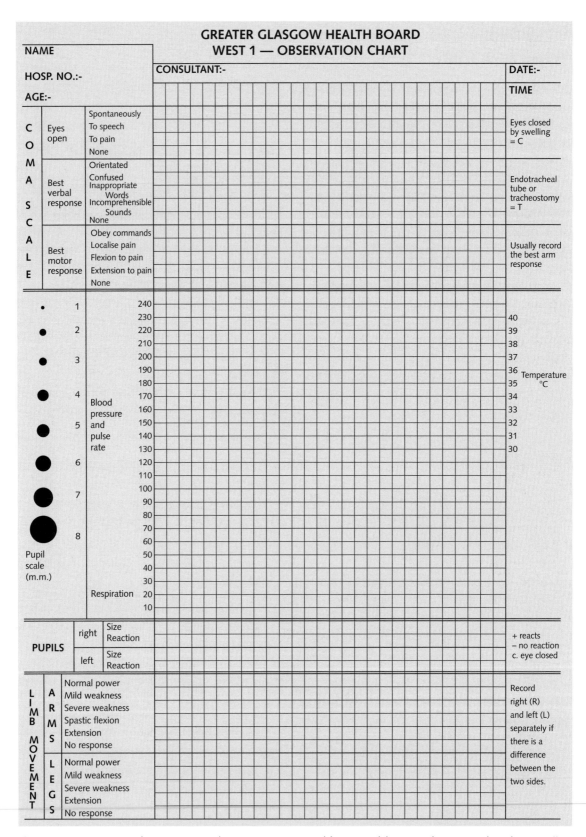

Figure 3.11 Assessment of coma & impaired consciousness. Derived from: Teasdale, GM and Jennett, B (1974) *Lancet*, **ii**, 81–4.

Neurological assessment of a patient

Key point: Where there is a rise in intracranial pressure (ICP), there will be a rise in blood pressure and fall in pulse rate and respirations. This is known as Cushing's reflex – this is a late sign of raised ICP and you should alert senior staff immediately.

Step	Rationale
1 Assess patient using Glasgow Coma Scale (see separate explanation).	This is a common way to assess the patient's conscious level and assesses eye opening, verbal response and motor response: E + V + M = GCS score.
2 Record pupil size and reaction (see separate explanation).	Pupil size and light reactivity and inequality may indicate pressure on the nerve supplying the eye or brainstem damage. The function of the optic nerve is tested by the reaction to light while the occulomotor nerve is tested by constriction of the pupil. A poor reaction indicates compression of the nerves. It is important that you ask the patient, family, or carers if there are any factors that may affect the eye. For example, cataracts, previous eye surgery, prostheses, and any drugs (legal or illegal) that may have been taken as some can affect the reaction or size of the pupil.
3 Assess limb movements (see separate explanation).	This can provide an accurate indication of the brain function. Any developing weakness or loss of movement can be caused by increased **intracranial pressure**. Intracranial pressure is the pressure exerted by normal cerebral components (brain tissue, blood, and cerebrospinal fluid, [CSF]) within the rigid structures of the brain. During some circumstances (for example, head injury) the pressure within the skull increases causing reduced cerebral perfusion (that is, blood supply) and, therefore, inadequate oxygen delivery to the brain tissues. The centres that control blood pressure, heart rate, temperature, and respiratory rate are located in the brainstem and can be affected by a raised ICP, causing changes to these vital signs.
4 Vital signs.	
5 Record respiratory rate and blood oxygen saturation (refer to Chapter 5).	You should record respiration observations first. The respiratory pattern provides the clearest indication of brain function (Dougherty and Lister 2008). See Section 3.3 and Chapter 5 for information on breathing assessment.

continued

6	**Record blood pressure (refer to Section 3.3).**	Blood pressure and pulse observations should also be carried out as these may change in response to a rise in ICP.
7	**Record pulse rate (refer to Section 3.3).**	
8	**Record temperature (refer to Chapter 9).**	Temperature fluctuations can be a sign of hypothalamic damage. During any rise in body temperature, the demand for oxygen to the brain cells increase and, therefore, it is desirable to keep the patient's temperature within normal limits where possible, especially where there is already suspected brain injury or damage. The use of prescribed medication (**antipyretic**), such as paracetamol or a fan or tepid sponging of the patient may be required to aid cooling. The procedure for measuring temperature can be found in Chapter 9.

Procedure: Using the Glasgow Coma Scale to assess conscious level

The three scores of the Glasgow Coma Scale (see **Tables 3.1** and **3.2**) are added to obtain a score from 3 to 15:

$$E + V + M = GCS.$$

- A score of 3 to 8 generally indicates a coma
- A score of greater than 9 indicates that the patient is not in a coma
- A score of 9 to 11 or 12 indicates moderate severity
- A score of 13 or greater indicates minor severity

It is essential that the use of painful stimuli within the GCS is addressed as an additional point here, because of the need for careful management. You should always inform patients, family, and carers of the reason for doing this procedure, as it can be distressing if the rationale for its use is unknown to them. The painful stimuli methods of sternal rub or nail-bed pressure are outdated and should not be used, owing to the risk of prolonged discomfort and bruising. The current recommended methods of carrying out painful stimuli are:

- Central painful stimulus:
  - Trapezius muscle pinch or squeeze,
  - Jaw pressure (pressure applied just in front of the earlobe),
  - Supra-orbital pressure (the groove or notch above the eye),

- Peripheral painful stimulus:
  - Lateral finger or toe pressure (a pen is rotated around the finger or toe and pressure applied).

The severity of limb movement is classified into six possible categories, as shown in **Box 3.6**.

Developing your skills

It is important that you can develop the skills required to take and record a patient's Glasgow Coma Score and

Box 3.6 Categories for limb movement	
Normal movement	There is no difficulty in the patient pushing against your resistance with the arm or legs.
Mild weakness	There is no difficulty in the patient pushing against your resistance with the arm or legs; however, this is easily overcome.
Severe weakness	The patient will be unable to push against your resistance with the arm or legs; however, the patient can move limbs unaided.
Spastic flexion	The patient flexes the arm or leg in response to painful stimuli.
Extension	The patient extends their arm or leg in response to painful stimuli.
No response	There is no limb movement even with painful stimuli.

Table 3.1 Glasgow Coma Scale (adult patient)

Action	Score	Response
Eye opening	4	Spontaneously opens eyes
	3	Opens eyes to speech
	2	Opens eyes to pain
	1	No response
Verbal response	5	Orientated
	4	Confused
	3	Inappropriate words
	2	Incomprehensible words
	1	No response
Motor response	6	Obeys commands
	5	Localizes pain
	4	Withdraws from pain
	3	Flexion to pain
	2	Extension to pain
	1	No response

Source: Reproduced from Teasdale and Jennett (1974) with permission from Elsevier.

Table 3.2 Glasgow Coma Scale (children under 5)

Action	Score	Response 0–23 months	Response 2–5 years
Eye opening	4	Spontaneously opens eyes	Spontaneously opens eyes
	3	Opens eyes to speech	Opens eyes to speech
	2	Opens eyes to pain	Opens eyes to pain
	1	No response	No response
Verbal response	5	Smiles and coos	Appropriate words or phrases
	4	Cries and consolable	Inappropriate words
	3	Persistent inappropriate crying or screaming	Persistent cries or screams
	2	Grunts or is agitated or restless	Grunts
	1	No response	No response
Motor response	6	Obeys commands	Obeys commands
	5	Localizes pain	Localizes pain
	4	Withdraws from pain	Withdraws from pain
	3	Flexion to pain	Flexion to pain
	2	Extension to pain	Extension to pain
	1	No response	No response

associated vital signs. Where possible, you should work with your mentor to practice using these skills and compiling the associated documentation as often as possible. You may also be able to practice these skills in a clinical skills laboratory. Repeated practice will improve your competence and confidence within this fairly complex skill.

Other factors to consider

Assessment of a child's neurological status

The Glasgow Coma Score is difficult to use on children, especially children younger than 5 years, owing to the

Assessing pupil size and reaction

Equipment
Pen torch,
A dimly lit room.

Step	Rationale
1 Wash hands.	To prevent cross-infection.
2 Explain the procedure to the patient, family, carer and give a rationale for completing the task.	To gain cooperation. To prevent embarrassment and maintain dignity.
3 Obtain patient's consent (if possible).	To facilitate informed consent.
4 Ask the patient to open their eyes or if not able, gently hold the eyelid open.	To gain cooperation.
5 Observe the size of each pupil (approximate normal size 2–5 mm).	To establish a baseline observation.
6 Are both pupils equal in size? If they are unequal, this can suggest a raised intracranial pressure.	To assess for signs of a raised ICP. Abnormal pupil size may be indicative of brain damage.
7 Are both pupils circular?	To assess for signs of brain damage.
8 It may be necessary to ask the patient, family, carer if there are any pupil or eye problems normally.	To establish a baseline observation.
9 Bring the pen torch in from the side of each eye and observe its reaction to light.	To observe the pupil's reaction to light.
10 Pupils normally react quickly to light and reduce in size.	To compare against the normal reaction you would expect.
11 Record the reaction to light (if there is one), and the intensity of the reaction (for example, brisk, sluggish, or absent) on a chart (see Fig. 3.12).	To ensure accurate documentation and continuity of care.
12 Inform patient and more senior staff of results.	To alert other staff to problems such that they can be managed effectively.
13 Ensure that the patient is comfortable before moving on.	To ensure that you demonstrate care and compassion.
14 Wash hands.	To prevent cross-infection.

Assessing limb movement

Step	Rationale
1 Wash hands.	To prevent cross-infection.
2 Explain the procedure to the patient, family, or carer, providing rationale.	To gain cooperation.
3 Obtain patient's consent (if possible).	To facilitate informed consent.
4 Make sure that the patient is lying flat.	To ease assessment.
5 Each limb is assessed and recorded separately.	To determine whether the patient has normal, mild, or severe weakness.
6 For the arms: while holding the wrist, ask the patient to pull you towards them and then push away.	To determine whether the patient has normal, mild, or severe weakness.
7 For the legs: while holding the top of the ankle, ask the patient to lift their leg off the bed and then while holding the back of the ankle ask them to pull their leg towards them.	To determine whether the patient has normal, mild, or severe weakness.
8 Record the level of the limb movement on the neurological chart.	To determine the level of weakness, see Box 3.6 for the levels of severity.
9 Inform patient and more senior staff of results.	To alert other staff to problems such that they can be managed effectively.
10 Ensure that the patient is comfortable before moving on.	To ensure that you demonstrate care and compassion.
11 Wash hands.	To prevent cross-infection.

inappropriateness of the verbal component of the score. Some rating scales have been developed for the use of facial expression (that is, a grimace) to score the child and it may be concluded that this is more reliable than the verbal response (Tatman *et al.* 1997). However, the NIHCE (2007) guidance on head injury and the SIGN (2000) guidance on early management of patients with head injury state that any of these scores should be interpreted with caution and that this scoring should be done by those with experience in working with young children and head injuries. If the assessment reveals that the child needs hospital care, the child may be referred to a specialist paediatric neurosurgical unit who specialize in head injuries, and should be transferred to that unit by a specialized transfer team.

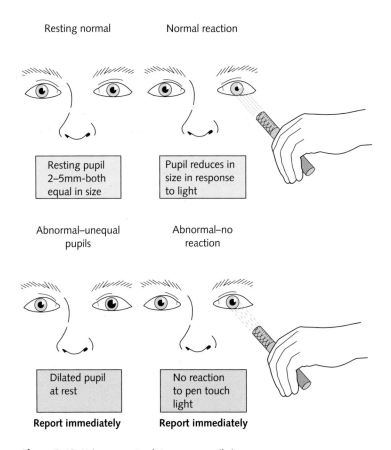

Resting normal   Normal reaction

Resting pupil
2–5mm–both
equal in size

Pupil reduces in
size in response
to light

Abnormal–unequal   Abnormal–no
pupils   reaction

Dilated pupil
at rest

No reaction
to pen touch
light

Report immediately   **Report immediately**

Figure 3.12 Using a pen torch to assess pupil size

Head injury

Guidelines on head injury (NIHCE 2007) state that both adults and children with the following risk factors should be admitted to hospital for close observation following a head injury:

- History of loss of consciousness
- Neurological abnormality or persisting headache or vomiting
- Clinical or radiological evidence of skull fracture or penetrating injury
- Difficulty in making a full assessment
- Suspicion of nonaccidental injury
- Other significant medical problem
- Not accompanied by responsible adult or social circumstances considered unsatisfactory

If the patient has no risk factors, but has had a history of a head injury, it is essential that families and carers are provided with relevant written and verbal information on the risk factors mentioned above. Any decision to discharge an adult or, particularly, a child (because of the difficulty in accurate assessment of children), will be made by experienced members of the multidisciplinary team following careful assessment and will be provided with detailed information on what to look out for after discharge. Assessment of the adult's or child's physical neurological status is essential, but so also is that of the adult's or child's social history (for example, is there a responsible adult within the household?) in order that a judgement can be made by the multidisciplinary team about the adult's or child's care.

There will be occasions where the child could be suffering from a nonaccidental injury, especially where the clinical findings of the assessment are not consistent with the information provided. Locally agreed guidelines and policies should be followed, including reporting and liaising with the multidisciplinary teams both within hospital and community setting (for example, social work, family GP). This should be done by an experienced member of the team.

Deterioration in adults or children with a history of head injury

The NIHCE (2007) recommend that anyone carrying out neurological observations should seek appropriate help at the most appropriate time. **Figure 3.13** lists changes to the patient's condition and shows an algorithm for patient review.

3.5 **Fall prevention and risk assessment**

Definition

Fall risk assessment aims to identify those patients at risk from a fall. Falls are more common in the elderly for many

Making observations

- If patient deteriorates to GCS < 15 after initial 2-hour period, revert to half-hourly observations and follow original schedule.

- Minimum acceptable documented neurological observations:
  - GCS (adult or paediatric, as appropriate)
  - pupil size and reactivity
  - limb movements
  - respiratory rate
  - heart rate
  - blood pressure
  - temperature
  - blood oxygen saturation.

Patient changes requiring review

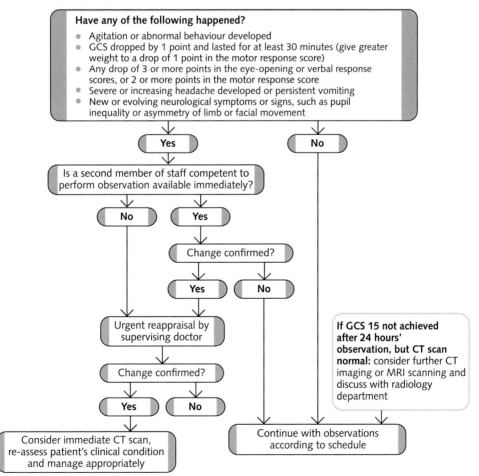

Figure 3.13 Patient changes requiring review. National Institute for Health and Clinical Excellence (2007) CG 56 *Head injury: triage, assessment, investigation and early management of head injury in infants, children and adults*. London: NICE Available from www.nice.org.uk/GG 56 Reproduced with permission.

reasons, to be discussed later in this section, but predominantly because of the ageing process. The consequences of a fall in an elderly patient can be significant both physically and psychologically. The most common injury sustained is a fracture to the neck of the femur, which is the large bone in the hip. This can be life-threatening in certain cases, because of subsequent surgery and limiting effects. Psychologically, falls can lead to depression, lack of confidence, and a reduced quality of life.

In many cases, these falls can be prevented. Nurses are ideally placed to assess and identify risks and to establish ways of reducing these risks.

There are many different fall risk assessment tools used in the clinical area. The choice of an appropriate tool will depend on how easy it is to use, how applicable it is to the patients in the particular setting, and its validity and reliability, that is, whether it measures what it is supposed to measure and whether it measures the same way each time it is used. Along with the fall risk assessment tool, there are many other tools or instruments that health professionals use to assess some of the influencing factors making up the full assessment. Some of these tools are mentioned in the procedure table; however, there are too many to mention them all. Some tools are more useful in certain healthcare settings and should be used as part of a comprehensive assessment by the multidisciplinary team. Many of the tools used to assess the risk of falls will have scoring systems. Often specialist knowledge is required to use the tools and score them. A typical risk assessment tool is shown is **Fig. 3.14**.

Background

Falls have serious consequences for the patient, the patient's family, the health service, and society as a whole. Falls are associated with injury and its consequences, as well as reduced patient function, confidence, and financial cost. Although they can occur at any time, the risks of a fall are greatly increased by admission to hospital. Falls are the most common patient-safety incident reported in inpatient areas: at least 40% of all accidents in hospital in the UK are related to falls. This may be because the patient has an illness or injury or has been subject to a change in medication regime, but is often a result of:

Environmental changes	Ward layout, lighting, toilet, signs, flooring, noise, and activity levels,
Changes to routine	Urinary voiding patterns, eating routines, diet, night or sleep pattern,
Personal changes	Lack of personal belongings, privacy, supervision, or company, separation from partner, family, friends, pets, confusion, cognition.

These causes can be further worsened at certain times of the day.

- During or immediately after mealtimes
- At night (often related to toileting needs)
- During staff handovers, when staffing or observation is poor
- During floor cleaning or other maintenance
- When bed rails are used
- During personal care and self-care

Balance relies on information from the eyes, the sensory organs in the inner ear (vestibular), and proprioceptors in the muscles and **tendons**. The elderly are at even greater risk of falls, because of age-related changes and diseases. With age, there is a reduction in the function of the sensory systems (visual, **proprioception**, and vestibular function), decreased muscle strength, changes in posture (a change to the curves of the spine alters the patient's centre of gravity; in women, the base narrows causing a change in gait), and reduced balance control, often resulting from problems with the musculoskeletal, cardiovascular, and urinary systems. Along with these factors, cognitive impairment and psychological factors, such as depression or anxiety, can exacerbate the risk even further. All of these factors should, therefore, be considered as part of the assessment of the patient.

Prevention of falls in the *community* is often more difficult, because of the numbers of potentially at-risk patients. Although the risk may be lower because they are more familiar with their surroundings; falls are still common in people's own homes. Because of the numerous causative factors, they can often be difficult to assess and prevent. For people over 65, most falls

Falls risk assessment tool

Age/sex	Score	Balance/Gait	Score	Mobility/Elimination	Score
Under 60 yrs (0) 60–70 (1) 71–80 (2) 80+ (3) Male (1) Female (2)		Immobile or gait/balance normal (0) Steady with aids (1) Unsteady-refuses aids (2) Parkinsonian gait (3)		Independent or chair/bed bound & continent (0) Weightbears/walks with assistance (1) Impaired balance / continent (2) Impaired balance/incontinent (3) Wandering/restless/continent (3) Wandering/restless/incontinent (4)	
Medication		**Physical**		**Systolic Blood Pressure**	
No meds (0) On meds but no relevant side-effects (1) Slight adverse reaction (2) Adverse response to meds (3) Unstable - PRN (4)		Physically fit relative to age (0) Weight loss/recent ill health (1) Marked frailty (2) Recent limb fracture/injury (3) TIAs/seizures (4)		No noted drop between lying and standing (0) Drop less than 20mmHg between lying and standing (1) Drop more than 20mmHg between lying and standing (2)	
Sleep Pattern		**Vision Status**		**Co-operation**	
Sleeps well (0) Broken sleep (1) Reversed day/night pattern (2) Minimal/no sleep (3)		Adequate (with or without glasses/lenses) (0) Poor (with or without) (1) Legally blind (3)		Fully cooperative (0) Regular reassurance and instruction (1) Verbally hostile (2) Unpredictable/variable mood (3) Physically aggressive/restrictive or reluctant (4)	
Consciousness/mental status		**Falls History**		**Diagnosis**	
Alert or comatose (0) Reduced alertness (1) Disorientated at all times/Sleepy (2) Intermittent confusiion/ Exhausted (3)		No falls known (0) Previous history (1) History or increasing frequency (2) Recent and uncontrolled (3)		Cognitively intact (0) Alzheimers (1) Vascular (2) Lewdy Body (3) Acute confusional state or unconfirmed/other (4) SCORE	
RATING SCALE			SCORE		
0–12 Low risk 13–20 Moderate risk 21–30 Significant risk 30+ High risk			Date:		
Review date:			Signature:		

Figure 3.14 A typical fall risk assessment tool, courtesy of Valerie Ness

occur when performing everyday activities. It is thought that about one third of these could be prevented, therefore, risk assessment tools specifically designed for community use should be chosen. Each local area will have its own fall risk assessment tool (FRAT), which may also include suggestions for further assessment, appropriate management strategies, and local referral options.

Falls are the most common cause of accidental injury to children of all ages. The cause of these falls often relates to the stage of development of the child, for example, young children may fall as a result of inexperience or unsteadiness.

When to assess the risk of a fall

The cause of falls is multifactorial, therefore, many approaches need to be used by the multidisciplinary team to facilitate prevention. There is no consensus about which tool is best at identifying people as high or low risk (Oliver *et al.* 2004); instead, it may be best to focus on identifying common, reversible risk factors in all patients and ensuring that if people do fall, they are fully assessed afterwards.

In the hospital, care homes, day centres, and residential care, staff should be trained in the assessment and analysis of falls to identify at-risk patients and problems and select appropriate solutions based on this assessment and the evidence base.

By being proactive in identifying at-risk patients and implementing multifactorial interventions, falls, and the impact that they have on the individual, the family, the health service, and society at large, can be reduced.

An individual risk assessment should be commenced at the very beginning of care and re-evaluated throughout the patient's stay and at discharge.

In addition to this, the NICE guidelines (NICE 2004) state that all older people who are under the care of a health professional should be assessed at least once a year. This may be carried out more frequently in patients with risk factors or after a fall.

After the assessment, preventative management interventions can be put in place to prevent falls. A multidisciplinary approach should be adopted, as

Fall risk assessment

Area to be assessed/questions to ask

Rationale

Area to be assessed/questions to ask	Rationale
History of falls: frequency, context, and characteristics.	This can establish risk factors and patterns.
Movement difficulties: gait, balance, mobility, weakness, dyspraxia, coordination, restricted movement, for example, arthritis, Parkinson's disease. Will patient benefit from strengthening exercises? Many tools are available to assess this, for example: Timed up and go test (Podsiadlo and Richardson 1991), Turn 180°, Tinetti scale (Tinetti *et al.* 1986), Functional reach (Duncan *et al.* 1990), Dynamic gait index, Berg Balance Scale (Berg *et al.* 2004). Is patient steady on feet? Does patient use aids and are they used appropriately?	This is useful in implementing management strategies.

Osteoporosis risk: **There are various tools, for example, the Black Fracture Index (Black *et al.* 2001) and tests that can be carried out, for example, DEXA scan. Functional ability.**	These patients are at greater risk of fracture following a fall.
Pain and disability: many scales exist to measure ability and pain.	Pain can be very distracting and influence the patient's ability to understand or participate in prevention programmes.
Fear in relation to falling: ascertain why, consider previous experiences.	Confidence can have a large impact on the risk of falling again.
Visual impairment; consider vision during daylight and at night and use of visual aids.	Inability to see edges, steps, or changes in floor covering can increase the risk of falls.
Cognitive impairment, neurological assessment: consider disorientation, memory difficulties, confusion, dementia. Many scales exist to aid in measurement, for example, Glasgow Coma Scale, Mini-Mental State Examination (MMSE) (Folstein *et al.* 1975), short orientation–memory–concentration test of cognitive impairment (Katzman *et al.* 1983).	May affect their ability to understand and may cause wandering and falls.
Communication difficulties: difficulty expressing or comprehending.	May affect ability to understand and participate in prevention programmes.
Psychological status: depression, mood changes, lack of motivation or awareness. There are many scales that can be used, for example, Hospital Anxiety Depression Scale (Zigmond and Snaith 1983).	May affect ability to participate in prevention programmes.
Urinary incontinence: a full incontinence assessment should be carried out if appropriate to establish the type and management options.	Patients hurrying to a toilet may be at greater risk of falling
Hazards and environment; make a home or hospital assessment.	The environment plays a major role in risk assessment.
Physical examination: cardiovascular, cerebrovascular, past medical history, for example, epilepsy. **Does patient have an acute physical illness?** **Does patient have an exacerbation of a chronic disorder, for example, unstable diabetes, hypotension?**	May cause an acute state of confusion.
Medication review: what is being taken, is patient actually taking it, how often, how much, and when?	There are many side effects and issues in relation to polypharmacy, which can increase the risk of falls.
Alcohol and substance misuse: many tests and tools exist to assess this, for example, CAGE (Ewing 1984) or AUDIT (Saunders *et al.* 1993) questionnaire	These can have physical and psychological effects that can increase susceptibility to falls.

continued

Diet and nutrition: is diet healthy? consider weight or recent weight loss; are there any special dietary needs, for example, diabetic, gluten-free	Nutritional deficiencies can increase the risk of falls.
Sleep pattern: is the sleep pattern disturbed? Are sleeping tablets being taken?	Poor sleep can increase the risk of falls.

many of these strategies will involve the entire healthcare team, from domestic staff cleaning the floors to doctors prescribing drugs. Many different management interventions are available. Often, these are used in combination with each other rather than on their own.

Aftercare

After a fall risk assessment has been carried out, it should be documented and kept with the patient's notes. This assessment will alert you to the risk of the individual patient and should then be used as a means of determining a suitable programme of prevention. Many of the interventions are listed in the table below and are based on the NICE guidelines (NICE 2004).

Both the results of the fall risk assessment and any strategies that are then adopted should be documented in the patient's notes, so that they can be reviewed regularly and evaluated. This should be documented and reviewed by all the relevant members of the multidisciplinary team.

It is not always possible to prevent falls from occurring. If a patient does fall, you should follow the guidelines in Chapter 10, which include completing an incident form. You should then investigate the possible causes by examining when and where the fall happened, who was involved, any activity that was taking place, and any possible causes. This may help to identify causes and patterns or evaluate the use of any interventions used.

Developing your skills

Assessment skills are vital for nurses, as will be highlighted throughout this book. You may get the chance to observe your mentor implement a fall risk assessment on a patient when you are on clinical placement. You should look at the various fall risk assessment tools available, especially if you are going to a placement involving care of the elderly. There will be specific tools that are used locally, so make sure you are aware of them and how to use them.

Other factors to consider

Each Community Health Partnership (CHP) or Primary Care Trust should have an appointed falls team or coordinator to tackle the prevention of falls in the community. Community nursing staff can identify patients who are at risk during a health screen or **opportunistically**, for example, if the patient presents with a fall or another problem or during a visit to the patient's home.

Strength and balance exercises can be recommended through community care or leisure and recreation services. Environmental changes can be made, such as improving pavements, lighting, and ensuring that public areas are safe.

The assessment and management of patients in primary and community care will involve a huge team comprising of both primary and secondary care, social work, housing, the ambulance service, community alarm services, and the voluntary and private sectors.

Multifactorial preventative measures to reduce falls

Intervention: how and when	Rationale
Strength and balance training Muscle-strengthening exercises, individually prescribed and monitored by an appropriately trained person. Involve a physiotherapist as appropriate.	Improves muscle tone, strength, balance, proprioception, and self-confidence.
Environmental hazard assessment and intervention Use of primary colours, better lighting including daylight, shock-absorbing floors, nonslip coverings, eye-level signs, good use of space, appropriate placement of nursing stations, lifts, and handrails; move badly positioned furniture, flexes, loose carpets; noise reduction and appropriate footwear (NPSA 2007). Should be part of discharge planning for at-risk patients in hospital. For those at risk living in the community this should be a regular assessment by trained health professionals Involve Occupational Therapist as appropriate.	Prevents falls due to poor visibility, slips, trips, and distractions.
Vision assessment and referral Regular ophthalmic check-ups should be arranged.	Poor vision can cause many falls.
Medication review with modification or withdrawal Reduction of the use of hypnotics and medication which calm anxiety or address psychosis where appropriate. It may be useful to involve the pharmacist.	Alternative drugs can be used (for example, antidepressants or herbal remedies) or other nonpharmacological strategies may be appropriate: these will not have the side effects likely to cause falls, for example, cognitive behaviour therapy, relaxation techniques, sleep hygiene.
Education and information for the patient, relatives, or significant others Discuss the changes that the patient is willing to make. Programmes should be flexible, provided by the multidisciplinary team and tailored to the patient.	To promote participation in the programme. To accommodate individual needs.
Hip protectors (Minns *et al.* 2004) Worn on the hip to prevent fractures if the patient falls and strikes the hip on a hard surface. Can be uncomfortable and need to be worn all day. Can also lead to episodes of incontinence if the user has difficulty removing them. The patient or carer may need to purchase them.	May be of use in older people living in extended care settings at high risk; however, there is no real evidence to show that they are effective and they are now rarely used in clinical practice.

continued

Close supervision of highly at-risk patients **Usually requires an increase in staffing, although this may be temporary.**	To prevent patients at high risk from independent activity that is deemed dangerous (must also consider therapeutic risk-taking, that is, the long-term effects, what will happen on discharge, do they have 24/7 care?)
Assistive technology **(Miskelly 2001) Only implemented after assessment of the appropriateness.** **Movement sensors or alarms.**	This alerts staff to the fact that an at-risk patient is mobilizing.
Fall detectors: these are bleep-sized devices worn around the waist or upper chest. They contain an accelerometer and a tilt meter and generate an alarm in the home and through the telephone if they detect impact or tilt.	Alerts a predetermined person when a person falls in the home.
Dawn or dusk lights, that respond to ambient light levels.	For people who get up at night to use the toilet – may prevent falls.
High-low beds or beds that can be adjusted to a very low level off the floor.	Less chance of injury if a patient falls out of bed.
Physical activity **Individual exercise and group exercise programmes can improve social contact and general mobility.** **Involve the physiotherapist, as appropriate.**	Can improve social contact, independence, quality of life, and general mobility. Can also improve levels of boredom, frustration, anxiety, depression, and aggression. Can improve self-confidence in patients who have already fallen.
Appropriate staffing levels **More staff may be required to supervise patients – this may only be on a short-term basis.**	Falls often occur at night and at busy times, when staffing is lower or staff are busy.
Vitamin D or calcium supplements **Involve dietician as appropriate.**	May be of use to reduce fracture rates, however, the evidence is still to be produced.

Bed rails

Bed rails are a controversial area. They are not recommended in patients with dementia or cognitive impairment because they are often associated with an increased risk, as the patient may try to climb over the rails or get out at the foot of the bed.

They may be used in certain circumstances but only after careful assessment by the multidisciplinary team and where there are no alternative strategies. Cot sides should certainly not be used to address problems with staffing or patient supervision or as a restraint (Mental Welfare Commission for Scotland 2006). In those exceptional circumstances where bed rails are deemed necessary, it is important to ensure that the sides are compatible with the make of bed and that you are complying with local policy.

Children

Preventative measures should be based on the assessment of the individual child. These include environmental measures to make the home safe, such as fireguards, safety corners, and gates and locks on windows. As children become older, they are less likely to injure themselves in the home but may be more likely to injure

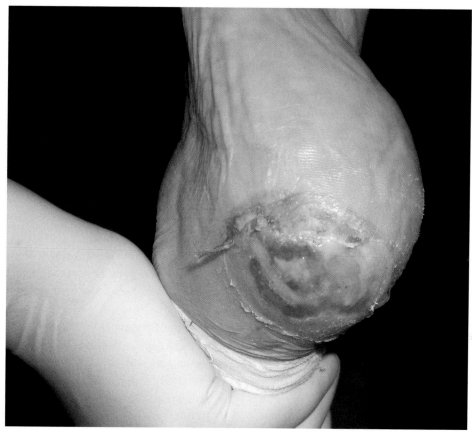

Figure 3.15 Grade II pressure sore on patient's heel. Permission from Aberdeen Royal Infirmary Department of Tissue Viability.

themselves outside of it, for example, falling from a height if climbing. Special surfaces can be used to prevent injury outside where children are running around (Child Accident Prevention Trust 2008).

When children are in hospital or visiting others in hospital it is important that they are aware of safety issues. Again many of these are environmental. It is also important that parents and visitors supervise any visiting children and are educated in safety measures if their children are patients, for example, suitable clothing and footwear, the effects of certain medications, and their ability to mobilize with or without support.

Scenarios

Consider what you should do in the following situations, then turn to the end of the section to check your answers.

Further scenarios are available at

 www.oxfordtextbooks.co.uk/orc/docherty/

Scenario 1

Mr Smith is a 50-year-old man who was diagnosed four weeks ago as having bowel cancer. Today, he has undergone bowel surgery and has returned to the ward area following a 2-hour operation. His vital signs are observed to be stable and he is making a good recovery. You notice on inspection of the sacral area of the heel that Mr Smith has a pressure ulcer, like the one shown in **Fig. 3.15**.

1 What grade of pressure sore do you think this is?
2 How might further deterioration be managed?

Scenario 2

Sophie, a 2-year-old girl, has been admitted for observation after a loss of consciousness (approximately one minute) following a fall from a toy. On a handover report, you are told that the child is being observed following this head injury. All observations indicate stable vital signs and her Glasgow Coma Score is 15. You are asked by her family why you want to look into her eyes for a pupil response.

1 What kind of explanation might you provide for this procedure?
2 You notice that one pupil is not responding as well to light as the other. What might this suggest?
3 Are there any other staff you want to involve at this stage?

 Scenario 3

You are on a placement with a community-based learning disability nurse. One of the patients on the caseload is a 23-year-old man called Jeffrey. Jeffrey was born with Down's Syndrome and has difficulty in various aspects of his learning. Your mentor has explained that Jeffrey often complains of pain, but that he, the mentor, finds it really difficult to assess Jeffrey's pain. Is there a pain assessment chart that might help you? Explain your choice.

 Scenario 4

Mr Brown was diagnosed with depression 16 years ago and has lived alone in the community with some input from his community psychiatric nurse (CPN). He usually complies with his medication regime but occasionally has episodes of severe depression that require him to be hospitalized. Your mentor has stated that he appears unkempt. You need to inspect his skin on admission to the acute receiving unit.

1 How will you gain cooperation and consent from the patient to assess his skin?
2 What are you observing and where will you document your findings?

Website

🌐 **www.oxfordtextbooks.co.uk/orc/docherty/**
You may find it helpful to work through our short online quiz and interactive scenarios intended to help you to develop and apply the skills in this chapter.

References

Adam S and Osborne S (2005). *Critical Care Nursing Science and Practice*, 2nd edn. Oxford University Press, Oxford.

Advanced Life Support Group (2005). *Advanced Paediatric Life Support: The Practical Approach*, 4th edn. BMJ, Oxford.

Berg KO, Wood-Dauphinese SL, Williams JI, and Maki B (2004). Measuring balance in the elderly: validation of an instrument. *Archives of Physical Medicine and Rehabilitation*, **85**(7), 1128–35.

Bird J (2005). Assessing pain in older people. *Nursing Standard*, **19**(19), 45–52.

Black DM, Steinbuch M, Palermo I, *et al.* (2001) An assessment tool for predicting fracture risk in postmenopausal women. *Osteoporosis International*, **12**(5), 519–28.

Braden B and Bergstrom N (1988). *The Braden Scale for Predicting Pressure Sore Risk*. www.bradenscale.com/braden.pdf.

Carter B (1994). *Child and Infant Pain: Principles of Nursing Care and Management*. Chapman and Hall, London.

Child Accident Prevention Trust (2008). *Factsheet: Falls in the Home*. Child Accident Prevention Trust, London. www.capt.org.uk/pdfs/factsheet%20falls.pdf.

Daut RL, Cleeland CS, and Flanery RC (1983). Development of the Wisconsin Brief Pain Questionnaire to assess pain in cancer and other diseases. *Pain*, **17**, 197–210.

Dawes E, Lloyd H, and Durham L (2007). Monitoring and recording patients' neurological observations. *Nursing Standard*, **22**(10), 40–5.

Dougherty L and Lister S, eds (2008). *The Royal Marsden Hospital Manual of Clinical Nursing Procedures*, 7th edn. Blackwell Publishing, London.

Duncan PW, Weiner DK, Chandler J, and Studenski S (1990). Functional reach: a new clinical measure of balance. *Journal of Gerontology*, **45**(6), M192–M197.

Ewing JA (1984). Detecting alcoholism: the CAGE questionnaire. *JAMA: Journal of the American Medical Association*, **252**, 1905–7.

Folstein MF, Folstein SE, and McHugh PR (1975). 'Mini-mental state,' a practical method for grading the cognitive state of patients for the clinician. *Journal of Psychiatry Research*, **12**(3) 189–98.

Gagliese L and Melzack R (2003). Age-related differences in the qualities but not the intensity of chronic pain. *Pain*, **104**(3), 597–608.

Giuliano KK and Higgins TL (2005). New generation pulse oximetry in the care of critically ill patients. *American Journal of Critical Care*, **14**(1), 26–37.

Horgan M, Choonara I, Al-Waidh Sambrookes J, *et al.* (1996). Measuring pain in neonates: an objective score. *Paediatric Nursing*, **8**(10), 24–7.

ILCOR (International Liaison Committee on Resuscitation) (2005). Part 4 Advanced life support. *Resuscitation*, **67**, 213–47.

Katzman R, Brown T, Fuld P, Schechter R, and Schimel H (1983). Validation of a short orientation-memory-concentration test of cognitive impairment. *American Journal of Psychiatry*, **140**(6) 734–9.

Kause J, Smith G, Prytherch D, *et al.* (2004). A comparison of antecedents to cardiac arrests, deaths and emergency intensive care admissions in Australia and New Zealand and the United Kingdom – the ACADEMIA study. *Resuscitation*, **62**, 275–82.

McCaffery M (1972). *Nursing Management of the Patient in Pain*. Lippincott, Philadelphia.

McCaffery M and Pasero C (1999). *Pain: Clinical Manual*, 2nd edn. Mosby, Philadelphia.

McHugh G and Thoms G (2001). Living with chronic pain: the patient's perspective. *Nursing Standard*, **15**(52), 33–7.

Melzack R (1975). The McGill Pain Questionnaire: major properties and scoring methods. *Pain*, 1: 277–99.

Melzack R and Wall PD (1965). Pain mechanisms: a new theory. *Science*, **150**, 971–9.

Merskey H, Albe-Fessard DJ, and Bonica JJ (1979). Pain terms: a list with definitions and notes on usage. *Pain*, **6**, 249–52.

Mental Welfare Commission for Scotland (2006). *Rights, Risks and Limits to Freedom: Principles and Good Practice Guidance for Practitioners Considering Restraint in Residential Care Settings*, Mental Welfare Commission for Scotland, Edinburgh. www.mwcscot. org.uk/web/FILES/Publications/Rights_Risks_web.pdf.

Middleton C (2004a). The assessment and treatment of patients with chronic pain. *Nursing Times*, **100**(18), 40–4.

Middleton C (2004b). Barriers to the provision of effective pain management. *Nursing Times*, **100**(3), 42–55.

Minns J, Dodd C, Gardner R, Bamford J, and Nabhani F (2004). Assessing the safety and effectiveness of hip protectors. *Nursing Standard*, **18**(39), 33–8.

Miskelly FG (2001). Assistive technology in elderly care. *Age and Ageing*, **30**, 455–8.

NICE (2003). *Pressure Ulcer Prevention*. Clinical Guideline 7. National Institute for Clinical Excellence, London.

NICE (2004). *Falls: the Assessment and Prevention of Falls in Older People*. Clinical Guideline 21. National Institute for Clinical Excellence, London. www.nice. org.uk/nicemedia/pdf/CG021NICEguideline.pdf.

NIHCE (2007). *Head Injury: Triage, Assessment, Investigation and Early Management of Head Injury in Infants, Children and Adults*. Clinical Guideline 56. National Institute for Health and Clinical Excellence, London. www.nice.org.uk/nicemedia/pdf/ CG56guidance.pdf.

NPSA (2007). *Slips, Trips and Falls in Hospital: Third Report From the Patient Safety Observatory*. National Patient Safety Agency, London. www.npsa. nhs.uk/patientsafety/alerts-and-directives/ directives-guidance/slips-trips-falls/.

NHS Quality Improvement Scotland (2005a). *Pressure Ulcer Prevention: Best Practice Statement*. www. nhshealthquality.org/nhsqis/files/21878%20 NHSQIS%20Ulcer%20BPS.pdf.

NHS Quality Improvement Scotland (2005b). *The Treatment/Management of Pressure Ulcers: Best Practice Statement*. www.nhshealthquality.org/ nhsqis/files/BPS%20Treatment%20Management%20 Pressure%20Ulcers%20(Mar%202005).pdf.

NHS Quality Improvement Scotland (2006). *Management of Chronic Pain in Adults: Best Practice Statement*. www.nhshealthquality.org/ nhsqis/files/BPSManage_chronic_pain%20_ adults%20(Feb06).pdf.

NMC (2005). *Guidance for Records and Record Keeping*. Nursing and Midwifery Council, London.

NMC (2007). *Advice Sheets: NMC Record Keeping Guidance*. Nursing and Midwifery Council, London.

Oliver D, Daly F, Martin FC, and McMurdo ME (2004). Risk factors and risk assessment tools for falls in hospital in-patients: a systematic review. *Age and Ageing*, **33**(2), 122–30.

Podsiadlo D and Richardson S (1991). The times 'up and go': a basic test of basic functional mobility for frail elderly persons. *Journal of the American Geriatrics Society*, **39**, 142–8.

Proctor WR and Hirdes JP (2001). Pain and cognitive status among nursing home residents in Canada. *Pain Research and Management*, **6**(3), 119–25.

Resuscitation Council UK (2006). *Immediate Life Support*, 2nd edn. Resuscitation Council UK, London.

Saunders JB, Aasland OG, and Babor TF (1993). Development of the alcohol use disorders identification test (AUDIT): WHO collaborative project on early detection of persons with harmful alcohol consumption. *Addiction*, **88**, 791–803.

Schofield P and Dunham M (2003). Pain assessment: how far have we come in listening to our patients? *Professional Nurse*, **18**(5), 276–9.

SIGN (2000). *Early Management of Patients With a Head Injury*, SIGN Publication No 46. Scottish Intercollegiate Guidelines Network, Edinburgh. www.sign.ac.uk/guidelines/fulltext/46/index.html.

Simon J and McTier C (1996). Development of a chronic pain assessment tool. *Rehabilitation Nursing*, **2**(1), 20–4.

Tatman A, Warren A, Williams A, Powell JE, and Whitehouse W (1997). Development of a modified paediatric coma scale in intensive care clinical practice. *Archives of Disease in Childhood*, **77**, 519–21.

Teasdale G and Jennett B (1974). Assessment of coma and impaired consciousness: a practical scale. *The Lancet*, **302**(7872), 81–4.

Tinetti ME, Willimas TF, and Mayewski R (1986). Fall risk index for elderly patients based on number of chronic disabilities. *American Journal of Medicine*, **80**, 429–34.

Twycross A, Moriarty A, and Betts T (1998). *Paediatric Pain Management: A Multidisciplinary Approach*. Radcliffe Medical Press, Oxfordshire.

Waterlow J (2005). *Waterlow Score Card*. www.judy-waterlow.co.uk/the-waterlow-score-card.htm.

White S (2004). Assessment of chronic neuropathic pain and the use of pain tools. *British Journal of Nursing*, **13**(7), 372–8.

Williams B, Poulter NR, Brown MJ, *et al.* (2004). British Hypertension Society guidelines for hypertension management 2004 (BHS-IV): summary. *BMJ*, **328**, 734–640.

Wilson M (2002). Overcoming the challenges of neuropathic pain. *Nursing Standard*, **16**(33), 47–53.

Wood S (2004). Factors influencing the selection of appropriate pain assessment tools. *Nursing Times*, **100**(35),42–7.

Zigmond AS and Snaith RP (1983). The Hospital Anxiety and Depression Scale. *Acta Psychiatrica Scandinavica*, **67**, 361–70.

Useful further reading and websites

Alcock K, Clancy M, and Crouch R (2002). Physiological observations of patients admitted to A & E. *Nursing Standard*, **16**(34), 33–7.
Provides more advanced reading around observations taken when the patient is showing signs of illness.

American Geriatric Society (2001). Guideline for the prevention of falls in older persons. *Journal of the American Geriatric Society*, **49**, 664–72.

Chaâbane F (2007). Falls prevention for older people with dementia. *Nursing Standard* **22**(6), 50–5.

Department of Health (2001). *National Service Framework for Older People. Standard Six: Falls*. The Stationery Office, London.

Hassen Fani-Salek M, Totten VY, and Terezakis SA (1999). Trauma scoring systems explained. *Emergency Medicine*, **11**, 155–66.
More advanced discussion on the use of scoring systems to identify patient's need.

Henderson Y (2007). Recognising dysfunctional breathing in asthma consultations. *Nursing Standard*, **22**(3), 40–1.
More advanced reading about respiratory patterns that are common in asthma – pertinent to acute episodes and day-to-day assessment.

Jevon P and Ewens B (2001). Assessment of a breathless patient. *Nursing Standard*, **15**(16), 48–53.
Consolidates the assessment of respiratory patterns.

Jevon P, Ewens B, and Pooni JS (2007). *Monitoring the Critically Ill Patient*, 2nd edn. Blackwell Publishing, London.
More advanced monitoring of the critically ill patient.

Kelly A and Downing M (2004). Reducing the likelihood of falls in older people. *Nursing Standard,* **18**(49), 33–40.

McCaffery M and Ferrel BR (1997). Nurses' knowledge of pain assessment and management: how much progress have we made? *Journal of Pain Symptom Management.* **14**(3), 175–86.

Morgan RJM, Williams F, and Wright MM (1997). An early warning scoring system for detecting developing critical illness. *Clinical Intensive Care*, **82**, 100–1. Comprehensive book on the assessment of pain.

Needham J (2004). Issues relating to effective pain management in young people. *Professional Nurse*, **19**(7), 406–8.

For those working in areas with young people.

O'Brien E, Asmar R, Beilin L, *et al*. (2003). European Society of Hypertension recommendations for conventional, ambulatory, and home blood pressure measurement. *Journal of Hypertension*, **21**, 821–48.

More advanced management of hypertension.

Resuscitation Council UK (2007). *Paediatric Immediate Life Support*, 1st edn. Resuscitation Council UK, London.

The British Pain Society (2004). *Recommendations for the Appropriate Use of Opioids for Persistent Non-cancer Pain*. The Pain Society, London. www.britishpainsociety.org/book_opioid_main.pdf. Best practice resources on a using opioids.

Woodrow P (1999). Pulse oximetry. *Nursing Standard*, **13**(42), 42–6.

More advanced discussion on pulse oximetry.

British National Formulary. www.bnf.org.uk.

A good reference source for any drug you may administer with supervision from your mentor.

National Institute for Health and Clinical Excellence. www.nice.org.uk.

Various best practice resources on a number of clinical issues.

Resuscitation Council UK. www.resus.org.uk.

A variety of best practice documents in relation to resuscitation.

Scottish Intercollegiate Guidelines Network. www.sign.ac.uk.

Various best practice resources on a number of clinical issues.

The British Pain Society. www.britishpainsociety.org. Various best practice resources on a number of pain issues.

Check **www.oxfordtextbooks.co.uk/orc/docherty/** for changes and new developments. Updated research, guidelines, or equipment will be added every four months.

 Answers to scenarios

 Scenario 1

1 The surface of the skin (epithelial layer) is slightly broken and there is redness on the skin. No underlying tissue appears damaged. Therefore, a grade 1/2 ulcer is noted.

2 Further deterioration be managed by:
- Further risk assessment: has the previous risk assessment been updated since Mr Smith came out of theatre?
- Change of position and early mobilization, as far as surgery will allow
- Pressure-relieving mattress
- Referral to physiotherapist for early mobilization and positioning
- Dressing to affected area if required
- Referral to tissue viability nurse specialist if further advice is required
- Assessment of nutritional status,
- Monitor continence; incontinence could cause further skin breakdown

 Scenario 2

1 You need to present this information in layman's terms to the family. You should explain that the eyes and the pupils' reaction to light can be useful in monitoring the brain.

2 You could ask whether Sophie normally has unequal pupils. If she does not normally have unequal pupils, this could be a sign of increase intracranial pressure and brain injury.

3 Inform your mentor immediately, as this sign may indicate the need for further medical intervention and closer observation of Sophie.

Scenario 3

Jeffrey would probably benefit from a pain tool that can be relatively easy to understand – avoid those with lots of writing. Perhaps a facial rating scale would be the easiest. You would need to perhaps test a few out and find out which you were able to use with Jeffrey. Remember that Jeffrey should rate his own pain so the scale should be used by the patient (not rated by the nurse).

 ## Scenario 4

1 Explain why it is important that you inspect the skin. Spend some time talking to Mr Brown before commencing the procedure. The procedure may require Mr Brown to undress and expose areas susceptible to pressure to you – you should ensure that his privacy and dignity are respected at all times.

2 The areas susceptible to pressure should be examined for signs of redness, blanching, broken skin, pressure ulcers, and any other skin problems (for example, **infestations** or skin disorders). You should document where you inspected, any areas of damage, and the date and time you completed this. Remember that this should be part of your initial risk assessment.

4 Communication

WILLIAM MCDONALD

Introduction

It is imperative that nurses demonstrate a professional approach in all of their communication and interaction with others, treating people with dignity, care, and respect. This chapter explores the skills associated with communication in nursing, and develops the previous discussion on communication contained in Section 2.1. It also links to Chapter 12, where the specific communication needs of dying patients are outlined.

This chapter provides an overview of some models of communication and then goes on to discuss the skills necessary to engage in effective communication within nursing. These are discussed in relation to **engaging** with patients, clients, families, carers, voluntary and statutory agencies, and colleagues within the multidisciplinary team. The following skills will be examined in detail: verbal and nonverbal communication, **active listening** and observing, the use of questioning, written communication, and the role of context and other factors that contribute to the efficacy of communication, for example, culture, age, and sex.

While this chapter predominantly discusses communication in relation to your role as a nurse, please keep in mind as you read it, that the way we employ our own communication skills is likely to have a significant impact on the communication approaches of those with whom we interact. The information in this chapter should, therefore, not only guide the development of your own communication skills, but it should also be used by you to support others to gain insight into how they may communicate more effectively.

In the case of patients, you may often encounter people who, for a wide range of reasons, including physical or mental health problems, may find communication extremely difficult, or almost impossible. By understanding all of the factors that contribute to effective communication, and by developing the skills involved in achieving this, you can compensate for your patients' compromised abilities and adapt your approaches to individual circumstances in ways that reduce communication difficulties for those involved.

Such awareness should enable you to minimize the impact of any potential barriers to communication in individual or specific situations. It is vital, therefore, that as part of your developing communication skills, you not only increase your own knowledge and understanding, but you are able to support your patients to become more effective communicators themselves. This may be best done by helping to raise their awareness of how they communicate, and helping them to identify and utilize their own strengths in relation to this.

Remember that you will be trying to develop your communication skills from your personal life, while also learning new skills to incorporate into professional contexts. This can take time to achieve successfully. You should not try to rush things: much of what you will learn is likely to occur over time from your ongoing nursing experiences. You are likely to make mistakes, but do not be disheartened by this. Instead, if you use reflection and the support of appropriately skilled senior colleagues to examine your communication skills, you can minimize the risk of errors and enhance your areas of strength. In doing so, you should ensure that you are able to demonstrate the highest quality in your communication with patients, families, and other professionals.

In addition, it is worth highlighting that while the information on communication in this book is often presented in relation to a specific setting or patient group, remember that the skills presented here are often transferable to other nursing contexts and environments. Nursing interventions now occur in a wide range of locations, for example, inpatient wards, community settings, clinics, and specialist centres, and the patients' own homes. You should consider each aspect and skill as part of a toolkit that you can keep in your 'mental tool bag' and select for use whenever and for whoever it would best be suited, thereby making yourself a more rounded, flexible, and effective nurse.

Many of the examples used in this chapter relate to the communication skills that you personally should employ, as a nurse. Please bear in mind, however, that as well as developing your own understanding of communication, you should apply your knowledge and skills to those in your care. Many of the people with whom you come into contact may have difficulty communicating. This can be for a very wide range of reasons, which may include physical impairment, psychological difficulties, or a lack of social skills or experience. You should strive to promote the strengths of those in your care, as in doing so, you will enable them to communicate and interact to the best of their ability, and facilitate their most effective participation in the process of communication.

Learning outcomes

The learning outcomes of this chapter expand on those of Section 2.1. It would be helpful to revise that section before proceeding with this chapter, as this will provide a more complete overview of this topic for you.

These outcomes relate to numbers 6 and 14 of the NMC's Essential Skill Clusters and specifically to Care Domains 1, 2, and 3 of the NMC's Standards of Proficiency for Pre-registration Nursing (outcomes to be achieved for entry to branch).

On reading the chapter and associated web pages and undertaking supervised activities, the student will be able to:

- Understand underpinning theories of communication
- Determine the potential impact of verbal and nonverbal communication skills on interpersonal interaction

- Effectively participate in all forms of communication, employing a variety of appropriate modes
- Document interactions accurately, recording aspects of communication that contribute to the understanding of particular circumstances
- Recognize factors that can have a positive or negative impact on communication
- Facilitate other people's use of effective communication skills to the best of their ability

Prior knowledge

As this chapter aims to develop the previous discussion on communication contained in the mandatory skills section within this book, you should reread that section to refresh your understanding of the key issues covered there, before continuing further.

Background

Thompson (2003) suggests that communication is so integral to our lives that it is most often taken for granted. He cites Fiske (1990), who stated that it is something that is widely recognized, but also something that few people can satisfactorily define. Communication is a concept that at first glance can appear quite simple and straightforward. In its most basic form, it can be described as a **linear** process involving a sender who sends a message to a receiver, using a method of communication, as shown in **Fig. 4.1**.

This model suggests that communication occurs when someone decides on a message that they wish to send, for example, choosing the words to say, the written text, or the **gestures** and expression to be used. This information is then transmitted through a chosen medium, for example, speech, email, signalling across a busy room, to the receiver, who interprets it based on their individual **perceptions** and understanding. Even at this simple level, however, it can be seen that there is a potential for difficulties. For instance, if the sender uses language or signals that are unknown to the receiver, there is a risk that errors

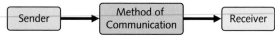

Figure 4.1 A basic model of communication

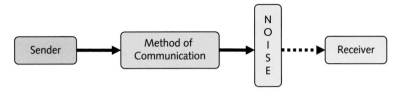

Figure 4.2 Barriers to communication in a linear process

could occur in translation, which may alter the interpretation of the message completely.

As communication theories developed, the effect of disruptions in the communication process was acknowledged. Often this is referred to as 'noise', which, in this context, refers to any interruption that hampers the message reaching the receiver and impeding their ability to interpret the message being sent (see **Fig. 4.2**). So while noise may refer to a more traditional definition of background sound that inhibits communication, in this context it also includes any distractions, **emotions**, or equipment failures that might impede clear channels of communication (Hargie and Dickson 2004).

It is difficult to find agreement on what communication actually is: numerous definitions of the term have been suggested. Many of these describe communication as a more complex process than this simple linear example. Nowadays, it is commonly recognized that communication involves an exchange of information between a sender and a receiver through a channel of communication, but the important role that feedback plays in the process is also acknowledged.

So while, as nurses, we may initially engage in interaction as a sender or receiver of information, we almost immediately adopt a dual role. We not only send out our own contribution to the process, but we also assess how this is impacting on the other participants and alter our approach according to the feedback they are consciously or subconsciously providing. If we are relating a story to a friend who starts yawning, we may wonder if they are tired of listening to us and try to inject more drama or excitement into our account.

When communicating with a patient, we should be continually aware of the feedback that they are providing, which may give us clues to their level of understanding, interest, or ability to retain the information we are sending. Feedback enables participants to assess more accurately the efficacy of their messages and the level of understanding of the recipient (see **Fig. 4.3**).

Such views, therefore, suggest that communication is more transactional in nature and involves an ongoing process, where participants both influence others and are influenced themselves by the continuing changes within their interactions (Ellis *et al.* 2003). It is important for us as nurses to be aware of this dual role, as patients, family, and indeed anyone with whom we communicate, are likely to be responding to the feedback that we are providing for them too. So, in effect, the participants in most communication processes work simultaneously as senders of information and feedback and receivers of information and feedback. Remember, too, that the impact of noise can influence the process during both the sending of the original message and the feedback being provided.

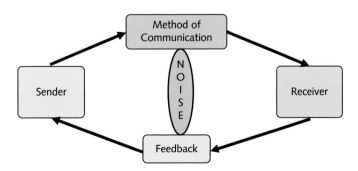

Figure 4.3 The role of feedback in the communication process

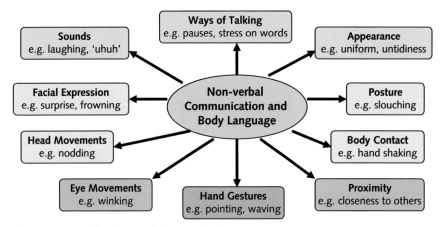

Figure 4.4 Examples of nonverbal communication

4.1 **Verbal and nonverbal communication**

Definition

Verbal communication involves the spoken word. Words are symbols we use to think about and express our thoughts, feelings, and perceptions of who we are and how we interact with the world and the people around us (Arnold and Boggs 2007). Verbal communication consists of several components, which can significantly influence or alter the meaning of the messages that we try to convey. Having an understanding of these components, therefore, enables us to enhance the messages we send, expressing our thoughts, feelings, and views more clearly and making our communication more effective.

Nonverbal communication refers to the aspects of our interaction that do not include spoken words (see **Fig. 4.4**). Hargie and Dickson (2004), however, wisely warn that the distinction between verbal and nonverbal communication is much less clear in the real world than in any discussion about communication. The reality is that communication involves a complex and continually changing set of methods, behaviours, and skills that are made additionally difficult, owing to the possibility of multiple interpretations of the message being sent and the intentions of those sending and receiving them. Remaining aware of these potential problems will enable you to take account of the changing interaction and adapt your communication style to one that best suits the needs of the situation at that particular time.

When to use nonverbal communication skills

Nonverbal communication enables us to enhance the information that we send in our messages to others and often offers cues that can contribute to a deeper understanding of interactions. Although there are times when these cues may seem very evident to us, remember that it can be easy to misinterpret what you are seeing, and you may have an inaccurate perception of what a person's nonverbal cues may indicate. For example, the facial expressions in **Fig. 4.5** could be misinterpreted without having fuller awareness of the context.

In reality the information presented nonverbally is often much more subtle. The nurse needs to demonstrate excellent observational skills and levels of awareness to identify and interpret these appropriately and effectively. It is unwise to rely solely on your interpretation of nonverbal communication and it is better to seek clarification of your views through discussion and confirmation with the other person.

As well as the words we use there are other aspects of our speech that help shape the meaning of those words. The term given to such characteristics, which includes using sounds like 'aha' or 'mmm', sighing, laughing, and so on, or the tone or inflection we give to the words that we say, is **paralinguistics**. As well as providing useful indicators of underlying thoughts, feelings or emotions, paralinguistics can be utilized to enhance communication when transmitting information. For example, by being consciously aware of maintaining good eye contact during a conversation we can demonstrate more clearly that we are eager to engage

Verbal communication

Communication approach	Rationale
Language **Choose terms appropriate to the receiver, for example, formal or informal language, consider the cultural perspective, for example use of local dialect.**	This makes it more likely that you will 'connect' with individuals and can enhance the receiver's understanding. It can help you to display a professional, respectful, and thoughtful approach.
Choose language relevant to individual's capabilities, for example, education, learning disability, whether English is the speaker's first language.	Enhances each person's understanding, reduces the likelihood of distress associated with lack of understanding, and shows consideration of the individual.
Avoid the use of jargon; choose terminology that is appropriate to individuals.	Enhances understanding, and minimizes confusion and frustration. Patients may not understand or be familiar with terms that are commonly used in nursing.
Content **Remain relevant to the topic. State what is intended unambiguously.**	Provides clarity and avoids confusion, reduces the risk of misunderstanding and misinterpretation.
Ensure that the amount of detail you give is appropriate: provide additional detail and description.	To aid understanding and clarify uncertainty.
Avoid giving too much information all at once.	To avoid overloading people or confusing them, especially if they have a **sensory** or **cognitive** impairment.
Volume **Ensure that the loudness of your voice is appropriate:**	To convey control and competence; to be reassuring when someone is upset or distressed.
Speak softly **Speak loudly**	To ensure confidential matters are not overheard. Can help convey a caring approach.
	To ensure you can be heard when addressing more people or in a noisy environment.
	Be aware that speaking loudly can be viewed as more **aggressive**, dominant, or demanding. Speaking loudly may also be an indication of stress, fear, or anxiety.
Tone **Keep the pitch and quality of your voice steady.**	This conveys control, concern, and approachability.
Alter the pitch to alter meaning.	Enables specific parts of a sentence to be emphasized.
Avoid using a sharp or abrupt tone.	This could suggest displeasure, irritation, being dismissive, or lack of interest.

continued

Rate

Ensure the rate of your speech is slow enough:	To aid the listener's understanding.
Avoid speaking too slowly.	Very slow speech may appear patronizing: it may also be perceived as deeper thinking, confusion, or boredom.
Avoid speaking too quickly.	There is a tendency to speak more rapidly when feeling stressed. It can be difficult to understand rapid speech, especially along with accents and dialects.

Emphasis

Stress specific words or phrases.	Can significantly alter the meaning of the words being used. Can be used to convey underlying emotions, for example, disagreement, disbelief, or support.

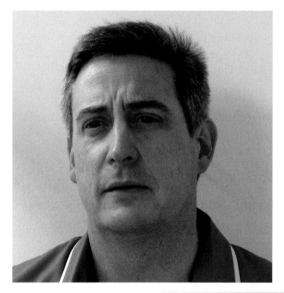
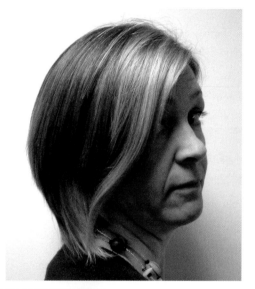
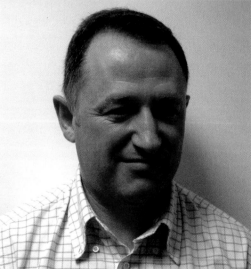

Figure 4.5 Ambiguous facial expressions

Nonverbal communication

Communication approach	Rationale
Posture Usually standing or sitting;	Choose appropriately for the situation, more formal or informal, what message is being conveyed, for example, authority, compassion, empathy.
	Consider the impact of room layout and physical barriers.
	If you are trying to communicate with children it is often best to get down to their level. There's nothing wrong with crouching or kneeling to talk to a child hiding under a table, for instance.
1. Erect, shoulders back, head held up.	Can convey confidence, being in control, empathy, the value being placed on the interaction, or status and dominance within it.
	Be wary of appearing arrogant or aloof.
2. Open posture—arms unfolded, held away from face, legs uncrossed.	Can suggest receptiveness, interest, positive frame of mind, and emotional state.
	Is nonthreatening and can show approachability and interest.
3. Postural mirroring.	Reflecting the posture of another person can help them feel that you are paying attention to them and are able to relate to them.
	Closed posture, that is, arms folded, legs crossed, can convey a lack of interest, willingness or ability to engage.
Orientation and proximity How we align ourselves to the other person:	Can convey attitude or apparent value placed on the interaction.
Face-to-face,	Can convey interest and enables better eye contact and connection with people.
Showing our back,	May suggest dissatisfaction or unease and is generally viewed as unacceptable or being rude.
Sitting at an angle	Can appear less direct or challenging for patients.
Distance or leaning forwards,	Can also convey interest and connection with what is being expressed.

continued

Awareness of appropriate interpersonal space.	This can change depending on the individuals involved and specific circumstances.
	Consider individual choice, sex, age, culture as these may affect what is viewed as appropriate.
Facial expression **This contributes significantly to meaning.**	Provides additional information about mood, emotion, state of mind.
Can involve the whole face.	For example, smiling, grimacing.
May be partial signals.	For example, raising an eyebrow, pursing lips.
Spontaneous reactions.	Be wary of spontaneous expressions, which may convey feelings of shock, disgust, or rejection, as this may be upsetting for patients.
Eye contact **Maintain good eye contact—not a fixed look or staring.**	Powerful way of establishing contact and monitoring feedback.
	Can convey a deep sense of interest, understanding, and connection between individuals.
	Can be used to regulate interaction by demonstrating when someone wants to say something.
Blinking and breaking eye contact.	Lack of eye contact can leave people unsure if the receiver is listening or has become distracted.
	Used excessively, eye contact can be perceived as threatening, challenging, or intimidating.
Gestures and movement **These can be categorized as fine and gross**	Provides additional information about mood, emotion, emphasis, and state of mind.
Fine—Smaller, more discreet, movements, for example, head nodding, shrugging shoulders	Provides indications of underlying thoughts, feelings, and emotions. Can be used to emphasize, enhance, contradict or replace what is being said.
Gross—large-scale, expansive movements, for example, running away, exuberant arm waving	Provides indications as above but in a more obvious, dynamic, or demonstrative way.

with the individual who is speaking. Additionally it can show the level of interest and attentiveness of the receiver to the message being sent. Similarly, as nurses, we can, by maintaining an even, controlled volume, rate, and tone in our verbal communication, convey an air of being competent, capable and in control of a situation in a way that may provide reassurance to someone who is feeling upset or distressed. This may be easier to do in routine circumstances, but in a demanding or stressful situation it can be difficult to remember to use these skills to reduce the level of tension.

Touch **Physical contact with others: hand on arm, holding hands when someone is upset or anxious**	Great care must be taken to ensure that touch is appropriate to sex, age, culture, and individual preference.
	Used appropriately, touching can offer comfort and empathy, demonstrates level of attention.
	Inappropriate touch can be seen as intrusive and beyond professional boundaries.
Paralinguistics, that is, aspects of language other than words	
This includes sounds and vocal inflection, for example, rate, tone volume, etc.	Can provide additional information by emphasizing, enhancing, contradicting or replacing what is being said.
	Can be subtle or obvious, for example, gently sighing, sniggering, laughing uproariously.
	Includes expressions like 'Aha!' and 'Mmmm'.
Autonomic responses **For example, blushing, sweating, breathlessness**	These are unconscious reactions which can occur in response to feeling under stress.
	As they can occur out with the person's control having an awareness of them enables the use of other methods of communicating to compensate.
General dress and appearance	Contributes to initial opinions and assumptions.
Refers to physical characteristics and attire	Clothing, jewellery, other adornments convey information about how we view ourselves.
Professional dress or uniform	Can convey status and role, relate to people's expectations of the individual wearing such attire.

If successfully practised, however, such skills can promote engagement with other people and help to defuse potentially difficult and challenging situations.

Relationship between verbal and nonverbal communication

So far it has been shown how verbal and nonverbal communication skills may impact positively and negatively on the communication process. By improving knowledge and understanding of these factors, nurses can improve the outcomes of their interactions, for example, choosing appropriate language and speaking clearly to enhance understanding; good eye contact to convey interest and caring; postural mirroring to encourage interaction; appropriate personal space to be nonthreatening. The verbal and nonverbal communication skills that we employ are closely linked and the impact of one on the other can be significant in the message that we transmit.

Developing your skills

So how do you use verbal and nonverbal communication skills together? Take a few moments to think about a

Relationship between verbal and nonverbal communication

Purpose	Rationale
Repeat or confirm	Reinforces the message being sent verbally, for example, 'He's over there,' while pointing in the right direction.
Contradict	Gives an opposite meaning to what is being said, for example, 'I'm happy to help,' while sighing and looking glum.
Add to; modify; compliment	Enhances the verbal information, for example, 'It was absolutely huge,' while using hands to demonstrate size.
Emphasize	Reinforces what is being said, for example, 'No, no, no! There's no way that I can go,' while shaking head and gesturing with hands.
Regulating	Dictating the tempo of speech or indicating a desire to talk, for example, banging a table as you emphasize important points, or opening your mouth and raising a finger when you want to contribute to a conversation.
Substitute	Replacing verbal communication completely, for example, replying to a question by nodding or shaking your head, or showing satisfaction by giving a thumbs-up sign.

situation where you have used nonverbal cues to enhance what you have been saying:

- What nonverbal cues or signals do you use to emphasize or contradict your oral messages?
- Are there some types of gesture that you would use in your private life but not in your professional role?
- If there is a difference, why might this be so?
- Are there situations where you would consider it inappropriate to use certain nonverbal signals?

When considering this, it is important to bear in mind that some gestures may have alternative meanings within particular groups or cultures. Signals that are acceptable to some may be considered meaningless, rude, or insulting by others. When using any signs, therefore, it is advisable to avoid possible confusion by checking that the receiver places the same meaning on the signal as the sender.

Other factors to consider

It is important to remember also that although the tables look at each aspect of verbal and nonverbal communication independently, in practice, these individual features overlap and there is often no clear boundary between them. When engaging in communication we are, in fact, likely to be utilizing a range of verbal and nonverbal skills simultaneously, in an attempt to ensure that our message is transmitted clearly and the risk of misunderstanding by the receiver is minimized.

Despite that, when carrying out our professional duties as nurses, we are often likely to be communicating with people who, for a variety of reasons, may not be able to interact or communicate with us in the way that we would hope or expect. For example, we may be talking to patients who are anxious, frightened, or in pain, younger children who are still developing language skills, or patients with sensory or cognitive impairment, mental health problems, or learning disabilities. Developing a deeper understanding of all aspects of communication, therefore, not only enables us to perform more effectively as transmitters of information, but it may also provide us with a clearer insight into the underlying meaning of other people's messages when we are trying to receive and interpret these. In addition it provides us with the ability to recognize potential barriers to all routes within the communication process.

4.2 **Listening and observation skills**

Definition

Two key components of good communication are active listening and observation. These skills provide nurses with valuable additional information, which can enhance their understanding and interpretation of specific circumstances.

Listening involves more than simply hearing what is being said. It is also important for nurses to be aware of other clues, verbal or nonverbal, that help provide a more accurate assessment of what someone is consciously or inadvertently communicating. As well as hearing, we need to observe the people we are communicating with to increase the likelihood that we will incorporate into our assessment all of the available signals and messages being sent.

When to use active listening and observation

Active listening and observing are skills that should be used continually as they can enable the identification of more overt or subtle cues to someone's emotions and state of mind – information that can be very helpful when trying to develop a **therapeutic** relationship. Whether specifically engaged in an activity with an individual or discreetly observing someone, maintaining and utilizing these skills can provide invaluable information to update your ongoing assessment and influence your decisions of how best to respond or act in your professional capacity.

Developing your skills

It is very important to understand the role of listening and observing during the communication process. As previously stated, the feedback provided from such interaction is crucial in the accurate interpretation of other people's underlying state of mind and emotions and in influencing your decisions on how best to proceed (Stickley and Freshwater 2006).

Try to be aware of how well you listen and observe what is happening when you are next engaged with patients or colleagues. How do you feel during silences? Are you uncomfortable? Are you easily distracted or do you find your mind wandering? Do you feel a desire or need to say something? What factors might influence this? For example, how well you know the other person, how capable you feel in the situation, whether you feel 'put on the spot' or out of your depth? Find time to reflect on your interactions with others with an appropriately experienced colleague.

Other factors to consider
Empathic linkages

The skills required to be an effective communicator include being able to use silence appropriately and you should not always feel that someone needs to be talking. Silence not only provides an opportunity for participants to reflect on what has been said and to plan how they want to develop discussion, but it can also provide the chance for people to create **empathic** linkages, which are the direct connection of feelings (Sully and Dallas 2005). Such connections can occur in circumstances when it may be difficult to know exactly the right words to say, for example, following bereavement. Simply by being with someone as a fellow human being, a nurse can provide feelings of support and sharing in their sorrow, which do not require any other form of communication to be expressed.

Empathy describes the ability to try to understand how someone feels in their given situation and circumstances, and the ability to convey that understanding to them. As such feelings are a result of a variety of factors that are unique to each individual, it is unlikely that we can know exactly how a person feels. But by trying to comprehend their emotions and points of view through active listening

Active listening and observation skills

Communication approach   Rationale

Communication approach	Rationale
Give undivided attention	Lets the individual know that you are paying attention and listening; that you value what is being said.
Do not interrupt	Breaking a person's flow can result in them losing their train of thought or confidence in what they are saying.
Remember what has been said	Accurate recollection conveys interest, allows for more accurate understanding, and enables the meaning of the sender to be checked.
Be aware of nonverbal cues	Listen to the 'baseline'; don't just focus on the words being said; think about what information is being sent through nonverbal communication channels.
Listen to yourself	As you listen, be aware of your own thoughts, which will be providing you with feedback on the interaction.
	Be wary of making assumptions, however, and ensure that any conclusions are based on what you have interpreted from your observations, not on supposition.
Use pauses and silence	Don't feel the need always to fill silences, sometimes people are using them to consider their next sentence or to reflect on how the interaction is progressing.
Try to be relaxed, comfortable, and calm	By conveying this approach, individuals may mirror it and feel more connected, becoming more relaxed and able to communicate.

and observation, we can gain a closer understanding of these and adapt our own contribution to the communication process to optimize the likelihood of success.

Barriers to listening and observing

How we communicate and what we say are external indicators of our internal thoughts and feelings. Being consciously aware of our thoughts and feelings during interactions, and having the ability to utilize this to enhance the situation, is indicative of a more expert practitioner who is able to reflect in practice. Don't be anxious, however, if you find that you are only able to reflect on your thoughts and feelings after events have occurred. You are

likely to develop your insight and awareness as you gain more practical experience of communicating in your professional role as a nurse. Although it is important to be aware of your own thoughts and feelings, take care to avoid becoming over-conscious of these, as this can lead to you becoming distracted, and can result in vital information being missed.

Other potential barriers to listening and observing include being preoccupied with one aspect of an individual's situation, thereby excluding others. In addition, **objective** interactions, care planning, and care delivery can all be hampered by feelings of disgust or dislike towards a patient, or by being **sympathetic** rather than empathic. These are all approaches which are likely to obstruct objectivity, and put our own needs in relation to the interaction before those of the patient.

Another barrier is in making assumptions about the individual and what they are trying to communicate. It is sometimes tempting to think that we have accurately assessed a patient based on the initial information communicated to us and, therefore, we fail to take the time to seek deeper understanding of the facts or clarification of our theories. There is a serious risk in arriving rashly at conclusions, and it is essential that patients are afforded the time to express themselves fully through verbal and nonverbal means.

Nurses should continually be assessing the patients' ability to communicate and take account of any potential barriers that may exist. There may be occasions when patients might be unable to express themselves as they would wish, which could be due to a range of reasons including physical illness, learning disability, mental ill health, or sensory impairment. In such instances, we need to be aware of possible alternative support available. This may be from a family member or specialist services for people with a particular condition. Some of these sources are discussed later in this chapter.

4.3 **Engaging skills**

Definition

To communicate effectively with other people, it is important to be able to engage with them. In these circumstances, engaging means stimulating an individual's interest and starting to communicate with them. Failure to make such a connection is likely to result in limited interaction of dubious quality with an individual who neither wants to participate in the process, nor wants you to do so.

Connecting with a fellow human being involves many of the skills you are likely to have developed throughout your life, and which you employ in your life on a daily basis. For example, adopting a closed or open posture (see **Fig. 4.6**) can send a message of how receptive you are to communicating at that time.

When to use engaging skills

While the skills that we have learned throughout our lives in relation to engaging with others may have some

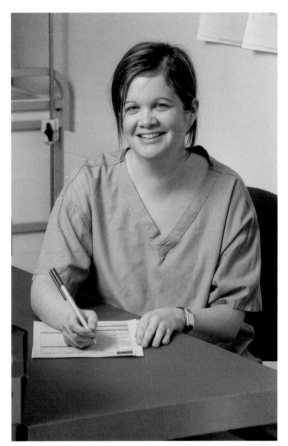

(a)

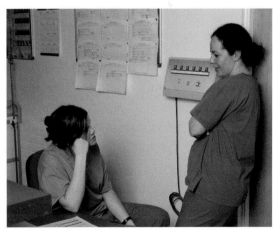

(b)

Figure 4.6 Open and closed body language. (a) Appearing approachable: looking up to make eye contact and smiling, despite being busy, (b) Appearing unapproachable: folding arms, turning away from patients, and focusing on a conversation with a colleague may discourage a patient or relative from asking a question.

Engaging skills

Communication approach	Rationale
Initial contact: be polite, open, clear, and professional.	Presenting a positive, competent, open, and approachable persona creates a good first impression and is known to enhance people's perceptions of quality of care.
Consider the nature of the topic being discussed.	Someone who has received upsetting news may require additional support and understanding.
	Someone who is trying to come to terms with life-changing news may be unlikely to be able to concentrate and participate in interaction as usual.
Use verbal and nonverbal communication skills effectively.	Enables the transmitter to address the purpose of the interaction most effectively and efficiently.
Ensure that your verbal and nonverbal communication are congruent with each other and the nature of the discussion.	This can demonstrate caring, sensitivity, and understanding. It would, for example, be inappropriate to discuss intimate, potentially embarrassing, or upsetting topics with a big smile and a jocular tone to your voice.
Discuss less threatening or distressing topics before gently introducing more challenging subjects.	This can make it easier for people to engage.
Continually assess the individual and adapt your communication style and the content of your discussion appropriately.	To meet their specific needs at a pace that is more suitable for each individual.
Provide information.	Can reduce feelings of anxiety and help anticipate areas of concern or potential problems.
	Do not overload with too much information, however, as this can prevent you from engaging effectively.
Provide support.	Demonstrates interest and empathy; this can reduce feelings of helplessness and confusion in the receiver.
	Be wary of offering false hope and do not commit to support that it is beyond your ability to provide.
Reflect content.	Demonstrates that attention is being paid to the receivers' perspective and offers the opportunity to check that this is being understood.
Reflect feeling.	Displays empathy and understanding.
Paraphrase.	Enables demonstration of understanding by repeating ideas using different words and phrases.

Use silence effectively.	Allows participants time to reflect on what has been said, how they are thinking and feeling, and how they might wish to proceed.
Be alert to excessive periods of silence and intervene either through verbal or nonverbal means, for example, touch, gesture, or eye contact.	To help avoid feelings of discomfort in the receiver.
Individualize input according to need, for example, age, sex, culture.	Shows that receiver's individuality is being acknowledged and respected.
	Enables communication to be tailored to suit the specific needs of individuals.
Assess abilities and needs on an individual basis.	While recognizing that certain groups of people may share similar skills and needs, individualizing the approach to communication chosen prevents stereotyping and over-generalizing.
Seek clarification and check perceptions.	Avoids the risk of making assumptions about messages being transferred and exchanged.
Summarize discussion.	Allows all parties to ensure meaning and understanding is shared by all.

relevance to what we do as nurses, it is important to remember that in this chapter we are considering our engaging with others from a professional perspective. When thinking about this facet of communication, remember to consider the different inpatient or community settings where nurses might try to engage with others, and the possible ways that these may influence this important aspect of the communication process.

As nurses, we are often trying to connect with individuals and build a rapport with them when they are in pain, distressed, or anxious. This can be very challenging, for example, some people, in particular younger people, may regress and display more childlike behaviour when they feel anxious, threatened, or confused. Developing your skills in this area will undoubtedly enhance your effectiveness as a nurse. The table highlights the skills that are necessary to engage with patients and build a rapport with them. This should help lead you to the development and maintenance of therapeutic relationships.

Developing your skills

Despite our best efforts, it may not always be possible to engage with others. However, by careful planning and continually assessing our interactions we can maximize the opportunity of success. To assist with this, nurses must balance an awareness of the possible needs of particular patient groups with the necessity to relate to everyone as an individual.

Other factors to consider

The following additional considerations suggest some common considerations regarding specific groups of people, which should be applied in appropriate situations in addition to those in the table on engaging skills. Nursing care for these groups is delivered in all care settings and individuals may be encountered wherever nurses practice. The information is generalized, so please remember that it will not apply to everyone within the identified groups. There are always likely to be individuals who do not conform to usual profiles associated with people within such groups. Once again it is each nurse's responsibility to ensure that everyone is assessed as an individual and avoid stereotypical thinking.

Older adults

Most older people are not confused and do not have **dementia**. Ensure that you treat individual older people with dignity and respect, and avoid talking to them in a patronizing or childlike way.

Remember that some terminology that is familiar to you may not be known by some older people. Terms that may be in common usage now may even appear overly familiar or disrespectful to some people from a different generation.

Be aware of possible physical or sensory health issues associated with ageing, which may affect communication, for example, difficulty hearing, poor eyesight.

When communicating with a confused person take additional time to talk and allow time for a reply. Try to recognize signs of apprehension or distress early to enable you to offer appropriate reassurance and support. Try to simplify your messages as this will improve the likelihood of being understood, but remember that you are not talking to a child and be wary of becoming patronizing. Do not use multiple questions, for example, 'Would you like a cup of tea? What do you take in it? Sugar and milk?' Instead, ask questions one at a time as this may be easier for the person to process and understand. If the individual has language difficulties, use gestures or objects to help convey meaning, for example, show someone a cup while asking if they would like some tea.

Begin by discuss nonthreatening topics with which the person is more familiar, as this can help build rapport and is less likely to **provoke** anxiety. It may then be easier to introduce gradually subjects that they find more challenging. You must not raise your voice, as this is disrespectful and is only likely to make an individual agitated, distressed, or frightened.

Young people and children

When communicating with children and adolescents, their developmental stage, chronological age, and level of cognitive development must influence your practice. It is important to communicate with young people at an appropriate level because if they are presented with information

they do not understand they may misinterpret, take things out of context, or simply feel worse because they are overwhelmed. Similarly, where young people feel that the communication style is too young for them, they may feel patronized and are unlikely to engage with you.

Communication in early childhood

Young children are fairly egocentric and it is hard for them to see things from someone else's point of view. They have a polarized view of themselves and the world, for example believing there are good and bad people in the world ('black and white thinking') and that if something happens it is irreversible. Young children find abstract concepts difficult to understand and need concrete examples to make sense of things. It is also difficult for them to retell a story coherently or elaborate on statements. As a consequence of this, the use of nonverbal techniques to engage young children is particularly useful, for example through play or drawing.

It is important to use simple language, short questions, and concrete examples of things from their own life experiences.

Communication in middle childhood

Between the ages of eight and eleven years, children are much more able to think about issues from another's point of view, for example, 'Kate thinks; John thinks.' They are much more able to give detailed cohesive accounts of things that have happened to them, although they still benefit from concrete examples. They have greater problem-solving skills and are able to self-regulate their emotions and behaviour. However, their thinking and behaviour is very much 'rule governed'. Verbal techniques are much more useful with this age group although it can help to give them the beginnings of sentences and allow them to complete them, for example, 'I feel sad when...,' 'I feel safe when...' Children of this age can also enjoy role play if they are given a concrete part to act out with clear instructions. At this age, children learn a lot through repetition.

Communication in adolescence

Between the ages of twelve and seventeen, young people are much more able to engage in abstract reasoning and can imagine and discuss what has never been encountered before. They are better able to solve problems and to explore possible ideas rather than thinking in 'black and white' terms. In adolescence, identity development is primary and family relationships become less primary than peer relationships.

When communicating with an adolescent, it is important to be respectful of their skills and their perceived adult status. They are much more able to reflect on their own beliefs and attitudes, although these may change over time. Adolescent communication style is often quite introspective; adolescents may appear egocentric, such is their preoccupation with their inner world. They may analyse the fine detail of social interactions.

General strategies for engaging with young people

Use closed questions to start young people talking and ask about less threatening topics initially, for example, friends or relationships. Try to give them something to do if they find it hard to talk, for example, draw a family tree. Offer to meet them without their family if they wish. Ask them to help you out. Ask others to tell their story, and then ask if they agree. Give lots of compliments for what they manage to do.

Younger children – and even some older ones – may respond to the use of, for example, puppets or telephones to say what they want, without speaking to you directly. The use of play is a topic within itself, but toys and other 'play equipment' should be freely available, in case the young person wants to 'act out' the communication. There are issues regarding **consent** and confidentiality when working with children therapeutically. Guidance and adherence to national and local policy should always be sought.

People with a learning disability

Communication problems in people with a learning disability can affect their comprehension and the way in which they express themselves. An individual's understanding and ability in self-expression can also be affected by many factors, including visual or hearing difficulties, attention, listening skills, concentration, confidence, and an inability to deal with new people or situations or anxiety levels. However, it is worth noting that where an individual has a dual diagnosis of a learning disability and mental ill health,

communication may also be affected by the individual's particular psychiatric condition.

People with a learning disability often experience difficulty in describing **subjective** feelings and internal emotional states. This can make it more difficult to detect mood changes or specific mental health symptoms, such as depressive ideas, in someone with limited expressive language skills. This can often lead to reliance on third-party accounts of behavioural signs, which can ignore the most vital source of information: the individual. The basic principles involved in communication with a person with a learning disability are the same as you would use for any client.

All of these factors can make it difficult for people to clearly understand what is expected of them. An individual may also require speech to be augmented by gestures, signs, pictures, or symbols, to aid comprehension. Many individuals who have a learning disability have limited or restricted literacy skills. In some cases they do not understand written information.

Specific issues, such as suggestibility, acquiescence, and confabulation can make communicating with an individual and interpreting a response more difficult. Suggestibility means giving in to leading questions and changing one's initial answer in response to negative feedback. Acquiescence is the tendency of an individual to answer 'yes' to a question regardless of the question's content. Confabulation is defined as problems in memory processing where people replace gaps in their memory with imaginary experiences that they believe to be true.

You can help minimize the influence of these factors by putting the person at ease. Keep your approach relaxed, informal, and conversational as far as possible. Start with easy questions to increase confidence of the respondent. Explain what the purpose of the conversation is and what questions will be asked. State who and what the information is for, why this is important, and, perhaps, how long the conversation will take. Use 'anchor events' as people with learning disabilities often have difficulties relating to time, number, and frequency. Therefore, you can ask the person to focus on events that have occurred in the past; for example, birthday, day out, Christmas.

Summarize the discussion. Attention and memory difficulties can make it important to recap and summarize what the person has said. This will allow you to check whether the conversation has been understood.

Be creative: use drawings or photographs. Find out from others who know the person well how you might best access their views. Bear in mind that communication is influenced by experience, environment, and cognitive ability. The principles involved in engaging people with a learning disability are *not* fundamentally different from those you would use when engaging with any other client.

People with a mental health problem

As individuals, there are aspects of our mental health that help us cope with our life circumstances, or undermine our ability to function as we would like. People with mental health problems are people like everyone else. Therefore, the general skills and approaches that we utilize to engage with someone with a mental health problem are very similar to those we would usually employ when trying to engage with anyone in our professional practice.

Mental illness can affect individuals in different ways. You must be careful not to stereotype a person, or how you expect them to behave, based solely on a confirmed or suspected diagnosis. Take the time to explore, with the individual if possible, how their mental health affects their life and acknowledge the strengths displayed by each person that help them to cope, not just the difficulties that they are experiencing.

It is impractical to list in this section all of the possible factors relating to mental health that you are likely to encounter or should consider. Rather, this section highlights some general perspectives of which you should be aware.

Anxiety

Anxiety can cause people to be preoccupied, unable to retain information, or feel panicky or overwhelmed. For some people, this can result in childlike behaviour. It is important that you maintain and project an air of calmness and control, remembering to speak in an even, calm voice while making use of eye contact and appropriate touch to give reassurance. You should be careful to ensure that the reassurance that you offer is realistic, for example, that you are there to help, not that you will be able to solve all of the individual's problems. Gently encourage the individual to try to gain awareness and control of their breathing, as this tends to become accelerated and shallow when someone is anxious. For example, encourage 'full cycle breathing', as described in **Box 4.1**.

Depression

People who are depressed or feel low in their mood are likely to be less communicative and may appear 'fed up' or uninterested. They are likely to have a bleak outlook of their situation and the future. It may appear that they do not want to engage with you. You should try to strike a balance between continuing to let the individual know that you are available to help, and becoming intrusive or overbearing. Communicating for shorter periods, but more often, may minimize the risk of them feeling overwhelmed. Depression can cause a slowing of thought processes, so it is important to allow such patients the time to formulate a response. By using silence and simply being with someone, you can demonstrate a caring attitude that may still promote a therapeutic relationship without having to engage in conversation. With time, this therapeutic relationship enables you to address the issues that are important to the individual person.

Box 4.1 Full cycle breathing

This exercise involves encouraging someone to take deep breaths to help reduce their level of anxiety.

1 Close your eyes and take a slow, steady breath in through your nose, letting your stomach extend.

2 As you do so count slowly in your head: 1…2… 3…4…5.

3 Now hold that breath for the same slow count: 1…2…3…4…5.

4 Now purse your lips and breathe out through your mouth slowly and in a controlled way, counting slowly: 1…2…3…4…5 and allowing your shoulders to drop.

5 Now do nothing for one second before repeating the exercise.

6 Do not repeat the exercise more than three times without breathing normally for at least a few minutes in between.

Psychosis

Patients with psychotic symptoms, for example, delusional thinking or **hallucinations**, may have a completely different view of reality from your perception of it. They may feel anxious, frightened, threatened, confused, angry, or suspicious. Be aware of any increased potential of risk to the patient, yourself, or others. Observe for any overt or subtle evidence that may suggest these and report them immediately to a more experienced colleague.

There is nothing to be gained in simply arguing with someone who holds a false, unshakeable belief. In fact, this is more likely to enflame a situation. You must continue to treat such individuals with respect and dignity. You should acknowledge the individual's view, which, although not the same as your own, and at times seemingly bizarre, will be as real to that individual as your own. Try not to reinforce such views but accept that they are those held by the individual and that the emotions associated with them are likely to be very real for that person. You can, therefore, work together towards finding a solution for these. It may help to tell them that while you may not share their interpretation of their circumstances, you are trying to understand how they feel in order to support them toward a solution. Remember that their feelings of distress, fear, anger, and so on, are very real.

Cognitive impairment

Patients may experience cognitive impairment for a variety of reasons, such as dementia, trauma, or infection, and this may result in them experiencing difficulty in understanding what is being said to them and expressing themselves clearly to others. Such patients may be disorientated to time, place or even who they, and those about them, are. This can be disconcerting, upsetting, and frightening. Review the section on older adults for advice on how to engage with such individuals.

People with sensory impairment or an inability to speak

People who are deaf, blind, deaf-blind, or unable to talk may view themselves as members of specific communities of people in similar circumstances. Some individuals may find it more difficult to engage with those outside of these communities. Take extra time to consider the individual needs of such patients and explore individual solutions to their needs and gain their consent before implementing any of the following suggestions.

Be aware of the potential for additional levels of consternation, anxiety, or distress. Often, the way deaf people communicate can appear aggressive to hearing people—they may use touch, make loud sounds, or use exaggerated gestures. You need to accept this as part of a style of communication. But remember not to stereotype individuals.

With the individual's consent, make use of specialist organizations and support services who may be able to compensate for some communication difficulties. Again with the individual's consent, perhaps a member of their family or circle of friends could assist. Be very aware of sensitive or confidential information about the patient or their care that the person may not want others to know.

Lip reading may help in some situations, but remember that some forms of communication for deaf or deaf-blind people, for example, sign language, **Makaton**, or hands-on signing, may not follow the same grammatical structures as spoken language. For deaf and deaf-blind people the use of interpreters can help, but requires additional consideration, for example, availability when most needed, trying to establish a rapport in a short time.

Patients who don't have English as a first language

Allow sufficient time to convey your message and for the person to reply. People may understand some words that you say: do not make assumptions about individuals and be careful not to be patronizing. Using written material with pictures or common phrases written in English and the individual's own language can enable two-way communication.

Nonverbal cues and some gestures may have different meanings in different cultures. Be sensitive and considerate to this and take care not to make assumptions about the way that people may communicate or act. Enquire about and respect views on matters specific to the individual's spiritual or cultural beliefs, for example, prayer times, or dietary issues.

While family members may offer to translate, remember issues of confidentiality or personal topics, which the person may not want to share. Also, consider how you can ensure that any translation is truly expressing the views of the individual and not the opinion of the family member, which may significantly differ from the patient's. There are translating services available, but there may be a cost involved in their use and they are likely to be able to offer only limited amounts of time. This makes it difficult for the individual to build rapport with the translator, and time should be planned carefully to maximize the benefit of their contribution.

Educating yourself about the cultural and spiritual needs of those in your care can enhance your understanding of how best to engage with people. Remember, though, that each person's individual views and how they choose to practice their religion, or how they regard their position within their culture, is likely to vary, and you should endeavour to identify such individual views.

Unconscious patients

Bear in mind that although unresponsive, a person may be able to hear, understand, and recall what is being said around them. You should avoid holding conversations with colleagues that ignore the unconscious person or are carried out as if they are not there. You must continue to offer reassurance to the individual while treating them with respect and dignity at all times. You should continue to inform an unconscious person of the care that you are planning and providing for them, recognizing that they may be able to comprehend what you are saying and doing, and recall this at a later date. The appropriate use of touch can be employed as another mode of communication to try to connect with an unconscious patient.

Relatives of patients

Use your knowledge and understanding of communication to try to assess the underlying thoughts and feelings of family members, for example, do they appear eager to help, anxious, frustrated, or frightened? At sensitive times, people will have mixed ability to take on information. They may fixate on one or two things and forget everything else. You need to select your words carefully and check understanding. Be sensitive to individual family's and family members' interpretation of the circumstances and offer support, education, and guidance as required.

Be aware that they may feel excluded or helpless in relation to the care and decisions being made about their loved one. To minimize the effects of this, you should frequently offer them updated information and seek and record their views and opinions. As with individuals, families behave in ways that may be particular to them. Behaviour that may seem unusual or strange to one person may be considered the norm by someone else. If you are concerned by any of your observations or assessment, seek advice from a more experienced member of staff. If the patient wants their family to be involved in their care, offer the family the opportunity to participate in caring and support that is appropriate to their understanding of the circumstances and their levels of skill and knowledge.

While including the views of family members can often be helpful in completing a **holistic** assessment, you must still respect your patient's right to confidentiality and remember not to divulge information to family members inappropriately, especially information that you have been specifically asked not to share with them.

Remember that family relationships may not be what they seem. There may be underlying tensions and emotions. The way that families interact in the company of others may be very different from interactions when on their own. Bear in mind that if someone divulges information that you consider indicates that they present a danger to themselves or others, then you must report this to a more senior member of staff.

Giving difficult or bad news

Sensitivity to the nature of the information being discussed can improve your awareness of an individual's feelings and behaviour. Consider the venue carefully, choosing somewhere that will allow privacy and the freedom to express deep emotions (see **Fig. 4.7**).

Be very sensitive to the potential impact of the information on the individual and try to convey that you are there to support them and that they are in an environment where it is safe to express their feelings. Be aware of the fact that individuals will react in ways that are specific to them and may not respond as you expect.

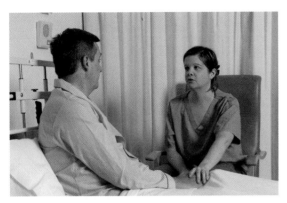

Figure 4.7 Giving bad news: ensure privacy, be at the same level as the patient, adopt an open posture, make direct eye contact and, if appropiate, use touch

Ongoing assessment of how the individual is responding is vital in enabling accurate adjustment of your input regarding the pace, content, and delivery of the news. Remember the importance of congruence between your verbal and nonverbal cues and the nature of the news being given.

Ensure that you have time available to spend with the person once the news has been given. This will allow them the chance to express themselves, seek clarification, and discuss how they might proceed. Be prepared to provide appropriate support, perhaps having a colleague available to assist you with this. Involvement in exchanges like this can be very challenging and demanding on you too, so make time to debrief and receive support from more experienced colleagues.

Communication in conflict

This subject is discussed in Section 2.3.

4.4 **Interviews and questioning**

Definition

Hargie and Dickson (2004) suggest that questioning is one of the most widely used approaches in any interaction. Whether in a formal interview or a more informal setting, it is certainly utilized in most activities where nurses try to engage with patients. These can occur as the result of a

spontaneous opportunity or as part of a planned and organized interaction.

Interviews tend to have a specific purpose and structure, sometimes incorporating the use of questionnaires or validated assessment tools. As well as providing information and support for patients, interviews can also provide nurses with detailed information to help develop and direct patient care planning, as well as evaluating the effectiveness of service delivery.

Background

This section explores the skills involved in questioning and interviewing as a planned interaction, rather than as a spontaneous one.

From the initial assessment, to the preparation for discharge, interviews provide opportunities to gather relevant information through communicating with patients. As has previously been stated, communication can happen at any time or place within the nurse's working environment, and nurses should take advantage of such opportunities as long as it is reasonable to do so, for example, considering issues of confidentiality and time available.

It would be inappropriate, for instance, to inform a patient that they are due to have a medical procedure and then, when they ask for details of what that will entail and when it is likely to happen, tell them that you have no time to answer as you have to go to a case conference. This is likely to result in the patient being left feeling anxious, frustrated, angry, or upset from the lack of knowledge and understanding of what is to happen. Such exchanges are better given when there is an opportunity for the patient to discuss their thoughts and feelings with you or another appropriate member of staff.

Preparation

Environmental factors are more easily managed when interviews occur within our own clinical areas. As care delivery is increasingly carried out in patients' homes, however, you may find that you are less able to arrange the environment in the way that you think best suits the purpose of the interview or interaction. This should not mean that you cannot still effectively engage in communication, but rather that you may need to adapt how you approach the situation, and the emphasis that you give to other aspects of the communication process.

It may be possible to make slight adjustments to your positioning or the furniture arrangements to enhance the room layout, but you must always seek permission from the home owner in a polite and professional manner before attempting this. Appropriate care should be taken with other people's possessions, you should not try to move heavy items of furniture and any changes that are made should be put back when the interview is complete.

Any difficulties regarding interruptions should be addressed in the same way as in any other setting, by politely requesting that other people in the house afford you some privacy, and perhaps answer any telephone calls during the interview. When planning to interview someone in their own home you should make clear arrangements, checking the dates and times carefully. On the day, make every effort to arrive on time and, should you be late for any reason, it is polite to call the person to inform them of this, apologizing, and making alternative arrangements if necessary.

Questions can be asked for a variety of reasons, including obtaining information, seeking clarification, expressing an interest, assessing another's understanding, and encouraging participation. The function of the question is influenced in part by the type of question asked and these are divided into closed and open questions. Examples of these are given in **Box 4.2**.

Closed questions tend to have a correct answer and come in the form of those with yes or no answers, those which offer a limited response, such as, 'Would you like a biscuit or a cake?' and those which seek a definite answer, for example, 'Where do you live?' Closed questions are useful for gathering specific information. As they are generally simpler to answer they can be used to initiate communication and encourage participation before advancing to open questions.

As the name suggests the answers to open questions are left open to the respondent and there are usually a variety of possible ways that can be chosen to respond. They, therefore, require more than a one-word answer. Examples are 'What do you like to do in your spare time?' or 'What has been happening since we last met?' Beginning with an open question enables the respondent more freedom in the answer, from which the nurse can then begin to seek more detailed replies using more closed questions.

Box 4.2 Closed and open questions	
Closed questions	**Open questions**
Do you like coffee?	What do you like about the taste of coffee?
Have you ever been to Greece?	What are your experiences of holidays overseas?
Is it still sunny outside?	Can you describe the weather to me please?
Have you seen your doctor today?	What did you discuss with your doctor at the review today?
Should smoking be banned in public places?	What do you think the key issues are relating to the banning of smoking in public places?
Do you have a job?	Can you tell me what your job is and detail your main duties please?

Developing your skills

Questioning requires understanding and communication skills, so as to be effective and not to appear interrogative or distressing for the patient. When considering what to ask in an interview, think about the purpose of what your question is. Are you seeking clarification, for example, 'When you say you feel depressed what does that mean for you?' or looking for an example; 'Can you tell me what happens to make you feel this way?' or encouraging the respondent to expand on their statement; 'Can you tell me some more about what happened?' Understanding the objective of the questioning enables you to utilize different types of question, to suit both the individual and the circumstances of the interview.

Other factors to consider

While reading the content of the procedure for interviewing and questioning, bear in mind the information and skills discussed earlier in this chapter. The table outlines key aspects in these areas and should be considered in relation to before, during and after the interview. As you read it, take time to think about how your communication

Interviews and questioning

Communication approach | Rationale

Environment

Communication approach	Rationale
Identify participants and purpose of the interview.	Ensures all relevant participants are ascertained and can be invited to attend.
	Provides clear understanding of the aim of the interview.
	Helps inform decisions regarding venue, resources required and approach to be used.
Identify and reserve available space.	Allows privacy and freedom from distraction and interruption.
Choose a nonthreatening venue, for example, the patient might find your office intimidating.	Indicates that the interaction is important and valued, warranting time and consideration.
	Informs colleagues of your whereabouts in case of emergency.
Room layout: consider the furniture, distance, lighting, temperature.	Comfortable surroundings may encourage participation.
	Layout can demonstrate status within the interaction, for example, higher seating suggests higher status, level seating is more equal. Remember the differences when interviewing someone in their own home.
They layout will be influenced by the approach chosen.	Can suggest more formal or informal intentions.
At the time of the interview, put a sign on the door that a meeting is in progress.	Indicates that the room is in use, ensures privacy, and avoids interruptions.
Consider risk factors, exit route, and alarm systems in use.	Awareness of any potential risk can ensure that these are minimized, for example, do not interview patients with a history of violence on your own.
Always position yourself between an exit and the person being interviewed to allow safe and rapid exit if necessary. Be mindful of any obstacles or trip hazards.	Even someone with no history of aggression can become violent, so observe for warning signs of all risks during any interactions.
	This is equally important when in someone's home. If entering a home for the first time, make sure that you do not increase the level of risk.
	Knowing where alarm points are situated and how they are activated allows for more rapid response from colleagues if required.

continued

Invitation and notice

Provide relevant parties with sufficient prior notice of their invitation.	Enables participants to check whether they are available.
	Allows preparation of information they may wish to bring to the interview, or questions they would like to ask.
Provide sufficient detail of the purpose of the interview.	Assists attendees with preparation.
	May help alleviate any anxiety or uncertainty about the purpose of the interview.

Choice of approach

Prepare yourself.	Allows identification of personal views on the purpose of the interview and any aspects that may raise strong opinions or feelings.
	The structure of the interview can then be decided, based on individual circumstances and needs.
Formal: structured; planned in advance.	Helps keep to the focus of the interview and can reduce bias if specific interview questionnaires are used.
Informal: no structure, more spontaneous.	May feel less interrogative, therefore, more relaxed and conversational.
Broad or funnel approach: initially takes a broad view then identifies the details of the individual's experience.	Allows the patient to introduce topics, for example, 'Where would you like to start?' or 'Is there something you'd like to discuss today?
Narrow or inverted funnel approach: initially asks about specific details, then broadens.	Begins by discussing specific experiences before expanding to look at the wider influences of these for the individual, for example, 'You said that you feel tired all of the time and have no energy; how does that affect your day to day life?'

Questions

Closed: seeking specific, short answers.	Answer required is limited and tends to be more focused.
	May help encourage responses initially.
	Provide a stepping stone for more open questions.
Open: question can be answered in many different ways.	Give more freedom to the respondent regarding answers.
	Encourage conversation and more detailed expression of the respondent's thoughts.
	Allow a broad approach, and then focus on specific areas within responses.

Verbal and nonverbal cues

As discussed previously in this chapter – includes reflecting content, reflecting feelings, providing information, seeking clarification, paraphrasing and checking perceptions.

Utilizing verbal and nonverbal cues enhances the role of the nurse as transmitter and receiver of information within interviewing and questioning.

Encourages and supports other attendees to participate to the best of their abilities.

Ensures clarity and understanding by all participants.

Listening and observing

As discussed previously in this chapter – includes using silence.

Employing active listening and observing skills enables the nurse to participate most effectively in interviewing and questioning.

Enables more accurate interpretation of other's contributions.

Terminating the interview

Clarification and summarizing.

Seeks to ensure that the interview has met the needs of all attendees.

Ensures all participants' understanding of the discussion.

Draws together all that has been said.

Links themes and topics in a succinct way.

Reduces the risk of misunderstanding.

Provide a clear indication of what will happen as a result of the interview.

Enables attendees to understand how information from the interview will be used to develop further discussion or care.

Recording the interview

Records should be kept as discussed in the written communication section of this chapter.

Records information vital to the planning, delivery, and evaluation of effective care.

Provides the necessary documentation to allow appropriate sharing of information.

Meets local, professional, and legal requirements.

---

skills might affect an interview. Think about potential barriers, including physical ones like desks, height, orientation to each other, and also psychological barriers, for instance, power within the relationship, knowledge, and familiarity between participants. Think about the types of environments that you as a nurse may find yourself delivering care in.

4.5 **Written communication**

Definition

Written documentation varies greatly between areas, so you should ensure that you make yourself familiar with the particular nursing paperwork used in any area in which you are working. The Nursing and Midwifery Council (NMC 2007) have produced an advice sheet on record keeping and you should also familiarize yourself with the content of this.

Written communication occurs in a variety of forms and has changed significantly with the development of electronic forms of sending messages (Cleary and Freeman 2005). Traditionally, letter writing consisted of two forms, business and personal, and there were specific rules regarding how these should be constructed and the language that was considered appropriate for each. Electronic communication, in the form of emails, chat rooms or texting now affords the sender a much greater choice of font styles, sizes and instantly accessible images to enhance, reinforce or reiterate the meaning of the words that they choose to use. While it is still not the norm for nurses to contact their patients by email or text messaging, these are increasingly becoming used in educational establishments as standard means of communication between academic staff and students. Having access to such a range of options does not mean that they can be used indiscriminately, however, and the generally accepted norms for letter writing should apply to electronic communication. So the style of an official email, for example, to a fellow professional or tutor, should reflect the more formal nature of such an exchange, and should not be written in the more casual form that you might use for a friend.

The term 'netiquette' is used to define the code of rules that apply to online communication and broadly refers to good behaviour while online. While there may be no official enforcement of these rules, there are still expected standards of behaviour when communicating electronically. As the number of users of these modes of communication increases, many people appear to be unfamiliar with netiquette or choose to ignore it. Nurses, however, need to demonstrate their awareness and skills when using electronic communication, by ensuring that they follow generally accepted guidelines, which reflect their professional behaviour.

Background

Bearing in mind that electronic communication is more likely between nurses and fellow professionals and, indeed, may rarely, if ever, be utilized with patients; it is,

nevertheless, a mode of communication employed by nurses in their professional role. It is, therefore, worthy of inclusion in this chapter, as there are aspects of this topic that are important to professional behaviour. Firstly, it is important to consider the intended receiver when deciding on the most appropriate mode of transmitting a message. For instance, the use of text messages and online sites may be very familiar – and the preferred choice of communicating for many of today's younger citizens – but they are likely to remain a source of frustration or mystery for many older members of the population. Be careful not to make assumptions about this, however, as there are increasing numbers of older people who are computer literate and may have become familiar with electronic communication systems through their working life or leisure activities. As with all aspects of nursing, be wary of stereotyping the people you must communicate with in any way. Instead look at each person as an individual and base your decisions about your interactions with them on their individual circumstances, preferences and needs. Remember, too, that although modes of communication are not governed by imposable, hard-and-fast rules, they are still subject to socially accepted patterns of behaviour, and people base at least part of their impressions of us on the way that we communicate.

Understanding the access that recipients may have to your written messages is vital to the successful transmission of communication. It is after all pointless sending an email to someone who has no Internet access or a letter to someone without a postal address. Written communication encompasses a variety of skills, not least influenced by the mode of communication chosen by or available to the sender.

Developing your skills

The more permanent nature of the written word provides nurses with a source of evidence to record the work that they do. Remember that such records are legal documents, whether on paper or electronic, and they are, therefore, admissible as evidence in legal proceedings. Even when deleted from personal sources, records are retained by service providers and these can be traced and made available for investigation by the authorities. The finality of this form of communication

Written communication skills

Mode of communication and key issues

Rationale

Mode of communication and key issues	Rationale
Nursing records Follow NMC Guidelines on record keeping; Become familiar with local paperwork; Writing must be in black ink and legible; Records should be succinct and to the point.	Patient care depends on accurate information being recorded relating to assessment, planning, implementation, and evaluation.
	Nursing records provide a legal record of nursing intervention.
	Records must be an accurate account of events to ensure that precise details are available to members of the inter-professional team.
	Enables meaning to be accurately interpreted.
	Do not assume that readers will understand the meaning of abbreviations or **colloquial** terms.
	Include all relevant information but avoid lengthy accounts with superfluous detail that does not add to the clinical picture.
	Remember that patients have access to their written records and the terminology used should always be professional.
Letter	Still a frequently used method of communication.
Format	Nowadays greater access to computers means that official letters should be word processed.
	Computer program offer advice and templates for the construction and layout of letters, but if unsure seek further guidance.
	Having letters proof-read by someone else helps identify any errors prior to them being sent out.
Time	Consider the time it will take for delivery; sometimes this may be extended by using internal mail systems.
	Is sufficient time allowed for any required response?
Electronic: email	Emails are becoming an increasingly used mode of communication in nursing, it is, therefore, important to understand how to access and send emails as they enable more rapid communication.

continued

Choose the format of emails and attachments.	Ensure attachments are in a form that can be read by the receiver's system.
Ensuring familiarity with local systems, traceability and copyright.	Appropriate training and guidance will promote efficiency and enable more effective working.
	Emails are legal documents and can be traced to the sender, even when apparently deleted from a personal computer or system.
	An awareness of local protocols and laws regarding copyright, file sharing, plagiarism, and confidentiality will reduce the risk of breaches and errors, for example, the contents of class handouts are the property of the issuing university and, therefore, should not be altered.
Ensure that you are identifiable, but be aware of risks.	Emails should inform your recipient of at least your name and your professional status; remember that sometimes your first name may not be enough to identify you. You may also include your contact details, student number, course details, or other information to identify who you are.
	Note: be aware of the potential risks, however, in inappropriately disclosing certain information, for example, your working hours, your address, or other personal details.
Consider the size and content of attached files, for example, images, emoticons. Inform the recipient first that you intend to send a large file.	Images and emoticons (character faces used to portray underlying emotions or tone, for example, ⊗) require greater amounts of memory. Large emails, of 5 megabytes or greater, use up the recipients electronic memory, filling their mailbox and preventing access to subsequent emails. Very large files may not be sent at all, especially with older systems.
	If you contact the recipient before sending a large file, they can quickly transfer the information to an alternative destination, leaving their mail system free to operate.
	Sending a link to a webpage, rather than the actual webpage itself, is one way to reduce the size of an email.
Tend to be less formal than letters.	Consider the recipient before choosing a formal or informal approach. Be aware that font size can alter meaning, for example, writing in CAPITALS is considered to be shouting.
Use of 'e-language' and images.	Avoid using abbreviated or amalgamated terms, for example, Gr8 for Great, B4 for before, these may not be known to your receiver, try to remain professional in the choice of language.

Avoid initiating or responding to flaming.	Be wary of using images or icons that denote emotion, for example, ☺ as these may suggest a more flippant or informal tone to your email, or may be misinterpreted by the receiver.
	Flaming is the term used for a personal attack via an email or a posted message.
	You should keep communication focused on the issues being discussed and not the personal qualities of those involved.
Refrain from adding kisses at the end of messages sent in your professional capacity.	Using upper or lower case, and the number of kisses used, can signify the level of friendship or affection towards the recipient.
	Kisses can be added as habit, but it is inappropriate for official communications (this has happened).
Electronic: clinical systems **When using a clinical information system, ensure that you log on personally to access or enter data and log off when finished.**	By law, you are limited to what you can access as a student and your use of a hospital system is monitored and audited. If you fail to log off, or if you access or enter data while another person is logged into the system, this breaks the audit trail and is illegal. Your password for logging on and off is secret and unique to you as an individual: you are accountable for its protection. Never share passwords or use the password of another person, this too is illegal.
Communication in clinical systems is highly structured and limits the freedom of the clinicians to express themselves.	Data needs to be in a form that is understandable not just to yourself, but to others reading the record who have little knowledge of the context. Thus, nursing interventions and nursing outcomes may use a specific terminology. Assessment tools may be limited to those approved and coded within the system. Behind the scenes of these information systems, are data dictionaries of standardized terms and concepts that allow healthcare practices in one institution to be aggregated and made available to governments to help decide policy, and to researchers and clinicians wanting to research the effectiveness of nursing practice. The use of a common 'language' is vital to this. Nurses, therefore, need to adhere to commonly agreed standards of communication, implicit within these systems.

continued

Electronic: texting	Tends to be used for more personal communication. While texting does not, at present, tend to be used by nurses to communicate with patients, this method of communication is increasingly being used by some academic organizations, as it is the mode most frequently accessed by many of their students.
Professional approach	As above with emails. It is considered impolite to text while conversing with or interviewing someone else (this has also happened). It is polite to ask if you can excuse yourself to take an expected important call, but this should only be in exceptional circumstances.
Consider the recipient's knowledge of this method of communication	The recipient may not be familiar with common text language and symbols. For example, does 'lol' - mean 'laugh out loud' or 'lots of love'. To many people <3 means less than three, not a heart shape.

means that great care should be taken when considering the content of written interactions, to try to minimize the risk of errors or the chance that messages may be misinterpreted. Some simple precautions include rereading any communications before sending them, having them proof-read by a colleague, and not writing when you feel angry, frustrated, or resentful. The latter can result in the expression of ideas and thoughts that can be quickly regretted, but not removed. You should always write showing respect for others, ask yourself whether you would be comfortable saying what you have written to their face. You should avoid personal attacks, know as 'flaming', and keep the focus of your communication on the issues being discussed rather than on the personal qualities of individuals. As with telephone communication, one of the inherent drawbacks of the written word is the lack of additional information available, for example, facial expression or gestures, which can be used to reinforce or alter the meaning of our messages during face-to-face interaction. Remember that a written message meant in jest may be interpreted as a serious communication, as the lighthearted intent of the sender cannot be reinforced by nonverbal cues.

4.6 **Telephone communication**

Definition

As in everyday life, the telephone enables rapid communication and feedback between people, often over long distances, and it has become an invaluable tool for nurses (Arnold and Boggs 2007). While the use of the telephone has undoubtedly made communication easier in many circumstances, one drawback of its use is, once again, the lack of opportunity to access additional data relating to the messages being sent. Much of the information available during face-to-face interaction through nonverbal cues is lost when this method of communication is employed. This necessitates, therefore, particular care regarding the verbal content and inflections in our voices to ensure that these do not alter or contradict our intended message.

Background

As with any communication, it is important that nurses maintain their professionalism when communicating over the telephone. When initiating a call, it is polite to start

Telephone etiquette

Communication approach	Example
Initiating a telephone call	'Good morning. My name is Alex Taylor; I'm a student nurse in Ward 62 in the City Hospital. I wonder if you can help me regarding ...'
Answering a telephone	'Good morning. Ward 39 City Hospital. Student Nurse McHugh speaking, how may I help you?'

with a greeting, state who you are, the position you hold, and where you are speaking from. When answering a call, similar information should be offered, along with a request of how you may help. Remember that the initial contact a person receives can greatly influence their overall perceived satisfaction with any service.

Developing your skills

Take a moment to think of situations you may have been in when using a telephone to communicate with someone in a professional or business capacity. How does it feel when someone does not offer you a greeting, identify themselves to you, or offer to help? How helpful is it to have a call answered by someone simply saying, 'Hello' or 'Yes'? How easy do you think that it is to assess someone's mood or attitude over the telephone? What difference does it make if the person is cheerful, polite, and seems eager to help? What impression does each approach give in relation to the person's interest or the organization's standards? The answers to these questions relate to every telephone communication that we participate in as nurses. People use their own knowledge and experiences and apply these to the situations in which they find themselves. By ensuring that you use a polite, helpful approach when first engaging with someone, the likelihood that future discussion and interactions will be carried out in a courteous, respectful manner is increased.

Other factors to consider

Another important consideration for communicating over the telephone is to try to remain focused on the conversation taking place. As we are unable to observe and assess any visual cues from the person on the other end of the phone, and we do not need to worry about them seeing our own posture, gestures, or facial expressions, we must be careful not to become distracted either by the environment in which the telephone is situated, or events happening around us. Failure to concentrate on the conversation can result in missed opportunities to hear and retain potentially important information being transmitted. Also, be wary of leaving messages with someone who answers the phone or on an answering machine; there may be confidentiality issues.

4.7 **Context in which communication occurs**

Definition

Communication can be greatly influenced by the context in which it occurs. Context refers to the aspects of an interaction relating to the physical location, the time that communication occurs, and other psychosocial factors that can influence the contributions of participants.

The role of context in communication

Context	Rationale
Physical location	People bring their personal views about locations based on individual experience; this influences how they believe that they ought to communicate in certain surroundings, for example, hospital ward, church, bar, relaxing at home, entertaining guests at home.
Timing of communication	People's participation can be influenced by the timing of interactions, for example, first thing in the morning, after a warm-up exercise, just before breaking up for a holiday.
Status within the relationship	People's perception of power or influence may alter their participation in communication, for example, feeling obliged to laugh at the boss's jokes, attending an event because they think that it will enhance their career rather than because they want to attend.
Level of closeness within the relationship	Having a more intimate or informal relationship with someone may enable a more relaxed attitude to communication. Shared relevance given to words or phrases within a close relationship may enable deeper levels of understanding than the terms seem to provide at an obvious level.
Value attribution	The perceived level of importance or worthiness of an interaction can lead to enthusiastic participation in something that is valued, or indifference in something that is viewed as worthless.
Medical conditions	Specific illnesses may result in individuals experiencing difficulties with communication, for example, deteriorating eyesight, cognitive impairment, delusional ideas.

Developing your skills

Our perceptions of the context in which communication occurs can significantly influence our behaviour and the phrases and terminology that we use. We may feel happy to use certain language with a group of our friends that we may not consider to be appropriate when we are communicating with people as part of our therapeutic role as nurses. Take a few moments to think about different ways that context influences the way that you communicate with others. For instance, how do you communicate with your line manager? Is it different if you also know that person socially? When recounting something that happened to you, would you use the same language, and verbal and nonverbal communication skills, to describe it to your closest friend, an elderly relative, or someone you have just met at a conference? What is it about these circumstances that may make you consider altering your method of communicating?

Additional considerations

Feature	Rationale
Personal understanding and values	Individuals place their own meanings and values on language, behaviour and what they regard as acceptable.
Assessment of others	This tends to be based on personal experience and expectations: committing time and effort to understand these can enhance the likelihood of better communication.
Awareness of self	Allows identification of any deeply held beliefs and prejudices that may influence our interaction with others. In nursing, this can be very important in ensuring that we care for everyone using similar standards.
Individual perception	Individuals can view or indeed participate in the same set of circumstances or the same set of behaviours and draw different and sometimes opposite conclusions from what has happened.
Assessment of others and awareness of self	Again, these opinions tend to be based on their own values and experiences of what is acceptable and what is not and can significantly impact on communication style.
	Understanding your own and the individual's point of view can aid comprehension of their messages during interactions.
Emotion	Emotional distress can play a considerable part in altering people's ability to understand their situation accurately, comprehend other's messages to them, and function as they would in more usual circumstances.
Awareness of emotional state	Providing realistic reassurance can help reduce levels of distress.
	Allowing extra time for understanding and being more careful when checking this can address some of the problems of emotional distress.
Age	Although communication styles may be influenced by a person's age, it is vital to avoid stereotyping people in relation to age.

continued

Awareness of the potential impact that age can have on communication	Individual assessment is vital.
	Be wary of using terms and phrases that may be unknown to people of a different generation.
	Be careful too, however, to avoid being patronizing or demeaning in tone, or using diminutive terms like 'Dear' or 'Sweetheart'. Do not say, for example, 'I'm just giving you this wee pill.'
Gender	There is evidence that, generally, men and women have different perceptions of the purpose of communication and the way each sex engages in this varies.
Awareness of the potential differences in male and female communication	As with age, however, nurses must avoid overgeneralizing and stereotyping, as such assertions cannot be applied to everyone.
Culture	There are too many possible cultural or religious influences to be listed here or to expect anyone to remember them all.
Awareness of cultural identity and aspects of culture that may influence communication	It is possible, however, to take the time to become familiar with the more general cultural aspects and customs of the groups you most frequently come into contact with, and this can demonstrate sensitivity and thoughtfulness.
	Remember that individuals may have differing views regarding culture, religion, and how it is practiced in their personal lives. By trying to establish this, you can identify how best to support and care for the individual.
	Maintaining a high level of awareness of the cultural issues and needs of those with whom we communicate reduces the risk of misunderstandings and causing offence.
Awareness of support services	Knowing where to access details of support services, for example, religious or community leaders, or translation services, enables rapid access to these services.
	Information can be obtained to support individuals in relation to their customs and practices:

It is vital that nurses consider context when choosing where to carry out communication and deciding on the language to employ when constructing messages.

As context can significantly alter the meaning of what is being said, nurses must endeavour to understand it and apply it to particular circumstances. For example, if someone exclaims, 'I could have killed him!' the meaning of their verbal message is very different if expressed in anger at, for instance, the actions of a neighbour with whom they have an ongoing feud, or if expressed in delight at the fact a colleague has organized a surprise birthday party. This statement may be further compounded, as even in the context of anger at the neighbour, it is unlikely that the person making the claim really intended to murder the other. It is more likely to be an attempt to indicate how strongly they feel about the particular situation. Because of the possible variance of meaning in what people say, nurses must try to clarify the aspects of context, which may be impacting on the communication. In so doing, they can gain a better understanding of the overt meaning of the message and the underlying intention of the person who is sending it. This can be achieved by observing and interpreting both verbal and nonverbal communication, and asking for clarification of the specific details of the situation and circumstances.

4.8 **Other factors that influence the success of communication**

As well as the aspects of communication discussed this far, there are other features of communication that relate to individuals as a whole, but which may play a significant role in our ability to communicate successfully with them. These are highlighted in the table on p. 195.

Summary

Possessing and understanding excellent communication skills is undoubtedly a key skill required of all nurses. As well as enabling us to engage with our patients and their families, and our colleagues, when used to their full potential, communication skills empower nurses in all professional settings to assess, plan, deliver, and evaluate the most appropriate care in the most effective way. In addition, effective communication skills can be used with clinical supervision to support, educate, and develop nursing practice. To remain effective, nurses are required continually to develop and utilize a range of communication styles and methods of transmission, from speech to the written word, and from the use of simple tools to the most modern technology. By understanding communication theory and recognizing the ways in which verbal, nonverbal, and emphatic communication can be employed to maximize the effectiveness of our interactions, nurses can communicate not only to those immediately in their care, but also in a wider forum to enhance services and advance the profession. The communication checklist on p.198 draws together important aspects that must be considered. Bear in mind, too, that as society evolves and technology advances, communication is happening in an ever-changing and dynamic environment. It is likely that language and its use will continue to develop and so, too, must nursing knowledge of communication if we are to remain effective in fulfilling the key elements of our nursing practice, as well as the many challenging and evolving aspects of our professional role.

 Scenarios

Consider what you should do in the following situations, then turn to the end of the section to check your answers.

Further scenarios are available at **www.oxford-textbooks.co.uk/orc/docherty/**

The following scenarios and the online scenarios are not branch-specific. The communication skills required to address each scenario are applicable across each of the branches, but, as before, it may be helpful to try to relate the information in each one to specific circumstances within your own branch.

 Scenario 1

You have been asked to assess Mrs Chen, who is here on holiday from China, and who has been referred to your service. She is 58 years of age and cannot speak or understand English. What are the main issues in relation to communicating with this woman? How might you try to address the potential language and cultural difficulties?

Communication checklist

Action	Rationale
Once aware of your target receivers, decide precisely what information you want to communicate. Or identify target receivers based on the information you want or need to transmit.	Ensures that the right people to be communicated with are identified and increases the likelihood that the intended message is transmitted accurately and in a succinct way, reducing the chances of misunderstanding.
Consider any factors that are specific to your chosen receivers, which may hinder the flow of information, for example, ability to understand language, cognitive impairment, sensory difficulties, medical conditions.	Individualizes the interaction: being aware of receivers' needs enables decisions to be made regarding the most appropriate mode or modes of communication.
Make any necessary adjustments to the mode of transmission to compensate for potential barriers, for example, provide hearing aid, use of interpreter, keep sentences short and to the point.	This minimizes the potential impact of barriers and optimizes the probability that messages will successfully reach and be understood by receivers.
Choose the most appropriate mode for sending your message, for example, speech, letter, email.	Enables messages to be transmitted using the most suitable methods of communication for individual circumstances.
Encode the message you want to send in clearly understood terms, appropriate to the decisions made regarding the above.	Minimizes the risk of messages being misinterpreted or misunderstood.
Remember to be professional and respectful in the language you use.	Ensures that professional expectations and requirements are maintained and demonstrates professionalism to receivers.
Be aware of additional information sent through nonverbal communication channels	Enables recognition of the possible impact of involuntary messages being transmitted.
Use your understanding of communication theory to enhance the message you send by using verbal and nonverbal skills to your advantage.	Increases the likelihood of successful transmission by reinforcing or supporting verbal messages.
Be congruent in your verbal and nonverbal cues, and relate these to the nature of the message being sent.	Minimizes the risk of mixed or confusing signals being sent and demonstrates sensitivity and understanding.
Monitor feedback from the receiver, for example, ask receiver to repeat information, ask supplementary questions.	Enables interpretation of the receiver's understanding, concordance, dissatisfaction, and so on.
	If recognized as being unsuccessful, allows the method of communication to be adapted.

Communication checklist

Evaluate the effectiveness of the interaction and decide if further communication is required.	Demonstrates whether or not the communication has successfully achieved its aim.
If unsuccessful restart the process from the beginning of this checklist.	Enables choices to be reviewed and altered where necessary, to increase the likelihood of successful communication
Once completed, follow NMC guidelines to record all of the appropriate details regarding the interaction according to local policy.	Provides written evidence of the communication and the evaluation of the outcome. This also allows for appropriate sharing of the information.

 ## Scenario 2

You are working as a member of a team in a busy unit. All other members of staff are involved in directly caring for patients when the telephone rings. You answer it to an irate relative, a Mrs McNab, who is demanding to know what is happening regarding her daughter's care. Mrs McNab insists that she 'has been told nothing' and is 'fed up at being palmed off!' How should you deal with this call? What are the important aspects of this situation regarding the daughter, Mrs McNab, and your own professional behaviour?

 ## Scenario 3

You have been asked to interview a male patient, Mr Howatson, who has just been given some very upsetting news about his condition. His prognosis is poor and it is likely that he will have to manage significant life changes. What would you consider to be the key issues in relation to preparing for and carrying out the interview?

 ## Scenario 4

While you are working in your clinical area you are approached by Maureen, a patient who appears upset and is asking for assistance to get home. From the information you received at the start of your duty, you know that she is confused and requires further treatment before discharge can be arranged. How should you approach this situation? What are the specific aspects of communication skills that you should consider and implement to assist in this situation?

Website

🌐 **www.oxfordtextbooks.co.uk/orc/docherty/**

You may find it helpful to work through our short online quiz and interactive scenarios intended to help you to develop and apply the skills in this chapter.

References

Arnold EC and Boggs KU (2007). *Interpersonal Relationships: Professional Communication Skills for Nurses*, 5th edn. Saunders Elsevier, St. Louis.

Cleary M and Freeman A (2005). Email etiquette: guidelines for mental health nurses. *International Journal of Mental Health Nursing*, **14**, 62–5.

Ellis RB, Gates B, and Kenworthy N (2003). *Interpersonal Communication in Nursing: Theory and Practice*, 2nd edn. Churchill Livingstone, London.

Fiske J (1990). *Introduction to Communication Studies*, 2nd edn. Routledge, London.

Hargie O and Dickson D (2004). *Skilled Interpersonal Communication: Research, Theory and Practice,* 4th edn. Routledge, Hove.

NMC (2007). *The NMC Record Keeping Guidance.* Nursing and Midwifery Council, London.

Stickley T and Freshwater D (2006). The art of listening in the therapeutic relationship. *Mental Health Practice,* **9**(5), 12–18.

Sully P and Dallas J (2005). *Essential Communication Skills for Nursing.* Elsevier Mosby, London.

Thompson N (2003). *Communication and Language. A Handbook of Theory and Practice.* Palgrave MacMillan, Basingstoke.

Useful further reading and websites

Ballard EC (2006). Improving information management in ward nurses' practice. *Nursing Standard,* **20**(50), 43–48.
Examines the ways in which information is utilized and suggests how systems can be adapted to maximize the management of clinical information.

Bateman N (2000). *Advocacy Skills for Health and Social Care Professionals.* Jessica Kingsley, London.
This text explores advocacy in relation to health and social care, offering definitions and rationale for its use. It includes information on assertiveness and negotiation.

Danet B (2001). *Cyberpl@y: Communicating Online.* Berg, Oxford.
This text does not relate specifically to nursing but provides a useful view of changing methods of communication, which are applicable within our profession.

Dhar J, Leggat C, and Bonar S (2006). Texting – a revolution in sexual health communication. *International Journal of STD and AIDS,* **17**, 375–7.
This article provides information on ways that developing technology can be utilized to enhance communication and services, to better suit the needs of service users.

Dunne K (2005). Effective communication in palliative care. *Nursing Standard,* **20**(13), 57–64.
This article highlights some of the issues that need to be considered when communicating in difficult circumstances. Although using the example of palliative care, many elements are transferable to other areas of nursing.

Gates B (ed.) (2003). *Learning Disabilities, Toward Inclusion,* 4th edn. Churchill Livingstone, London.
This text includes a chapter relating specifically to communication. This will allow nurses to consider the additional needs of people with a learning disability and assist in identifying ways to improve communication and the delivery of care.

Jack K and Smith A (2007). Promoting self-awareness in nurses to improve nursing practice. *Nursing Standard,* **21**(32), 47–52.

This article examines the benefits of increased self-awareness in both personal and professional development for nurses, with advice on portfolio development.

NMC (2007b). *Essential Skills Clusters (ESCs) for Pre-registration Nursing Programmes.* Nursing and Midwifery Council, London.

NMC (2008). *The Code.* Nursing and Midwifery Council, London.

O'Carroll M and Park A (2007). *Essential Mental Health Nursing Skills.* Mosby Elsevier, London.
Although this text is aimed at mental health nurses, it covers many aspects of mental health nursing, including communication, which would be of benefit to nurses from all branches.

Pattee C, Von Berg S, and Ghezzi P (2006). Effects of alternative communication on the communicative effectiveness of an individual with a progressive language disorder. *International Journal of Rehabilitation Research,* **29**, 151–3.
This study explores alternative methods of communication with individuals who have lost the ability to communicate verbally. It highlights the possibility of communicating using a variety of alternative methods.

Perry J, Galloway S, Bottorff JL, and Nixon S (2005). Nurse-patient communication in dementia: improving the odds. *Journal of Gerontological Nursing,* **31**(4), 43–52.
Explores the use of conversational strategies to improve communication with individuals with cognitive impairment.

Rogan Foy C and Timmons F (2004). Improving communication in day surgery settings. *Nursing Standard,* **19**(7), 37–42.
This article highlights the need for effective communication and engaging skills even when supporting patients in settings that permit only brief contact.

Slaven A (2003). Communication and the hearing-impaired patient. *Nursing Standard,* **18**(12), 39–41.
This brief article explores the role that the sender, receiver, and environment can play in promoting or hampering communication.

Thompson J and Pickering S, eds (2002a). *Meeting the Needs of People Who Have a Learning Disability.* Bailliere Tindall, London.

This text considers the notion of addressing bad health and promoting good health among people with learning disabilities and their right to be treated with the same respect as everyone else. Sections include general political and professional factors that impinge on health, and specific strategies for assisting individuals to improve health and reduce high-risk behaviours.

Thompson N (2002b). *People Skills*. Palgrave Macmillan, Basingstoke.

Videbeck SL (2006). *Psychiatric Mental Health Nursing*, 3rd edn. Lippincott Williams and Wilkins, Philadelphia.

Although written specifically for mental health nurses this text has information relating to communication and engaging that should be valuable to all nurses, and that can be adopted in the full range of practice settings.

Welch M (2005). Pivotal moments in the therapeutic relationship. *International Journal of Mental Health Nursing*, **14**, 161–5.

This research study explores nurses' views on key moments within therapeutic relationships and considers how this information may be used to guide future interactions to be more effective.

Williams K, Kemper S, and Hummert L (2004). Enhancing communication with older adults: overcoming elderspeak. *Journal of Gerontological Nursing*, **30**(10), 17–25.

Nurses must maintain awareness of their preconceptions and attitudes, as these may influence the way that they interact with patients. This may happen inadvertently, often through the language and terms that we use. Many of the issues in this article are applicable to communicating appropriately and with respect with individuals across the lifespan.

Winbolt B (2002). *Difficult People: A Guide to Handling Difficult Behaviour*. The Institute for Social Relations, Seaford.

This text offers valuable information to help develop strategies for communicating in difficult situations or with people who may not want to engage. It examines difficult behaviour in a variety of individual circumstances.

Check 🌐 **www.oxfordtextbooks.co.uk/orc/docherty/** for changes and new developments. Updated research, guidelines, or equipment will be added every four months.

 # Answers to scenarios

 ## Scenario 1

- After establishing what language Mrs Chen speaks, you should access an official interpreting service to enable her to participate in care planning and discussions about her care
- As there is likely to be a cost involved, this should be discussed with an appropriate manager
- Try to access written material in Mrs Chen's language to assist her understanding of her circumstances
- Try to establish any specific cultural requirements for Mrs Chen, for example, diet, religious practices
- Family, friends, or an appropriate person who speaks both the patient's language and English could be asked to write a list of common terms and phrases in both languages. For example, 'Good morning,' 'Thank you,' 'I would like a drink,' 'I would like to use the toilet.' This will enable two-way communication and can help with engagement, as it is likely to be nonthreatening
- Communication boards with pictures or images may help convey messages for both you and Mrs Chen
- If possible, learning a few words of Mrs Chen's language may also help engage with her and displays sensitivity and caring
- Remember that there is a risk in using unofficial interpreters. You cannot confirm the accuracy of the translation or identify mistakes, and the interpreter may be expressing his or her own views rather than those of the patient
- You can utilize nonverbal communication, for example, through facial expression, gestures, the use of objects, to try to convey meaning to Mrs Chen. Be aware that cultural differences may, from the patient's viewpoint, alter the significance of your actions or your intended meaning, and remain sensitive to the patient's perspective and needs
- Be aware of the likelihood of frustration for both you and Mrs Chen, and take extra time to compensate for language difficulties

Scenario 2

- When answering any telephone call, it is polite to offer a greeting, then clearly identify the area you are working in, your position, and who you are, before asking how you might help. For example, 'Good morning, Student Nurse Periin, Accident and Emergency Unit. How can I help you?'

- If a caller does not identify him- or herself you should politely ask who you are speaking to. For example, 'Hello, could I ask who this is calling please?' or 'Mrs McNab, thank you. What can I do for you?'

- Speak clearly and slowly, maintaining a professional approach throughout the interaction. Do not lose your temper or engage in an argument with Mrs McNab.

- Using Mrs McNab's name at intervals during the call can help her feel that you are trying to engage and connect with her.

- As Mrs McNab cannot see you, you should use verbal cues, for example, 'Uhuh... yes... I see.' to let her know that you are still listening and understand what she is saying.

- Consider ways that you may be inadvertently making the situation worse. For example, does your tone of voice or the phrases that you use suggest disinterest, impertinence, or annoyance on your part? Might you come across as being impatient and unhelpful?

- Reassure Mrs McNab that you understand that she feels frustrated or angry and that you wish to help resolve the situation.

- If Mrs McNab becomes verbally abusive, you should ask her to stop using an offensive style of communicating, reinforcing that you are trying to help her resolve the situation.

- Listen attentively to what is being said. This should help you to empathize with Mrs McNab and perhaps understand the underlying circumstances that have led to her frustration. Her feelings of irritation and dissatisfaction may well be justified.

- It is very important to remember issues of confidentiality. Patients' personal details should not be discussed over the telephone, especially if you do not know who is on the other end of the line, or if a patient has asked that particular circumstances are not discussed with relatives. This can be difficult for some people to accept and may add to their frustration, therefore, your approach and explanation is paramount in preventing a situation like this deteriorating.

- If you believe that you are unable to help, you should inform Mrs McNab that you are going to pass her on to someone who is more able to be of assistance to her.

- Be honest. If it is likely that someone will only be able to speak to Mrs McNab in one hour's time, apologise but tell her truthfully. If you say, 'Someone will call you right back,' when it is unlikely that this will happen, any delay is only likely to further infuriate Mrs McNab and inflame the situation.

- Record details of the call on paper to ensure that you can pass on correct information to senior staff. This will not only enable them to deal more effectively with Mrs Jackson, but also ensures that you record and share the information accurately.

 Scenario 3

- Have a clear understanding of the purpose of the interview, the information you hope to provide and obtain, and the method or tools that you intend to utilize.

- Arrange for an appropriate room to be available to carry out the interview, for example, with adequate lighting, heating, and space.

- Ensure that the layout and furniture are suitable for your requirements. For example, whether you need a desk, and the positioning and height of chairs.

- Inform colleagues of your whereabouts to enhance safety and if appropriate ask for someone to attend the interview with you.

- Based on your assessment of Mr Howatson, you would decide when best to inform him of the pending interview, offering him reassurance, and the opportunity to ask questions about what it will entail.

- Use verbal and nonverbal communication skills to try to engage with Mr Howatson and reduce any levels of distress or anxiety.

- Escort Mr Howatson to the interview room, offering appropriate reassurance.

- Prior to commencing the interview, remember to ensure that you have access to alarm buttons, and a safe and direct route of exit in case you need to leave quickly.

- Once in the interview area explain the purpose of the interview, the proposed format, and the expected timescale.

- Observe for signs of anxiety, distress, or agitation and offer Mr Howatson the opportunity to ask any questions about worries that may be contributing to this.
- During the interview continue to assess the situation and use communication skills to try to connect with Mr Howatson and put him at his ease.
- Try to identify Mr Howatson's perspective of the situation by using active listening skills, demonstrating your interest, and encouraging his participation.
- Recap what has been said to confirm that you have understood Mr Howatson and to give him the chance to ask further questions, offer clarification, and correct any errors or misunderstandings.
- Discuss how the interview will inform further planned care and how this will be influenced by Mr Howatson's contribution.
- Thank Mr Howatson for his participation and escort him away from the interview room.
- Record the findings from the interview in appropriate documentation and inform other members of the multidisciplinary team of significant information.

Scenario 4

- Adopt a gentle, compassionate approach, as this is likely to encourage engagement and reduce anxiety.
- Treat Maureen with respect and dignity; avoid being patronizing.
- Avoid appearing impatient and allow additional time for Maureen to express herself.

- Reassure her that you will try to help.
- Offer to discuss the situation with Maureen in private and escort her to an appropriate area.
- Be aware that Maureen's confusion may be making her frightened, frustrated, or distressed.
- Be aware of potential risk and consider your safety should Maureen become hostile or aggressive.
- Simplify your language and seek clarification of Maureen's concerns and her understanding by asking simple questions.
- Avoid complex questions that require several answers, as they can be difficult for a confused person to understand and respond to.
- Do not offer false promises, for example, saying that you will arrange for Maureen to go home when you know this is not possible.
- Acknowledge that you understand Maureen's concerns and try to orientate her to her current situation, but be aware of information that may cause her additional distress.
- Choose terms that are less likely to upset Maureen and gently use diversion to encourage communication about less distressing topics.
- You must be very careful that you do not ignore Maureen's main concerns, as this can add to her feelings of frustration.
- If you are unable to resolve Maureen's distress, seek assistance from more experienced staff.
- Report the interaction to staff to enable the information to be appropriately recorded and shared.

Breathing

5

JACQUELINE MCCALLUM AND ELLEN MALCOLM

Introduction

This chapter introduces the fundamental skills of assessing the patient's respiratory status and using different techniques to aid breathing. This includes the observational and clinical skills required in detecting change or abnormality in the patient's ability to breathe normally, and related documentation. As with most aspects of healthcare, respiratory care is constantly evolving and changing. To ensure that patients get the best and most appropriate care, nurses need to be aware of current and new therapies that are available.

As a student nurse, you will encounter patients in the community and acute care setting who have respiratory problems. These can be found at any age and can be acute, such as in bronchiolitis in children, or chronic, such as in emphysema in adults.

Learning outcomes

These outcomes relate to numbers 9 and 10 of the NMC's Essential Skill Clusters and specifically to Care Domains 2 and 3 of the NMC's Standards of Proficiency for Pre-registration Nursing (outcomes to be achieved for entry to branch).

On reading the chapter and associated web pages and undertaking supervised activities, the student will be able to:

- Understand normal breathing patterns and identify abnormal breathing patterns
- Assess the patient's respiratory rate
- Be aware of validated tools that measure vital signs for example early warning scoring charts (EWS)
- Document the patient's respiratory rate and quality of breathing

- Recognize and report changes in the patient's respiratory status and understand the resultant consequences of these changes
- Identify and apply the appropriate breathing equipment necessary to support and monitor the patient's respiratory status
- Obtain a sputum sample

Prior knowledge

To carry out the skills in this chapter it is important that you have a good understanding of the anatomy and physiology of the respiratory system. This can be found in a large range of textbooks. To support the patient's respiratory function, an understanding of the following anatomy and physiology is necessary:

- Normal physiology of the lung
- Physiology associated with oxygen transport and delivery
- Factors that effect changes in breathing both in patients with normal physiology, and in those with lung disease
- The respiratory centre in the brain
- Normal control of respiration

Background

Breathing is the process of moving air into the lungs, called **inspiration**, and then out of the lungs, called **expiration**. Inspiration requires work by the body and uses energy; this means that it is active. Normally expiration uses no energy and is, therefore, called **passive**. Expiration is then followed by a short pause before the next breath is taken. The main muscles used are the diaphragm and the intercostal muscles.

The respiratory system's function is to supply the body with the required amount of oxygen and to remove carbon dioxide. The basic rate, rhythm, and depth of breathing is controlled by the respiratory centre in the brain to meet the changing needs of the body at times of rest (where demand for oxygen and production of carbon dioxide are both low), and at times of exercise when oxygen demand and carbon dioxide production are very high. However, other factors can affect this normal control mechanism in a large number of different diseases, such as pneumonia (inflammation and infection of the lungs), chest trauma, such as fractured ribs, and even neurological diseases, such as **motor neuron disease**.

Where oxygen intake is too low or when carbon dioxide excretion is inadequate, the patient is described as being in 'respiratory failure'. This can be severe and sudden, requiring emergency care, or it can be a progressive long-term condition.

In healthy breathing, when an individual is at rest, chest movement should be equal: both sides of the chest should rise and fall at the same rate and depth. Respiratory rate in the relaxed resting patient is approximately 12–18 breaths per minute (Ahern and Philpot 2002). This rate is much quicker in infants; around 40 breaths per minute. Normal chest movement is equal, bilateral, and symmetrical during both inspiration and expiration. The patient does not display signs of **cyanosis** (lack of oxygen) or **pallor** (pale colour of skin).

Recording respiratory rate, assessing the patient's colour and determining how well the skin is receiving oxygen by measuring oxygen saturation are important nursing skills that do not stand alone. Understanding the patient's respiratory state and recent changes in their respiratory condition allows assessment of breathing to be used to plan and adjust any treatments or interventions that the patient requires (Jevon and Ewens 2001).

You should familiarize yourself with the terminology in **Box 5.1**. You should be able to explain the rate of breathing and types of breathing and be able to distinguish between similar terms.

In addition, there are a lot of causes of breathlessness (see **Box 5.2**). You should be aware of this and start to learn about these conditions and how they are best treated.

These can be put into specific categories, but as well as these, any problems with any part of the respiratory system can cause breathlessness. This involves the nose, pharynx, larynx, trachea, bronchi, and lungs (see **Fig. 5.1**).

Using observation skills, the nurse can assess for cyanosis in a patient. Cyanosis occurs when there is severe respiratory failure and the saturation of haemoglobin (SpO_2) with oxygen falls below 70%. However, severe respiratory failure generally happens when the saturation of haemoglobin with oxygen falls to 85–90%. Pulse oximetry allows the nurse to assess the patient rapidly for hypoxia. An SpO_2 of below 92% would indicate the need for supplemental oxygen. When the SpO_2 falls below 90%, this is indicative of respiratory failure (Woodrow 1999).

To interpret saturation levels, the patient's haemoglobin level must also be known. An anaemic patient has a low concentration of haemoglobin. So a 'normal' oxygen saturation measured in an anaemic patient through pulse oximetry may be misleading, and does not mean that the overall amount of oxygen in the blood is good. It means that the anaemic patient has less haemoglobin and although this is well saturated, overall there will be less oxygen being transported and insufficient oxygen will reach the tissues. The student nurse must, therefore, understand the physiology of the blood to understand this and be aware of some of the complexities involved in interpreting the reading: when in doubt, seek confirmation from a more experienced nurse.

5.1 **Assessment of breathing**

Definition

Nurses are in a key position to recognize and treat breathing dysfunction. To do this, however, they must first recognize that there is a problem with the patient's breathing. This requires an understanding of the anatomy and physiology of the respiratory system (Simpson 2006). There are three things involved when carrying out an assessment of a patient's breathing.

1 Patient history.
2 General appearance of the patient: the patient should be observed for altered mental status, anxiety, confusion, and drowsiness due to hypoxia (lack of oxygen in

Box 5.1 Breathing terminology

Apnoea	is the cessation of breathing and occurs on suppression of the drive or ability to breathe.
Bradypnoea	(less than 12 breaths per minute). This can indicate severe deterioration in the patient's condition. Possible causes include fatigue, **hypothermia**, central nervous system depression, and drugs, such as opioids, and infection. Very fit individuals, at rest or sleeping, may normally have a low respiratory rate in the bradypnoea range.
Biot's pattern	describes a few respirations varying in volume with long periods of apnoea (no breathing).
Cheyne–Stokes respiration	is a period of apnoea followed by sudden resumption of normal breathing that gradually reduces in frequency, becoming **bradypnoeic**, slower and slower, until respirations cease again, and the cycle continues. Causes include left ventricular failure and brain injury. It is frequently seen at the end stage of life.
Cyanosis	can be a symptom of a severe lack of oxygen. Haemoglobin molecules in red blood cells are normally pink when they carry oxygen from the lungs to the tissues. If there isn't much oxygen available for transport, haemoglobin reverts to a shade of blue similar to 'cyan'. So someone suffering from a lack of oxygen in the blood is 'cyanosed' and tissues assume a blue or purplish colour. Central cyanosis is evident on the lips, tongue, and mouth, is more significant and more likely to represent lack of oxygen than **peripheral** cyanosis, which can be seen on the fingers, ears, and could be a symptom of poor circulation, perhaps through exposure on a cold day, so more investigation is needed if a patient appears 'cyanosed'.
Dyspnoea	is defined as a **subjective** (the patient's own) experience of breathing discomfort (Bennett 2003). It is considered one of the most frightening and disturbing physiological symptoms. Dyspnoea is when the patient displays signs of shortness of breath and needs to use 'accessory muscles'. These muscles are not normally used for breathing. However, they do contract during strenuous exercise or when there is an obstruction to normal breathing. When this happens, they pull the rib cage up. The accessory muscles of respiration primarily consist of the scalene muscles and the sternocleidomastoid muscle. When these muscles contract, the upper ribs and the sternum are pulled to aid respiration. When breathing becomes difficult, for whatever reason, the patient can use the muscles to supplement those already working to full capacity. The patient exerts extra effort in breathing both during inspiration and expiration and can tire very quickly.
Hyperventilation	is fast shallow breathing. It is often associated with anxiety: this relationship can sometimes obscure causes and effects in some respiratory disorders, for example, someone suffering from asthma can be very anxious, and it may be possible for the inexperienced to confuse an asthmatic attack with an anxiety or panic attack. Hyperventilation may be a symptom of an increased need to get rid of carbon dioxide that is accumulating in the blood. We hyperventilate normally with exercise, but some disease conditions cause hyperventilation at rest.
Hypoxia	is a shortage of oxygen in the body.
Kussmaul's respirations	are rapid and very deep.
Orthopnoea	is positional breathlessness. It is at its worst when lying down, and relieved when sitting upright.
Tachypnoea	(greater than 20 breaths per minute for the adult and older children, but greater than 40 breaths for the infant and 30 breaths for young children). This is an abnormally rapid rate of breathing. It is usually one of the first indicators of respiratory distress.

Box 5.2 Causes of breathlessness

Obstructive disorders of the airways

These cause narrowing or obstruction of the airways (Bennett 2003). This can commonly be caused by:

- Chronic obstructive pulmonary disease (COPD)
- Bronchitis (inflammation in the bronchi of the lungs)
- Bronchiolitis (inflammation of the small airways in the lungs, the bronchioles)
- Asthma (a condition that causes narrowing of the bronchiole airways)
- **Aspiration** (of fluid) into the lungs
- Tumour in the lungs
- Cystic fibrosis (a hereditary disease causing thick mucous production in the lungs).

Restrictive disorders

These result when there is less room for the lungs to expand in the thoracic cavity (Bennett 2003). Common causes are:

- Scoliosis (deviation of the spine)
- Respiratory muscle dysfunction
- Pleural effusion (fluid within the pleural space)
- Pneumothorax (a collapsed lung)
- Pulmonary fibrosis (thickening and stiffening of the alveoli)

Pulmonary vascular disorders

These result from problems of the blood supply to and from the lungs. Common causes are:

- Pulmonary **hypertension** (raised blood pressure in the blood vessels supplying the lungs)
- Pulmonary oedema (accumulation of fluid within the air spaces of the lungs)
- **Pulmonary embolism** (an **embolus**—usually a blood clot—becomes lodged in the blood vessel in the lungs and obstructs blood flow)

Infection

A number of infections that can occur in the respiratory tract can cause the patient to become breathless.

- Bacterial (for example tuberculosis)
- Viral (for example croup in children)
- Aspiration (fluid getting into the lungs, commonly from vomit)

Trauma

This can be direct trauma to the lungs or chest, or indirectly, to the brain:

- Crushing injury to the chest
- Rib fractures
- Flail chest (all ribs fracture off the sternum)
- Penetrating chest wounds (stabbing)
- Head injury
- Toxic substances (drugs)

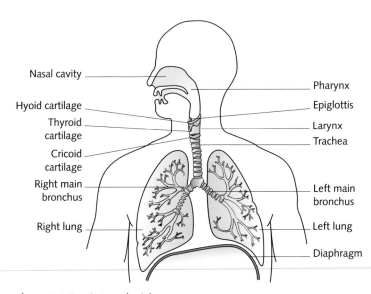

Figure 5.1 Respiratory physiology

the cells) or **hypercarbia** (high level of carbon dioxide in the blood).

3 Observations:

- Respiratory rate
- Temperature (Chapter 9)
- Heart rate (Chapter 3)
- Blood pressure (Chapter 3)
- BMI (**body mass index**, height and weight, Chapter 6)

Key point: It may be necessary to make the observations first and then provide treatment before taking the patient history and observing the patient's appearance. This will avoid greater respiratory distress through the patient attempting to engage in conversation.

When to assess a patient's breathing

A patient's breathing is assessed for a number of reasons:

- To obtain a baseline for later comparisons
- To monitor any changes to respiratory rate
- To evaluate any changes due to treatment

Assessment, documentation, and interpretation of physiological information are essential for the nurses' ability to identify patients at risk of adverse events related to respiratory dysfunction. The optimum frequency of vital sign measurement has yet to be defined; however, there is a need for an individualized assessment of patient's respiratory rate and vital signs. If the patient is acutely breathless and you find any abnormalities in the history, general appearance, or observations related to the patient's breathing, then you will be carrying out respiratory assessments more frequently.

Procedure: Taking a patient history

Preparation

To carry out an assessment of the patient's breathing, it is important to ensure that there are no distractions, and a

quiet, well-lit warm private room will ensure this. Using the 'look, listen, and feel' approach (see Chapter 3; Resuscitation Council UK 2005) can help with the assessment. The best position for the patient is to be sitting upright (high Fowler's, as shown in **Fig. 5.2**). This will aid lung expansion.

You should assess if the patient is breathless or not. At rest, there may be no evidence of breathlessness, so you should ask if the patient is ever breathless. If the patient is obviously, or claims to be, breathless, you need to assess the level of their breathlessness.

A breathless patient may find it difficult to answer your questions fully. If this is the case, it is helpful to use closed questions, requiring only a very limited response, such as yes or no, to gain information (Bennett 2003). This type of communication makes it easier for the patient and requires little respiratory effort. You can also help by prioritizing questions. Ask the most important questions first and finish the assessment after treatment, when the patient is less breathless. You could also get information from

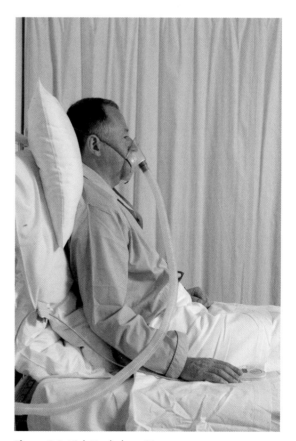

Figure 5.2 High Fowler's position

sources other than the patient, for instance a GP, community nurse, or relative.

Procedure: Assessing a patient's general appearance

Assessing the patient's general appearance starts at the bottom of the bed, or as you approach the patient, and by listening at the bedside. Normally, breathing is quiet; noisy breathing can alert you to a problem (Jevon and Ewens 2001). The common noises are shown in **Box 5.3**. The student should use observation skills to identify other alterations in appearance that can indicate breathing problems.

Box 5.3 Common noises indicating a problem with breathing	
Stridor	usually occurs on inspiration and is a high pitched sound commonly caused by an obstruction in the larynx or pharynx, such as a foreign body (for example, an inhaled peanut), a tumour, or croup in children.
Wheeze	usually occurs on expiration and is commonly associated with some disorders, such as asthma.
A rattly chest	can be the result of a build-up of fluid in the lungs and is generally associated with pulmonary oedema or a build-up of sputum.
Grunting	is associated with neonates. This usually indicates that their respiratory function is deteriorating and expert help should be sought immediately.
Snoring	sounds in the healthy normal patient when they are sleeping is very common and not generally life-threatening or of concern. However, in the semi-conscious patient it can be caused by the tongue occluding the airway and can lead to respiratory arrest (the cessation of breathing) and death.

Procedure: Observing and documenting respiratory rate

The patient's respiratory rate is assessed usually in conjunction with and as part of an ongoing assessment and monitoring of all the vital signs of the patient (Butler-Williams et al. 2005). It is important that the patient has rested prior to measuring the respiratory rate. It is also important for the student nurse to be aware that the patient may have tachypnoea (fast rate of breathing) as a result of certain disorders:

- **Anaemia**
- Heart disease
- Severe haemorrhage
- Respiratory disease

You should also be aware that tachypnoea can be expected in some cases:

- After exercise
- Fear or anxiety
- Pain
- Fever
- Infants and young children have a faster respiratory rate than older children and adults

There are also certain circumstances where the patient may have **bradypnoea** (slow rate of breathing):
- Sedation and opioids
- Excessive alcohol

Aftercare: recognizing deterioration

It is extremely important to document the respiratory rate on the vital signs assessment chart. In many hospitals, this is done on the Early Warning Scoring (EWS) chart, which has been described in Chapter 3. The EWS, in association with a call-out algorithm, is a useful and appropriate risk-management tool that should be implemented for all patients admitted to the acute care setting.

Early warning scoring systems are widely used to identify the deteriorating patient and to activate emergency response systems as well as to identify those who require a higher level of care and observation.

Taking a patient history

EQUIPMENT

- Watch with a second hand
- Vital signs documentation chart or EWS chart
- Pen
- Nursing admission documentation

Typical questions to ask	Rationale
1 **Physical** **Are you breathless at rest?**	To highlight if breathlessness is related to activity.
2 **Can you carry out a conversation?**	To highlight the extent of the patient's breathlessness.
3 **How far can you walk before becoming breathless when you are well?**	This can help judge the extent of the breathlessness.
4 **Can you climb a flight of stairs?**	This can help judge the extent of the breathlessness
5 **Has this happened before? If so, how long did it last?**	To highlight any previous incidents or medical history.
6 **Have you been on any medication for this breathlessness?**	To highlight any previous remedies.
	To highlight any medications that could be causing the breathlessness.
7 **Do you have a family history of respiratory disease?**	There is some genetic link in certain respiratory conditions.
8 **Do you have a cough? How long have you had a cough? Is it productive or dry?**	To highlight the possibility of infection.
9 **If the patient coughed up sputum, ask:** **What colour was it?** **Did it have blood in it?** **Was it frothy?** **What was its consistency?** **Was it foul-smelling?** **Has a specimen been collected?**	To highlight the possibility of infection, inflammation, injury, or oedema in the lungs.
10 **Psychological** **Try and determine whether the patient appears anxious.**	Anxiety can exacerbate respiratory problems.

continued

11	**Sociocultural** **Do you smoke?** **If so, how many per day?**	To highlight underlying risk factors to respiratory disease.
12	**Environmental**	
13	**What factors seem to influence your breathing (for example, positioning, medication)?**	To highlight underlying risk factors of respiratory disease.
14	**Any history of allergies or recent travel?**	To highlight underlying risk factors of respiratory disease.
15	**Politico-economic** **Are there any housing problems (for example, dampness)?**	To highlight underlying risk factors of respiratory disease.
16	**Ask about the patient's occupational and social history.**	To highlight underlying risk factors of respiratory disease.

The EWS is a tool for bedside evaluation based on five physiological assessments:

- Respiratory rate
- Systolic blood pressure
- Pulse rate
- Temperature
- Urinary output

This tool, therefore, identifies patients who are at risk of becoming very unwell at an early stage and is used to try and prevent further deterioration in the patient's condition. The respiratory rate is an extremely important part of this and should not be ignored.

Procedure: Assessment of blood oxygen saturation using pulse oximetry

A pulse oximeter is a small piece of monitoring equipment that works by measuring the transmission of a beam of infrared light through an area of tissue, such as a small finger or an earlobe, or the bridge of the nose, where there is blood circulating (see **Fig. 5.4**). It measures and digitally displays the (peripheral) oxygen saturation (SpO_2) in the patient's blood, and the patient's pulse rate (Allen 2004). Many models of pulse oximeter are available.

In acute care, such as intensive care, pulse oximeters form part of comprehensive monitoring equipment. They

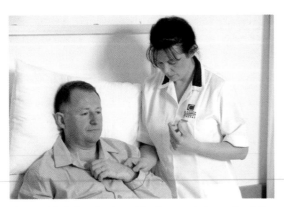

Figure 5.3 Pulse check and feeling respiratory rate at the same time

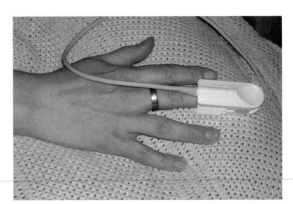

Figure 5.4 A pulse oximeter

Assessing a patient's general appearance

Step	Rationale
1 **Look** at the patient's general colour: look at the lips, ears, arms, and legs, as well as the central part of the body. Does the patient feel warm and look pink, as opposed to feeling cold and looking cyanosed?	This will identify if the patient is getting enough oxygen.
2 **Look** at the patient's facial expression.	Facial expressions, such as grimacing, can alert you to any discomfort due to breathlessness.
3 **Look** at the patient's posture.	The patient's posture can alert you to any discomfort due to breathlessness.
4 **Look** at the patient's hands.	Tremor in the hands can be a result of using high doses of **bronchodilator** drugs (used to expand the airways) and carbon dioxide retention. The hands can also show nicotine staining, indicating that the patient is a smoker, and there can be evidence of 'finger clubbing'. Finger clubbing is an enlargement, thinning, and alteration of the finger and nail bases, which can result from hypoxia over many years.
5 **Look** at the shape of the patient's chest.	Looking at the chest can alert you to any abnormal shape, such as a 'barrel chest' or whether the patient is using additional accessory muscles to help breathing.
	In babies and children who have an increased work of breathing you will see drawing in of the chest between the ribs (recession) and at the top of the sternum (tracheal tug).
	Many patients will sit upright and have their hand outstretched supporting them in front (like a tripod) when they are struggling to breathe, for example, patients with chronic obstructive pulmonary disease (COPD): this is called an orthopnoeic position.
6 **Listen** to the patient's breathing.	The breathing should be quiet; any noisy breathing could alert you to a problem.
7 **Feel** the patient's chest movement by holding the wrist as if you are checking the pulse and laying the patient's hand and your hand over the patient's chest, as shown in Fig. 5.3.	To feel the chest wall rising *without the patient knowing*: this is important, to prevent the patient from altering the respiratory rate.

can also be an adjunct to electronic blood pressure machines. However, pulse oximeters can also be small portable hand-held machines, which are particularly helpful to the community nurse. They are designed to be used for both single and continuous measurement.

In general, the sites used for monitoring have to be easily accessible; the finger or earlobe is a common site for adults, while in infants and neonates the probe can be wrapped around the wrist or foot. It is important in infants and neonates to select the correct size of probe. If the patient's pulse is weak in a particular area, or if the patient is cold peripherally indicating poor circulation then a pulse oximeter cannot be used reliably.

Normal saturation levels are between 94% and 100%. The student must remember that equipment can give false readings and the patient should also be examined for any physical signs of cyanosis.

Developing your skills

In acute and community care the nurse's knowledge, skills, and actions in assessing the patient can have a huge influence on the patient's outcome. It is, therefore, important that, as a student nurse, you practice and become competent in these skills. It is also important to keep your knowledge up to date at all times. It is vitally important in assessing the patient's respiratory status, since there is a very close link with respiratory dysfunction and adverse events and **mortality** (Considine 2005).

It is essential that you become accustomed to and practice the skill of assessing a patient's breathing and providing assistance depending on what the assessment shows the patient's requirements to be. You will see patients' breathing being assessed with patients in acute care, community, and care homes. It is also highly important that the patient is assessed and re-evaluated at appropriate times depending on their illness and their recovery or deterioration. You should try and practice the skill of assessing a patient's breathing on your next placement. Remember that if a patient presents with numerous problems you will need some expert help from the qualified nursing staff and the multiprofessional team to help address these.

For the more advanced student, and for the qualified and expert nurse, there is more that can be assessed, but these are advanced skills and not expected of the first-year student. These are:

- **Palpation** (using the hands to feel the part of the body) of the chest wall
- **Percussion** (tapping on the chest wall to estimate the amount of air in the lungs) of the chest wall
- **Auscultation,** which is listening to chest sounds with a stethoscope
- **Peak flow**, which is the highest rate of air blown out during a forced expiration

Other factors to consider

Effects on eating

It is very common that the breathless patient becomes malnourished due to loss of independence and physical problems. It is very difficult to chew and swallow if you are very breathless; try eating while running! The nurse must identify this. Chapter 6 explains how to assess a patient's nutritional status.

Some simple steps can help the breathless patient with eating and drinking. Giving them longer to eat their meal will help, since they will have to eat between taking breaths. Therefore, having a meal that is not hot will mean that it will remain palatable for longer, for instance, having sandwiches for lunch. Also if a patient is having a hot pudding or other dessert, you can wait and serve this later.

Investigations

There are a number of investigations that can also be carried out to help in the assessment of patients breathing and to assist in diagnosis. These include, chest X-rays, spirometry, monitoring arterial blood gases, electrocardiography (ECG), and measuring peak expiratory flow rate (PEFR). When you are on clinical placement, it would be beneficial to visit the lung-function laboratory to see these tests being carried out.

5.2 **Positioning the patient to facilitate breathing**

Definition

You can advise the patient about positions that will help breathing as well as help the patient find a comfortable position to help them breathe more easily.

The purpose of turning and positioning patients is to:

Observing and documenting respiratory rate in adults

Key point: It is advised that a stethoscope is used to listen to the air moving in and out of the lungs of a baby under 12 months old to measure the respiratory rate. For an older child, the same procedure is followed as for an adult.

 Step   **Rationale**

Step	Rationale
This assessment is best carried out without the patient's knowledge.	If the patient becomes aware that the respiratory rate is being assessed, this can cause the rate to change.
1 Ensure privacy.	To prevent embarrassment and maintain dignity.
2 Gain patient **consent**: provide information that you will be assessing respiratory status, without explaining how you intend to count respirations.	To gain the patient's approval and cooperation.
3 Cleanse hands prior to assisting.	To prevent cross-infection.
4 Ensure correct seating or positioning of the patient in an upright position (**supine**).	To ensure best position for breathing.
5 Ensure correct seating or positioning next to patient.	To ensure best position for measuring the respiratory rate.
6 Ensure the patient has rested for five minutes.	To bring patient's breathing rate down to a resting normal rate.
7 Ask the patient not to speak or distract you as you measure the pulse.	Speaking interrupts normal breathing. Answering the patient distracts you from your task.
8 The patient's breathing should be observed: • Mouth or nasal breathing • Rate of respirations • Bilateral movement of chest wall • Depth of respiration • Pattern of respiration **Signs of respiratory distress:** • Pursed lips • Use of accessory muscles **Other observations:** • Patient's colour • Associated noises	To identify whether normal respiratory rate pattern and depth are present. To determine if the patient is experiencing any degree of respiratory distress. To determine if wheeze, stridor, or rales are present.
9 Measure breathing rate by continuing to hold the patient's hand after checking the pulse, by putting it across the patient's chest (see Fig. 5.3).	This allows you to count the number of times your hand move up and down with their breathing.

continued

10	Count the respirations for 60 seconds by observing the rise and fall of the patient's chest. One respiration consists of an inspiration and expiration.	Assessment for 60 seconds enables the student nurse to observe the patient for long enough to determine depth, pattern, and any signs of respiratory distress in addition to rate.
11	Report the rate and any abnormal findings to a more senior member of staff (registered nurse or doctor).	To allow remedial action to be taken immediately if necessary.
12	Ensure that the patient's record is updated.	To ensure that the patient's details are kept up to date and also to ensure that information is available to ensure continuity of care.

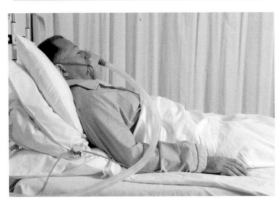

(a)

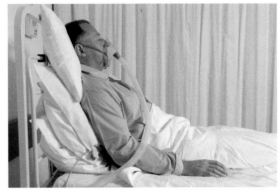

(b)

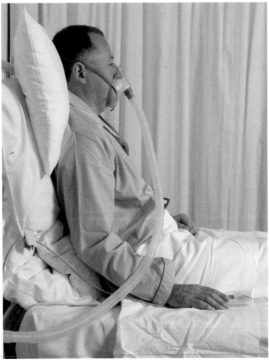

(c)

Figure 5.5 Different Fowler's positions: (a) low, (b) mid, (c) high from top to bottom.

- Relieve pressure
- Improve patient comfort
- Facilitate comfortable respiration, and
- Help the patient to **expectorate** pulmonary secretions

The patient's position and posture can affect the work of breathing. A stooped or slumped position can cause rib compression, limiting the volume of air entering the lungs and the ability to expel air out of the lung effectively. If a breathless patient on bed rest should be nursed in an upright position. Pillows for support will aid adequate breathing, but avoid putting pillows into a position that can limit chest movement and worsen the situation.

There are a number of positions that can help the patient to breathe more easily. The Fowler's position literally means the semi-sitting position, therefore, sitting upright. There are three stages of the Fowler's position, as shown in **Fig. 5.5** from top to bottom:

1 Low Fowler's, where the head and torso are raised by 30°,

2 Mid Fowler's, where the head and torso are raised by 45°,

Assessment of blood oxygen saturation using pulse oximetry

EQUIPMENT

- Pulse oximeter
- Appropriate pulse oximeter probe
- Pen
- Assessment chart (EWS or medical records)

Key point: Care must be taken when choosing the site. If the finger is the choice then it has to be free of nail polish or artificial nails (the light may not be able to pass through), be free of tremor and not be on the same arm as the blood pressure cuff.

Step	Rationale
1 Ensure privacy.	To prevent embarrassment and maintain dignity.
2 Gain patient consent.	To gain informed consent.
3 Ensure that the patient is comfortable and warm.	To maintain comfort. Shivering may interfere with the device.
4 Cleanse hands prior to assisting.	To prevent cross-infection.
5 Explain procedure to the patient.	To gain cooperation and keep the patient informed.
6 Assess patient for pulse sites: fingers, earlobe in adult; fingers, toe, forearm in child; earlobe in infants.	To find a good pulse site in order to gain an accurate reading.
7 Collect pulse oximeter and probe.	To obtain correct equipment.
8 Make sure probe and machine are clean and in good working order.	To minimize cross-infection and ensure that equipment is fit for use.
9 Ensure that the pulse site is dry and the probe is not causing excessive sweating.	To gain an accurate reading.
10 Switch on pulse oximeter, attach the probe to the chosen site, and place probe as directed by the manufacturer's instructions. Wait until reading is displayed.	To gain reading.
11 Encourage patient to keep pulse site still, especially if the finger is used.	To gain accurate recording.
12 Ensure that the pulse sensor is detecting the patient's pulse.	To gain accurate recording.

continued

13	Take the SpO₂ reading and record this in the patient's notes.	To ensure that information is available.
		To ensure complete and accurate assessment.
14	Ensure that any abnormal reading or observation is reported to the medical team.	To ensure that any problems are communicated.
15	If the monitoring is to be intermittent, remove probe, and ensure that the patient is comfortable.	The pulse oximeter probe and machine only need to be on when the reading is required.
16	If monitoring is continuous, regularly change the site (30 min–2 hr); change from one finger to another or use different ear lobes.	To prevent any trauma to the area where the probe is attached.
17	When finished, clean, and return equipment to storage.	To minimize cross-infection. Proper storage, including charging or replacing any battery, will ensure that the equipment is ready for use next time.

3 High Fowler's, where the head and torso are raised by 60° to 90°.

The low and mid Fowler's position may not be good enough for the breathless patient: the high Fowler's position is the best choice to assist breathing. The reason for this is that in this position the abdominal organs are free to hang from the diaphragm, relieving upward pressure and helping the chest to inflate during inspiration, facilitating lung expansion and providing more oxygen.

There is one other position that many breathless patients find beneficial and this is called the orthopnoeic position. The patient is seated with the arms in front, supported on pillows on a table, as shown in **Fig. 5.6**. The patient can then lean forwards and rest the head on the pillows. This position again allows expansion of the lungs, but can be very good if the patient is tired and wishes to sleep or rest.

When to reposition a patient

You should ensure that any patient for whom you are providing nursing care is in a comfortable position with reduced risk of developing pressure sores. If a patient has breathing problems, then helping them to move into particular positions can improve their breathing. It is also important to find out which positions are most comfortable. Some patients will prefer to move from one

position to another, to ease their breathing, while at the same time helping to relieve pressure on their sacrum.

Developing your skills

It is essential that you become accustomed to and practice the skill of positioning patients to assist their breathing. This is applicable for breathless patients in acute care and community settings. At home, the patient may be more comfortable in a chair with a high back. You should try and practice the skill on your next placement. Remember to make a risk assessment first for manual handling and to follow these guidelines to move the patient into the high Fowler's position or the orthopnoeic position.

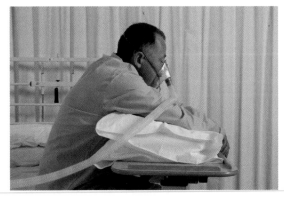

Figure 5.6 Orthopnoeic position: the patient can lean forwards and rest on the pillows

Positioning the patient to facilitating breathing

Step	Rationale
1 Ensure privacy.	To prevent embarrassment and maintain dignity.
2 Gain patient consent.	To gain informed consent.
3 Cleanse hands prior to assisting.	To prevent cross-infection.
4 Explain procedure to the patient.	To gain cooperation and keep the patient informed.
5 Discuss with the patient the Fowler's position and the Orthopnoeic position.	To gain insight into the patient's preference.
6 Position the patient into the patient's position of choice. Remember to follow manual handling guidelines (Section 2.2 and Chapter 10).	To move the patient into the position safely.
Fowler's position can be achieved by putting pillows behind the patient. Two or three pillows are piled up and then two pillows are placed in front using an upside down V, with one more pillow on top.	To ease breathing by positioning into the Fowler's position.
Orthopnoeic position: the patient sits at the side of the bed with feet on the floor. The bed table is put in front of them with a pillow on top. The patient can then lean forwards with the arms on the pillow. This can also be done with the patient sitting in a chair.	To ease breathing by positioning into the orthopnoeic position.
7 Ensure that the patient is comfortable.	The patient will not relax in an uncomfortable position.
8 Ensure that the nurse call button is accessible to the patient (the telephone if in the community).	To ensure that the patient can contact the nurse if required.
9 Ensure that the patient can reach a drink.	To ensure adequate hydration of the patient.
10 Ensure documentation completed when task complete.	To ensure that the patient's details are kept up to date and also to ensure that information is available to ensure complete and accurate assessment.

Other factors to consider

Quitting smoking is the greatest single step that smokers can take to improve their health. The body then has an opportunity to repair the damage that smoking causes. Although long-term damage may be caused by smoking, some benefits to the patient's breathing can happen within weeks. These can improve breathing through loss of a smoker's cough and reduction in sputum. It is, therefore, an important role for the nurse to provide health promotion to assist the patient to stop smoking. In the community, many practice nurses run smoking-cessation clinics and there are smoking-cessation nurses for community and acute care.

Although there is no evidence that using a fan or opening a window helps, patients who are extremely breathless usually find these helpful in that the fan or open window allows them to feel better, and by allowing excess body heat to be dissipated through convection currents. A hand-held fan can be very beneficial.

Relaxation techniques can also help the breathless patient. This can be very effective if the patient is breathing very fast. The nurse can get the patient to focus the attention on breathing. Instruct the patient to breathe in deeply and then let the breath out. Do this with the patient and get them to count their breaths, and say the number of the breath as they let it out (this gives them something to concentrate on other than their breathing). You can then take control of the rate of the breathing and get the patient to slow down to your normal rate. You can also get breathing relaxation tapes that the patient can listen to.

Deep breathing techniques can assist the breathless patient by maximizing ventilation. To teach this to a patient; instruct the patient to take in as much air as possible, hold the breath briefly and slowly exhale. This can help to reduce the respiratory rate, particularly if the patient is breathing very quickly.

Patients will tell you that breathlessness is extremely frightening and isolating, and can make any other disability worse. Many patients feel as if they are suffocating and are going to die. It is important, therefore, to provide **emotional** and psychological support to the patient. Many hospitals and community nurses provide pulmonary rehabilitation. This is aimed at supporting patients, providing education, helping patients to manage their breathlessness, and encouraging social networks.

Sometimes patients with breathing difficulties can be very uncooperative and disorientated. This can be because of cerebral hypoxia (a lack of oxygen to the brain). It is important to calm the patient, be reassuring, and try to get them comfortable.

5.3 **Using oxygen therapy to support the patient's breathing**

Definition

Oxygen therapy is used to correct hypoxia and is considered a drug (Bennett 2003). A doctor should prescribe oxygen for patients. Oxygen therapy can be life-saving. However, if administered at the wrong dose oxygen can be toxic and life-threatening. Therefore, oxygen prescriptions should include the flow rate, number of hours of daily use, the type of oxygen system to be used and the method of delivery.

Carrying out an assessment of the patient's respiratory function will provide the nurse and doctor with information to determine whether the patient requires oxygen therapy to support breathing. This will involve assessing the patient's history, general appearance, and breathing. This may include monitoring respiratory rate and saturation levels using a pulse oximeter, but more advanced tests may also be used, such as taking a chest X-ray, measuring peak expiratory flow rate, and arterial blood gas analysis.

Background

Room air consists of 21% oxygen, 78% nitrogen, and 1% of other gases (including carbon dioxide). The administration of a known concentration of oxygen is an important part of routine care for patients both in the hospital setting and at home. There are many devices currently available (Dunn and Chisholm 1998). Regardless of the device chosen, oxygen delivery to the lungs depends on the patient's ability to tolerate the oxygen delivery system, and the patient's respiratory rate and depth of breathing.

The method of delivery will be dependent on the concentration of oxygen required, the patient's compliance with the therapy, and the underlying cause of their breathlessness. There are various methods of oxygen delivery and they are put into two categories, fixed performance devices and variable performance devices.

Methods of oxygen delivery

Fixed performance devices

Venturi system

A venturi system (see **Fig. 5.7**) is a face mask with a valve to mix oxygen and air. It provides a specific oxygen percentage at a specific oxygen flow rate. Different masks are available with different settings to provide different oxygen concentrations. To make this safer, each particular type of mask, capable of providing a different percentage of oxygen, is colour coded, and the amount of oxygen provided is clearly labelled. Oxygen concentrations from 24% to 60% can be delivered in this way.

Variable performance devices

Nasal cannula

A nasal cannula is a length of tubing that sits over the ears and comes round to divide into two outlets, each designed to sit in the entrance to a different nostril (**Fig. 5.8**). The other end of the tubing is attached to the oxygen supply. Patients like this, especially if they have felt claustrophobic with a facemask. It also allows them to eat and drink while continuing to receive oxygen.

Nasal cannulae can, however, cause pressure sores to the nostrils and ears if applied too tightly. There may also be dryness and damage to the **mucosa** within the nasal cavity, as oxygen is being administered as a dry gas without humidification. Nasal cannulae can deliver oxygen concentrations of 24–44% at flow rates of 1–6 litres per minute. However, high flow rates above 4 litres per minute can cause the patient discomfort and nasal mucosa damage, as described. In an infant or neonate, a lower flow of about 1–2 litres per minute is used.

Hudson mask

A plain Hudson mask is not designed for long-term or accurate use, as it delivers an unpredictable level of oxygen depending on the patient's respiration pattern, and on how much mouth breathing occurs. These are, therefore, not suitable for patients who have chronic respiratory disease where an accurate, continuous low concentration has to be ensured. In acute care, the nonrebreathe mask has mainly superseded the Hudson mask.

Nonrebreathe mask

Nonrebreathe masks (see **Fig. 5.9**) allow for the delivery of very high concentrations of oxygen therapy. For this

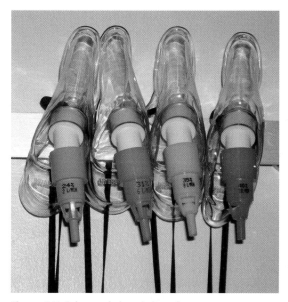

Figure 5.7 Colour-coded venturi masks

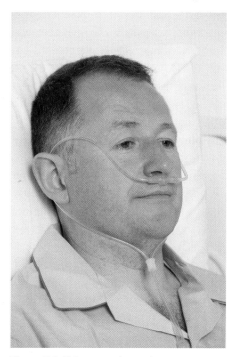

Figure 5.8 Using a nasal cannula

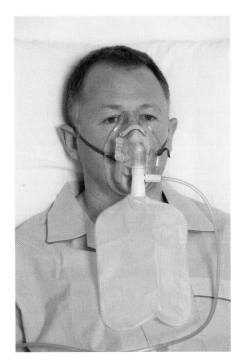

Figure 5.9 Nonrebreathe mask

reason, they are used in acute care in such situations as a heart attack or respiratory failure, such as acute asthma. They can deliver concentrations of 95% at a flow rate of 12 litres per minute. This happens because there is a reservoir bag attached to the mask, which has a one-way valve to prevent exhaled air re-entering the patient's lungs. The facemask should be securely attached to the patient's face. This can be uncomfortable for patients and is generally only used for short-term therapy.

Blow-by-blow oxygen

In past times, an oxygen tent or hood was used for children, especially if they could not tolerate a mask or nasal cannula. Now, with advancing technology, blow-by-oxygen is used, whereby oxygen is blown into the **incubator** of the neonate or infant, and is designed to provide a prescribed ambient concentration of oxygen.

Incubator

Incubators are used for the sick baby or for a baby who is born early (preterm). They are also used in the very ill neonate. The amount of oxygen in the air, as well as the temperature, can be controlled.

When to use oxygen therapy

Oxygen therapy (**Fig. 5.10**) is used for the patient who is breathless in an attempt to maintain oxygen levels in the blood and, thus, to the major organs (Casey 2001). The correct administration of oxygen therapy can be a life-saving procedure for breathless patients. Safe delivery depends on flow rate, the delivery system, duration of delivery, and continuous monitoring.

Many conditions that cause breathlessness can be treated with oxygen. The conditions can be acute or chronic. Some examples are:

- Cardiac arrest
- Heart attack
- Shock
- Chest infection
- Asthma
- Chronic obstructive pulmonary disease (COPD)
- Chest trauma

Patients may be on oxygen therapy for a short time, usually if they are in acute care and treated for an acute illness causing breathlessness, which can be treated. But many patients receive long-term oxygen therapy (LTOT). These patients are typically treated at home or in care homes. Long-term oxygen therapy usually refers to 15 hours or more per day of treatment. Domiciliary (home) oxygen cylinders can provide this. However, Dunn and Chisholm (1998) suggest that more commonly an oxygen concentrator is used. This machine uses room air and removes nitrogen from it, thus providing the patient with a relatively larger percentage of oxygen. These devices can be portable, usually allowing the patient to get out of the house using a wheelchair.

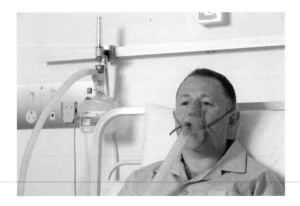

Figure 5.10 Humidified oxygen system

Administration of oxygen

EQUIPMENT

- Patient drug prescription chart
- Oxygen supply, either from a wall outlet, an oxygen cylinder, or oxygen concentrator
- A flow meter: this will allow the oxygen supply to be set in litres per minute
- Oxygen delivery tubing
- Delivery device, that is, nasal cannula or face mask
- Humidifier bottle
- Distilled water

Key point: There are dangers with oxygen therapy. The most common danger is that oxygen can enhance combustion. Therefore, the oxygen, or oxygenated air, should not come into contact with a naked flame or a spark from electricity. Care has to be taken to educate patients of these dangers, particularly if they smoke. Smoking has been banned in hospitals and should, therefore, not be a problem; however, with domiciliary oxygen therapy, the patient may be tempted to smoke, or there may be other smokers in the home.

	Step	Rationale
1	Ensure privacy.	To prevent embarrassment and maintain dignity.
2	Gain patient consent.	To gain informed consent.
3	Cleanse hands prior to assisting.	To prevent cross-infection.
4	Explain procedure to the patient.	To gain cooperation and keep the patient informed.
5	Check the patient prescription chart for flow rate, dose, length of use, and delivery system.	To ensure correct prescription provided.
6	Collect the equipment required.	To obtain correct equipment.
7	Attach the oxygen tubing to the flow meter and the oxygen mask (or nasal cannula).	To set up equipment.
8	Attach face mask (or nasal cannula) to the patient's face.	To ensure correct fitting.
9	Set the flow meter at the correct prescribed rate in litres per minute.	To ensure correct dosage.
10	Ensure that the patient is comfortable.	To maintain patient's comfort.

continued

11	Check regularly to ensure that the patient is receiving the correct dose.	To maintain correct administration of medicines.
12	Sign for prescription with countersignature from registered nurse.	To ensure correct procedures for administration of medicines.
13	Ensure that documentation is completed.	To ensure that the patient's details are kept up to date and also to ensure that information is available to ensure complete and accurate assessment.

Humidification can warm and moisten oxygen during administration. This should be considered in anyone who is receiving high concentrations of oxygen for more than a few hours. Humidification can help to prevent the mouth and the mucous membranes of the respiratory system drying out. It can also prevent sputum from becoming very thick and tenacious, which can prevent the patient from being able to expectorate.

Other factors to consider

The prolonged use of humidification equipment can cause problems in infection control. The moist oxygen-rich environment is ideal for the incubation of microorganisms. Therefore, sterile water is used. This needs to be changed regularly, sometimes as often as daily. The equipment must be changed according to the manufacturer's guidelines.

Patients who are receiving oxygen therapy because of breathlessness are generally affected in other activities of living and will require nursing care for these. Generally, they have reduced mobility, difficulty in washing and dressing themselves, and impaired eating and drinking functionality.

5.4 **Observation of cough and sputum and collection of a sputum sample**

Definition

Normally healthy people continuously produce mucus in the lungs but this is in small enough quantities to go unnoticed, and is either swallowed or reabsorbed. When this is in sufficient quantities to become noticeable as 'sputum',

which is coughed up into the mouth for swallowing or spitting, it is associated with respiratory disease and therefore, indicates something abnormal (Bennett 2003).

Observing sputum and reporting on its colour, amount (as well as if this has increased recently), consistency, and smell, can help medical staff diagnose a respiratory condition. Additionally, if the patient is producing sputum, a sample should be collected. This can then be examined and cultured in the laboratory for organisms, bronchial casts, eosinophils and cancer cells. Tests can be carried out to find which **antibiotics** the organisms are sensitive to and which, therefore, will kill them. This can help to decide which treatment is best to reduce the sputum.

Background

The linings of the airways leading into the lungs produce secretions that are wafted upwards by cilia and eventually coughed up as sputum. When lung cancers develop in these airway tissues, the sputum that forms near the growth will often contain cancer cells. By collecting and examining that sputum under a microscope using sputum cytology, lung cancer can now be diagnosed from a sputum specimen. If you are asked to collect a specimen of sputum you must find out if it is for cytology (cancer) or bacteriology (infection).

If active tuberculosis is suspected, then it is important to find out if tuberculosis mycobacteria are, in fact, present. Once a sputum sample is collected, this is stained in the laboratory to examine under a microscope and an attempt can be made to culture the organisms. If tuberculosis is suspected, it is important that the patient is kept away from other patients due to the risk of infection; especially if the patient has a productive cough.

Administration of humidified oxygen

Step		Rationale
1	Ensure privacy.	To prevent embarrassment and maintain dignity.
2	Gain patient consent.	To gain informed consent.
3	Cleanse hands prior to assisting.	To prevent cross-infection.
4	Explain procedure to the patient.	To gain cooperation and keep the patient informed.
5	Check the patient prescription chart for flow rate, dose, length of use, and delivery system.	To ensure correct prescription provided.
6	Collect the equipment required.	To obtain correct equipment.
7	Fill the humidifier with distilled water to the marked level.	To put water into the humidifier to moisten the oxygen.
8	Attach the humidifier to the flow meter.	To set up equipment.
9	Attach the oxygen tubing to the humidifier and the oxygen mask (or nasal cannula).	To set up equipment.
10	Attach face mask (or nasal cannula) to the patient's face.	To ensure correct fitting.
11	Set the flow meter at the correct prescribed rate in litres per minute.	To ensure correct dosage.
12	Ensure that the patient is comfortable.	To maintain patient's comfort.
13	Check regularly to ensure that the patient is receiving the correct dose.	To maintain correct administration of medicines.
14	Check regularly to see if the humidifier requires more distilled water.	To ensure that the humidifier does not dry out.
15	Sign for prescription with countersignature from registered nurse.	To ensure correct procedures for administration of medicines.
16	Ensure that documentation is completed.	To ensure that the patient's details are kept up to date and also to ensure that information is available to ensure complete and accurate assessment.

Observation of sputum

EQUIPMENT

- Sputum carton and lid
- Tissues
- Patient medical records
- Disposal bag and polythene bag

Action	Rationale
Ensure privacy.	To prevent embarrassment and maintain dignity.
Gain patient consent.	To gain informed consent.
Cleanse hands prior to assisting.	To prevent cross-infection.
Explain procedure to the patient.	To gain cooperation and keep the patient informed.
Look inside sputum carton and assess for colour, amount, consistency, and smell.	To assess the sputum.
Remove old sputum carton and replace lid.	To ensure no spillage of sputum.
Place sputum carton into disposal bag and polythene bag and tie in a knot.	To prevent spillage of sputum.
Dispose in accordance with local infection control policy; usually yellow waste bag for incineration.	To prevent contamination.
Provide patient with fresh clean sputum carton and lid.	To collect sputum for the next 24 hours.
Cleanse hands after the procedure.	To prevent cross-infection.
Ensure documentation into patient's records of colour, amount, consistency, and smell.	To ensure that patient's details are kept up to date and also to ensure that information is available to ensure complete and accurate assessment.

Obtaining a sputum sample

EQUIPMENT

- Dry wide neck specimen jar
- Pen
- Request form
- Hazard bag
- Patient's records
- Tissues
- Disposal bag

Key point: Some patients may find it unpleasant to have to cough up sputum into the jar. They should be offered a drink, mouthwash, or to brush their teeth afterwards to cleanse the mouth.

Action	Rationale
Ensure privacy.	To prevent embarrassment and maintain dignity.
Gain patient consent.	To gain informed consent.
Cleanse hands prior to assisting.	To prevent cross-infection.
Explain procedure to the patient.	To gain cooperation and keep the patient informed.
Ask the patient to take a deep breath and cough.	To assist with coughing up some sputum.
Ask the patient to expectorate any sputum coughed up into the dry wide specimen jar.	To collect the sputum in a sterile uncontaminated jar.
Offer the patient tissues to wipe any residual sputum from the face.	To help clean the patient after coughing up the sputum.
Seal the specimen jar.	To make sure that no sputum can come out of the jar.
Complete all the details on the specimen jar, including the ward, patient's name, identification number, and date of birth.	To record all the patient's details accurately on the jar and, therefore, not mix patients or samples up.
Insert specimen into biohazard bag and seal.	To prevent any harm to anyone while the specimen is in transit to the laboratory.
Complete the request form accurately.	To ensure that all the patient's details are recorded correctly and the laboratory are aware of the instructions.
Send the sputum specimen and request form to the laboratory.	To ensure that the laboratory receive the specimen quickly.
Cleanse hands after the procedure.	To prevent cross-infection.
Note in patient's records that a sample has been collected: record the date and time of collection.	To ensure that patient's record is kept up to date and also to ensure that information is available to ensure complete and accurate assessment.

To be able to assess sputum, the student nurse must be able to describe it using standard terminology, as listed in **Box 5.4**.

When to collect a patient's sputum

If a patient is coughing and producing sputum, then it is important that the nurse recognizes this and ensures that the patient always has a sputum carton, tissues, and a disposal bag. Coughing and deep breathing will aid the expectoration of mucous and, therefore, improve breathing, and so should be encouraged.

The best time to collect a sputum sample is first thing in the morning. There is more likely to be a large amount of organisms, since they may have been accumulating overnight in the lungs when respirations have been shallow and coughing minimized. Once the person begins to mobilize and breathe deeply, these secretions begin to loosen and can be coughed up and expectorated readily.

Generally sputum cartons (see **Fig. 5.11**) are collected for disposal from patients in a ward area once a day. This will differ from ward to ward, but is usually in the morning, before the day shift commence duty.

You should provide the patient with a fresh sputum carton, tissues, and disposal bag. The old sputum carton

Box 5.4 Terminology to describe sputum

Saliva	is clear watery fluid and is produced in the mouth. It has no respiratory significance.
White mucoid	is opalescent or white. This sputum is produced in the lungs and coughed into the mouth for expulsion: this can indicate asthma or bronchitis.
Mucopurlent sputum	is slightly discoloured mucus and **pus**, but not frank pus. Infection is normally present.
Purulent	is thick, viscous, and green or yellow. This can indicate a severe respiratory infection.
Haemoptysis	is bloodstained and can be bright red or dark brown in colour. It can indicate cancer, infection, such as tuberculosis, and sometimes localized trauma, for example, following a general **anaesthetic**, where an endotracheal tube was required.
Thick viscid	sputum can indicate asthma.
Frothy	is thin watery, is pink or white, and can indicate acute pulmonary oedema.

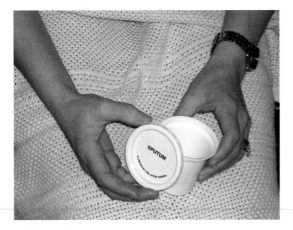

Figure 5.11 Sputum container

should have the lid securely in place and be put into a disposal bag and a clear polythene bag and tied in a knot. This should then be disposed according to the health and safety infection control regulations of the area in which you are working. This generally means that infected material, such as tissues and sputum cartons, should be collected in a yellow bag for incineration.

Aftercare

It is extremely important to document the colour, amount, and consistency of the sputum in the patient's record. Some patients will produce a large amount of sputum and, therefore, will require frequent checking if the sputum carton needs to be changed.

It is also important to document when a sputum sample has been collected and sent to the laboratory. It is equally important to check that the results return from the laboratory and that these are seen by medical staff when available. Normally, laboratory information systems report findings electronically. Only when the type of organism is known and its sensitivity to different antibiotics tested can the most appropriate treatment be prescribed.

Developing your skills

Some nurses find it extremely difficult to observe sputum for colour, amount, consistency, and smell, especially first thing in the morning after a night shift. However, it is a very important procedure to do and report on. Therefore, you will need to practice this skill to recognize the abnormal from the normal, as well as to cope with observing it.

Other factors to consider

Some patients can find it very difficult to expectorate very thick, viscous sputum. Providing the patient with a warm drink can help this. Also a **nebulizer** (see Section 2.6) with normal saline can assist in loosening the sputum from the lungs.

Sputum specimens can also be collected after physiotherapy treatment. Alerting the physiotherapist to the fact that a specimen is required will help to gain a specimen quickly. It is also possible to collect a sputum sample from the unconscious patient using suction equipment; however, this is a more advanced skill.

Scenarios

Consider what you should do in the following situations, then turn to the end of the section to check your answers.

Further scenarios are available at

🌐 **www.oxfordtextbooks.co.uk/orc/docherty/**

Scenario 1

You are assessing a gentleman who is 52 years old. He has been admitted for a number of reasons, but he is unwell and a full assessment is required. This means that you need to make a respiratory assessment. You observe that he has a pulse of 90 beats per minute, blood pressure of 105/60 mmHg and a respiratory rate of 24 breaths per minute. On general assessment, you note that he has nicotine-stained fingers and cold extremities (hands and feet). Your mentor suggests that you use pulse oximetry to record his oxygen saturation. Which would be the best site for pulse oximetry in this gentleman and why?

Scenario 2

You are working in the Accident and Emergency unit at a children's hospital. Maya, who is 20 months old, has been admitted with breathing problems. When you observe her in the single cubicle, she is highly distressed, screaming, acutely breathless, and sobbing, and her face is flushed. How best can you help to reduce Maya's anxiety to carry out a respiratory assessment?

Scenario 3

You are working on a medical ward and a young man, Rob, has been admitted from a community supported-living flat with aspiration pneumonia. He is very anxious, confused, unable to communicate with staff, and unable to tolerate any treatment. He needs oxygen therapy, but will not tolerate this. How are you going to help communicate with him in order to reduce his anxiety and assess his respiratory function?

Scenario 4

During the night a 55-year-old woman, Mrs White, was admitted with suspected pneumonia. She also has **dementia**. She is breathless, with a respiratory rate of 26 breaths per minute and an oxygen saturation of 90%. She has been commenced on oxygen therapy, but is not tolerating this well and keeps pulling the face mask off. How could you improve her tolerance of the oxygen therapy?

Website

🌐 **www.oxfordtextbooks.co.uk/orc/docherty/**
You may find it helpful to work through our short online quiz and interactive scenarios intended to help you to develop and apply the skills in this chapter.

References

Ahern J and Philpot P (2002). Assessing acutely ill patients on general wards. *Nursing Standard,* **16**(47), 54–7.

Allen K (2004). Principles and limitations of pulse oximetry in patient monitoring. *Nursing Times,* **100**(41), 34–7.

Bennett C (2003). Nursing the breathless patient. *Nursing Standard,* **17**(1), 45–51.

Butler-Williams C, Cantrill N, and Marton S (2005). Increasing staff awareness of respiratory rate significance. *Nursing Times,* **101**(27), 35–7.

Casey G (2001). Oxygen transport and the use of pulse oximetry. *Nursing Standard,* **15**(47), 46–60.

Considine J (2005). The role of nurses in preventing adverse events related to respiratory dysfunction: literature review. *Journal of Advanced Nursing,* **49**(6), 624–33.

Dunn L and Chisholm H (1998). Oxygen therapy. *Nursing Standard,* **13**(7), 57–64.

Jevon P and Ewens B (2001). Assessment of a breathless patient. *Nursing Standard,* **15**(16), 48–53.

Resuscitation Council UK (2005) *Resuscitation Council Guidelines 2005.* Resuscitation Council UK, London.

Simpson H (2006). Respiratory assessment. *British Journal of Nursing,* **15**(9), 484–8.

Woodrow P (1999). Pulse oximetry. *Nursing Standard,* **13**(42), 42–6.

Useful further reading and websites

British Thoracic Society (BTS) (2001) *The Burden of Lung Disease*. British Thoracic Society, London. www.brit-thoracic.org.uk/Portals/0/Library/BTS%20Publications/burden_of_lung_disease.pdf.

This document explains the prevalence of lung disease in the UK compared with Europe and the rest of the world.

Cuthbertson BH, Boroujerdi M, McKie L, Aucott L, and Prescott G (2007). Can physiological variables and early warning scoring systems allow early recognition of the deteriorating surgical patient? *Critical Care Medicine*, **35**(2), 402–9.

This article provides background to the use of early warning scoring charts and how they can help the nurse recognize a patient whose condition is deteriorating.

Department of Health (2000). *Guidelines for the Management of Acute Respiratory Failure in Normal Infants and Children (Excluding Upper Airway Obstruction)*. Department of Health, London

This government document provides guidelines for nurses who are providing care for children with respiratory diseases.

NICE (2006). *Clinical Diagnosis and Management of Tuberculosis and Measures for its Prevention and Control*. National Institute for Health and Clinical Excellence, London.

This NICE document provides detailed information on dealing with tuberculosis.

Scottish Executive (2004). *People with Learning Disabilities in Scotland: Health Needs Assessment Report*. Scottish Executive, Edinburgh.

This government document details care for patients with learning disabilities, no matter what physical illness they have.

Action for Smoking and Health (ASH). www.ash.org.uk/.

This site provides you with lots of information about stopping smoking and ways to give up. It also provides statistics about smoking.

British National Formulary. www.bnf.org/bnf/.

This site provides you with information on the drugs administered to patients. This can be found as a paper copy, but also on this online site.

Check 🌐 **www.oxfordtextbooks.co.uk/orc/docherty/** for changes and new developments. Updated research, guidelines, or equipment will be added every four months.

 # Answers to scenarios

 ## Scenario 1

This gentleman has cold hands and feet, so he probably has poor peripheral pulses here; this could also indicate vascular disease. Because of this and the obvious nicotine staining to his hands, his fingers and toes would not be the best site for pulse oximetry. The best site would, therefore, be the bridge of his nose.

Remember that the pulse oximeter could provide false readings with this man and you should use observation skills to check for cyanosis.

 ## Scenario 2

You need to calm Maya down before you can carry out an accurate assessment. It is best if someone Maya knows can comfort her. This might be her mother, father, a sibling, carer, and so on. Also if her family have brought with them Maya's favourite soft toy, or a comfort blanket, then she should have this.

 ## Scenario 3

Patients with a learning disability who are in assisted housing should have some record including details about how to communicate with them. This record should have come into hospital with Rob. It would be extremely helpful to get a carer or family member to come in and speak to the staff on how best to communicate with Rob. Additionally, if someone could stay to help with communication and encourage Rob to accept treatment this would be ideal.

 ## Scenario 4

Changing to a nasal cannula could help. Many patients do not like the face mask because they feel claustrophobic. Additionally, you might allow Mrs White's family or carers to be present at all times and not restrict them to visiting times. A familiar face may encourage her to continue with the treatment.

6 Eating and drinking

JACQUELINE MCCALLUM AND BRIDGET READE

Introduction

This chapter introduces the fundamental skills associated with eating and drinking and helps you assess and recognize any patients who are malnourished (which can be taken to mean either under- or overweight), dehydrated, or overhydrated.

Maintenance of a patient's nutrition and hydration are important both for physical and psychological well-being. Everyone needs nutrients so that the body can work properly and stay healthy. We need to take in nutrients in the form of calories, vitamins and minerals, carbohydrates, fats, vegetables, and protein by eating a balanced diet. A balanced diet includes a combination of food types: carbohydrates, proteins, certain fats, vitamins and minerals, and, of course, water, and fibre.

Having an inadequate or poorly balanced diet can lead to **malnutrition**. This can mean not eating enough, commonly referred to as protein–energy malnutrition (PEM) (Johnstone *et al.* 2006a). But it can also mean eating a lot of food that is low in nutrients, such as some 'fast foods'. In fact, it is possible to be obese and malnourished at the same time. Malnutrition leaves you prone to illness, and when you become ill, your body needs even more nutrients to help you recover.

Learning outcomes

These outcomes relate to numbers 9, 27, 28, 29, 30, and 31 of the NMC's Essential Skill Clusters and specifically to Care Domain 2 and 3 of the NMC's Standards of Proficiency for Pre-registration Nursing (outcomes to be achieved for entry to branch).

On reading the chapter and associated web pages and undertaking supervised activities, the student will be able to:

- Explain factors that can affect nutrition and hydration
- Describe the assessment of nutrition and hydration
- Explain the nurse's role in ensuring that adequate nutrition and hydration are maintained
- Recognize how to identify whether a patient has feeding requirements
- Describe how to help in feeding children and adults who require minimal and maximal assistance
- Provide details of special diets and how to ensure that the patient receives these
- Explain how to care for the patient who is nauseated or vomiting
- Define fluid balance and the factors that influence it
- Explain the importance of accurately completing a fluid balance chart
- Describe the problems that inadequate dentition causes for eating and drinking

Prior knowledge

To perform the clinical skills in this chapter it is important that you have related knowledge and understanding. This is obtainable from reference books that specialize in the sciences associated with nursing, such as biology, physiology, and chemistry. Key areas to learn for eating and drinking are

- The gastrointestinal (GI) system: how the normal GI system works from the mouth to the anus, in detail, including the swallowing **reflex**. You will need to know normal physiology in order to understand how it is affected by disease

- The renal system: how the kidneys filter blood to remove waste products and produce urine. The kidneys also have a role in maintaining a balance between **dehydration** and fluid overload. This is vital for **homeostasis**; the process of maintaining a stable environment inside the body
- Normal urea and electrolyte values: to recognize irregularities
- Muscle **contraction**: this relies on elements in the bloodstream that are derived from the diet, such as glucose and salts
- Wound healing: this requires a diet rich in nutrients, such as protein and the vitamins essential for tissue repair
- The body's response to stress, and how this can influence the way food is digested, absorbed, and used within the body

In addition to learning about the relevant physiology, it is also important to know what makes a balanced diet and the different constituent food groups.

Background

Nutrition has an impact on all areas of patient care. It has been estimated that between 20% and 40% of hospital patients in Europe are at risk of malnutrition (Kondrup *et al.* 2003). It is not unusual for people to lose their appetite when they are unwell. This may be because of the illness itself, the treatment, or the patients' fears and anxiety of being in hospital and what is wrong with them. In addition to this, being a hospital inpatient and having to conform to set mealtimes and set menus is not always easy. In addition to feeling less inclined to eat, patients will have a higher demand for energy, protein, vitamins, and minerals, as they attempt to recover from illness.

People of any age may suffer from eating and drinking problems, whether through acute life-threatening or chronic illnesses. As a student going to different placements in both hospital and community settings, you will encounter many patients who have problems with eating and drinking.

Some patients you encounter will have breaks in the integrity of their skin, either through their illnesses or as part of their treatment, such as surgery. A key factor in wound healing is nutrition: even in previously healthy individuals, extra protein, carbohydrate, and fats are required for collagen synthesis and repair. There is also a requirement for additional vitamin C, iron, and zinc, for scar tissue to develop and strengthen. These factors become increasingly important when caring for someone who is unwell or has had a chronic illness for some time. Remember, too, that in some illnesses, there are no external signs of tissue damage or the extent of the healing process required by the body, and that assessing appropriate dietary requirements requires knowledge of both the patients and their ailments.

Providing nutrition for patients has become something of a lower-priority nursing skill and this has received much publicity, particularly in the care of older adult patients. It is reported that many of these patients leave hospital more malnourished than when they entered. This concern extends to patients who are living in care homes, nursing homes, or residential care, where dietary inadequacies are sometimes reported. Additionally, many people living with learning disabilities live in their own homes but may still require support with nutrition.

The skills and knowledge related to eating and drinking have assumed less of a priority in nursing, as nurses have increasingly conflicting demands for their time. New roles for nurses have appeared in the past few years, requiring competence in technical skills, such as venepuncture and **cannulation**. In this context, assisting patients to eat has sometimes been regarded as a more humble activity that could be delegated to support staff. In fact, some care homes do not even have nurses on the staff. All of this can affect a patient's nutritional state. Despite this, assisting patients to eat remains one of the fundamental nursing skills and is vitally important. It is, therefore, imperative for the student nurse to learn about and gain the skills required to perform a nutritional assessment as well as the practicalities of how to feed a patient, how to record and evaluate dietary intake, and how to help patients gain an adequate balanced diet.

In the UK, the British Association of **Parenteral** and **Enteral** Nutrition (BAPEN 2003) help by providing ways of increasing the standards of assessing patient's nutrition as well as suggesting ways that the nurse can assist the patient to maintain an adequate dietary intake and prevent malnutrition in both hospital and community settings. There are equivalent organizations in America (ASPEN) and Europe (ESPEN) (Kondrup *et al.* 2002). This chapter will, therefore, help you acquire the skills to recognize patients who need assistance with eating and drinking, and to intervene effectively to help correct any tendency towards malnutrition.

6.1 **Nutritional assessment**

Definition

A nutritional assessment is an in-depth evaluation of both **objective** and **subjective** data related to the patient's food and nutrient intake, as well as lifestyle, and their medical or nursing history. The nutritional assessment is used to collect information on the patient's nutrition and identify individuals who require instruction or support to improve or maintain their nutritional status.

Once the information is collected, and the individual's nutritional status is assessed, this should then lead to a plan of care, featuring interventions designed to help patients to maintain their current nutritional state or, where necessary, to move towards a healthier nutritional state. Nutritional assessment also identifies 'at-risk' patients, who require a more in-depth assessment, perhaps including referral to specialists from the multidisciplinary team. For these reasons, it is important to carry out a nutritional assessment as early as possible so that appropriate treatment is carried out.

Background

Malnutrition can cause problems with the body's functioning. You may notice that the person slows down or does not perform activities as well as usual. It can take longer for wounds to heal and to recover from infections. The individual may find it harder to stay warm, and may feel tired or depressed.

The following problems may be caused by malnutrition:

- Impaired immune response (and susceptibility to disease)
- Reduced muscle strength and fatigue

- Breathing difficulties as a result of muscle fatigue
- Depression, self-neglect and impaired social function can lead to malnutrition, but malnutrition can also lead to these problems
- Poor wound healing through lack of essential components, such as vitamins and proteins
- Poor **libido** (sexual drive), fertility, and pregnancy problems
- Water and electrolyte disturbances, such as dehydration or oedema
- Impaired **thermoregulation** (regulation of body temperature by the brain)
- Vitamin deficiencies that can cause diseases such as rickets and scurvy

In children there can be:

- Failure to achieve maximum growth potential (referred to as **stunting**)
- Developmental delay
- Increase in **morbidity** and **mortality**

It is helpful to use more than one method of assessing the patient's nutritional status. The data required for completing a nutritional assessment fall into four categories (NHS Quality Improvement Scotland 2003):

1 Anthropometric (height and weight = **body mass index**, BMI),
2 **Biochemical** (can be obtained by a nurse, doctor, or phlebotomist),
3 Clinical features and verbal history,
4 Dietary history (for example, food or activity diary).

When to perform the nutritional assessment of a patient

In the UK, it is mandatory for every patient admitted to hospital or a community care setting; or on a first visit to a general practitioner or NMPDU 2002; consultant, to have a nutritional assessment carried out (NMPDU 2002; NHS Quality Improvement Scotland 2003; NICE 2006). Admission to a care environment can be a distressing time for any patient. It is especially important with children and people with a learning disability that you carry out an initial assessment to obtain a baseline assessment on their nutritional status.

Recording anthropometric measurements (body mass index)

Anthropometric measurements are measurements of the human body (Johnstone *et al.* 2006b) that can provide information on current nutritional and growth status. There are a number of tools to take such measurements. An example of such a tool is the Malnutrition Universal Screening Tool (MUST), which is shown in **Fig. 6.1** (BAPEN 2003; Todorvic *et al.* 2003). This consists of five steps, providing a score identifying the patient's risk of malnutrition and whether they are under- or overweight.

The most common tool is the body mass index (BMI), which is a function of height and weight. The BMI provides a quick and easy way to interpret the patient's nutritional requirements. References are used to standardize the measurement by comparing the person's measurement with the median or average measure for a reference population of healthy people of the same age and sex. The BMI can be used to identify patients who are underweight, at desirable weight, overweight, or very overweight (see **Fig 6.2**).

It must be noted, however, that the BMI is used differently in children and adults. In adults, the BMI is calculated from the weight and height. In children, age-related growth and body fat gain must be acknowledged. There are separate charts for adults and children.

Ensure that all the required documentation and the appropriate version of the assessment tool are available. Hips and waist can also be measured to calculate the patient's hip:waist ratio.

The World Health Organization (WHO) classifies patients into different categories according to their BMI, as shown in **Box 6.1**. A BMI of between 20 and 25 is the most desirable and appropriate weight for most people.

Procedure: measuring and recording a patient's height

It is important to measure a patient's height rather than just taking the patient's word for it. When people become older, they can lose centimetres (or inches) from their original height. This can occur through **osteoporosis** and the spine shrinking and pushing downwards, as well as a result of the effect of gravity. Thus, adults will be shorter when older than when they were in their teens or twenties and may not have measured their height for a long time. Similarly children can grow quickly and may not know their current height with any accuracy. It is, therefore, important to take the time to measure height.

Other factors to consider

Some patients may be bedbound, either at home or in hospital, and, therefore, it becomes very difficult to measure their height. Some patients may have asymmetrical body shapes that can make it difficult for them to stand straight, however, it is still equally important to record height for these patients. There are a number of ways that this can be achieved.

Measuring arm span

One method is by measuring arm span (Johnstone *et al.* 2006b) to achieve an estimate of a person's height. This can be achieved using a measuring tape. The patient's arm is extended. The length from the notch in the sternum to the tip of the fingertips is measured, and this measurement is doubled (**Fig. 6.3**). Although this is an *estimate* of height it may be the best option to obtain height for some patients in some circumstances.

Supine measurement

Another option is to carry out a **supine** (lying flat) measurement. To do this, position the patient on a bed without pillows. The patient should lie as flat as possible with body and limbs straight. Mark the surface at the tip of the head and base of the heels. Move the patient and measure the length of the flat surface.

Measuring an infant's length

An infant's length (it is referred to as height when the infant can stand) can be measured using a simple tape measure at home, although this can be unreliable. A supine measuring device should be used when available (Corkins *et al.* 2002). To obtain a correct measurement, it will be necessary to lay the baby on his or her back. Position the baby's head against the top of the board, as shown in

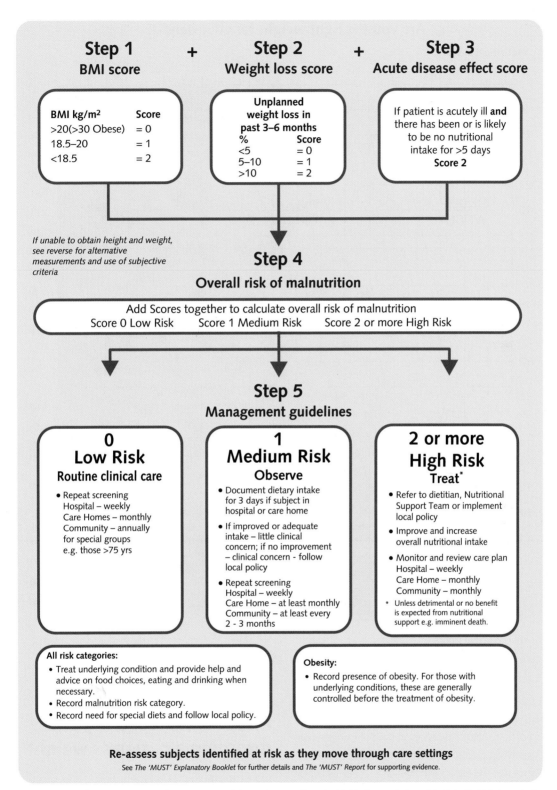

Figure 6.1 Malnutrition Universal Screening Tool (MUST). Reproduced with kind permission of BAPEN (British Association for Parenteral and Enteral Nutrition)

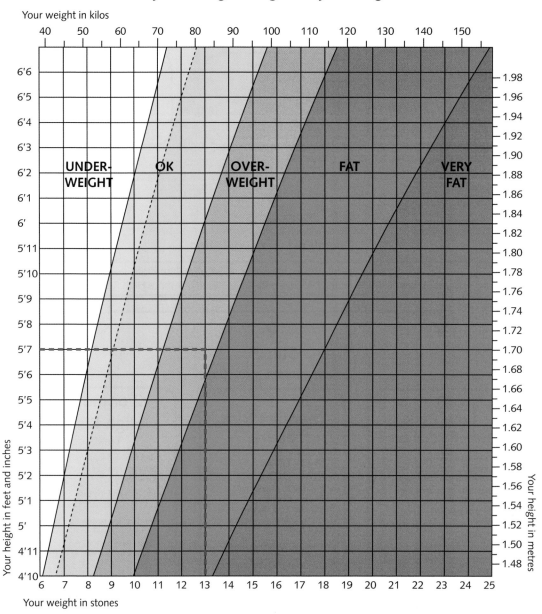

Figure 6.2 Body mass index (BMI) chart for adults. Courtesy of the Food Standards Agency.

Fig. 6.4. The baby's knees are held together and pressed down gently. It may be necessary to have one person hold the infant while another measures. The child must be completely aligned and flat against the board. Check with local policy, since in some areas students must have the measurement checked by a qualified nurse. Your mentor would be an ideal person to watch you perform this task.

Procedure: Measuring and recording a patient's weight

Just as height can vary, so too can a person's weight. This is very important to note, especially if the patient has been unwell for some time, since he or she may not be obtaining the correct nutritional support that is

Box 6.1 WHO classification of BMI

BMI range, kg/m2	Weight category
<18.5	Underweight
18.5–20	Underweight
20–25	Desirable weight
25–30	Overweight
>30	Very overweight

required when unwell. Children grow quickly and may not know their weight. Again check with local policy, since in some areas students must have the measurement checked by a qualified nurse. Your mentor would be an ideal person to watch you perform this task.

It is important for the nurse to measure the patient's weight rather than recording the patient's estimate. This can be done on standing scales, chair scales, bed scales, ramp scales, or hoist scales, depending on the patient's physical condition.

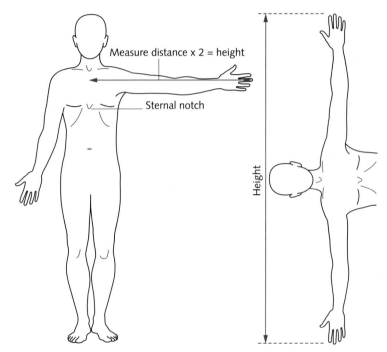

Measure distance x 2 = height

Sternal notch

Height

Figure 6.3 Measuring arm span

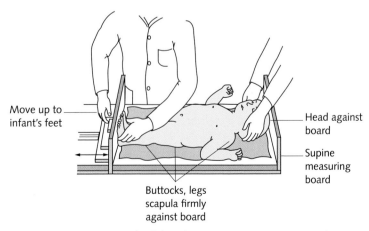

Move up to infant's feet

Head against board

Supine measuring board

Buttocks, legs scapula firmly against board

Figure 6.4 Measuring an infant's length using a supine measurement device

Measuring and recording a patient's height

EQUIPMENT

- Height stick (stadiometer) positioned against a wall or tape measure
- Pen

Key point: Height and weight are used to calculate a patient's calorie, protein, and fluid needs. If data are inaccurate then these calculations will also be inaccurate.

Step	Rationale
1 Cleanse hands prior to the assessment.	To prevent cross-infection.
2 Explain the assessment to the patient.	To facilitate informed **consent**.
3 Gain patient consent.	To gain cooperation.
4 Ensure privacy.	To prevent embarrassment and maintain dignity.
5 Ask the patient to remove shoes.	To ensure correct height measurement.
6 Ask the patient to stand upright against the height stick or wall.	To ensure accurate measurement.
7 Ask the patient to look straight ahead.	To ensure that patient is standing up straight.
8 Read the documented height in metres and centimetres.	To take the measurement.
9 Inform the patient of the measurement.	To keep patient informed.
10 Cleanse hands after the assessment.	To prevent cross-infection.
11 Record the height in notes or assessment tool.	To document the measurement accurately.

Other factors to consider

Weighing patients in wheelchairs, or who are bedbound, can be more challenging. There are mechanical scales that wheelchairs can be wheeled onto, allowing an accurate calculation of the patient's weight. You must also remember to take the weight of the wheelchair off the total weight of the patient in the wheelchair. There are also devices that can be attached to mechanical hoists: these weigh the patient when the hoist and patient are lifted.

Procedure: Calculating the BMI

The BMI of the patient can be calculated from the height and weight, or using a BMI chart.

Measuring and recording an adult's weight

EQUIPMENT

- Clinical scales (make sure that they are calibrated to zero)
- Pen

Key points: Medication doses are often prescribed based on weight. An inaccurate weight could result in an over- or underdose of medication.

In some cases, daily weights might be indicated, therefore, time of day and timing in relation to eliminating and eating or drinking should be consistent.

Step		Rationale
1	Cleanse hands prior to the assessment.	To prevent cross-infection.
2	Explain the assessment to the patient.	To facilitate informed consent.
3	Gain patient consent.	To gain cooperation.
4	Ensure privacy.	To prevent embarrassment and maintain dignity.
5	Ensure that scales are set at zero.	To prevent inaccurate reading.
6	Weigh the patient in light clothing without shoes.	To prevent clothing from adding additional weight.
7	Read the weight in kilograms.	To take the measurement.
8	Cleanse hands after the assessment.	To prevent cross-infection.
9	Inform the patient of the measurement.	To keep patient informed.
10	Record the weight in notes or assessment tool.	To accurately document the measurement.

$$BMI = weight\ (kg) \div height\ (m)^2$$

Example: if a patient weights 65 kg and has a height of 165 cm, the BMI will be BMI = $65/(1.65)^2$ = 65/2.72 = 23.9 (which can be found from the chart in **Fig. 6.2** to be within the normal range).

This calculation should then be recorded in the patient's clinical notes or the nutrition assessment tool.

Recording biochemical measurements

Laboratory tests based on blood and urine samples can help determine the patient's nutritional status or any deficiencies (lack of something) in specific vitamins and minerals. For example, it is useful to measure iron levels when the patient has **anaemia** (lack of red blood cells), since

Measuring and recording an infant's weight

EQUIPMENT

- Clinical scales (make sure that they are calibrated to zero)
- Pen

Key points: It is important to check the local policy about weighing a baby who is wearing a nappy. Some areas state that the nappy should always be removed. Other areas stipulate that keeping the nappy on will protect dignity and privacy for the infant. Remember the nappy has to be weighed and this weight taken off the weight obtained for the infant wearing the nappy, to obtain the correct weight.

Step	Rationale
1 Cleanse hands prior to the assessment.	To prevent cross-infection.
2 Explain the assessment to the infant and parent.	To relax the infant. To facilitate informed consent.
3 Gain parental consent.	To gain cooperation.
4 Ensure privacy.	To prevent embarrassment and maintain dignity.
5 An apron should be worn, since the infant will be lifted.	To prevent cross-infection.
6 Check local policy, but usually the nappy is taken off.	To gain an accurate weight.
7 Ensure that the scales are set at zero.	To reduce inaccurate reading.
8 Weigh the infant with no clothing or nappy (check local policy).	To prevent clothing from adding additional weight.
9 Read the weight in kilograms.	To take the measurement.
10 Cleanse hands after the assessment.	To prevent cross-infection.
11 Inform the parent of the measurement.	To keep family informed.
12 Record the weight in notes or assessment tool.	To document the measurement accurately.

iron in the diet is required by the bone marrow to help make red blood cells. Testing the patient's red blood cell count (RBC) is carried out with a test called 'full blood count' (FBC), which tests for white and red blood cells, haemoglobin, and platelets. Haemoglobin is the molecule that gives blood its colour and is essential to oxygen transport: the major constituent of haemoglobin is iron.

When some major organs of the body malfunction, this can cause nutritional and dietary problems. Common examples are the **thyroid** gland and pancreas. The thyroid gland, located in the neck, regulates metabolic rate through the hormones it produces. Overproduction can cause weight loss by causing an increase in the patient's metabolic rate: energy is expended through increased activity and heat production. Conversely, underproduction can cause weight gain as a result of the metabolism slowing down.

The pancreas, located in the abdomen, has two broad functions: firstly it secretes enzymes that help with digestion. Secondly, the pancreas has an endocrine function in producing insulin, a hormone required to metabolize carbohydrate, fat, and proteins. To put it simply, if the pancreas reduces its secretion of insulin, this can lead to the chronic disease diabetes mellitus and this has serious consequences for health.

It is, therefore, important that you learn the normal and abnormal physiology associated with the major organs of the body. Additionally, learning the normal levels of components of the blood will help you to quickly recognize when blood test results are abnormal and can help you understand diseases that can affect the patient's nutrition and health.

Electrolytes are chemical compounds that are obtained from food and drink. They commonly exist as solutions of acids, bases, or salts present in the body fluids, and their concentrations are closely regulated. Determining the levels of these chemicals in the bloodstream is a commonly performed blood test. It is usually carried out on admission to hospital as a routine test, especially when it is suspected that the patient might be dehydrated. Electrolytes are measured in the serum of blood specimens. The chemicals routinely tested are shown in **Box 6.2**.

It is essential to maintain electrolytes at their correct concentrations, and homeostatic mechanisms exist for this purpose. If there is too much or too little of some of these electrolytes, problems can develop. An extreme example is that if potassium is dangerously low or high then cardiac **arrhythmia** (irregular heartbeat) can be

Box 6.2 Normal ranges for electrolytes in blood serum		
Urea		2.5–6.4 mmol/l
Creatinine		60–120 mmol/l
Sodium	Na	135–145 mmol/l
Potassium	K	3.5–5.3 mmol/l
Calcium	Ca	2.1–2.6 mmol/l
Magnesium	Mg	0.75–1.0 mmol/l
Chloride	Cl	97–106 mmol/l
Phosphate	PO_3, PO_4	0.8–1.4 mmol/l
Bicarbonate	HCO_3	35–45 mmol/l

These figures may vary, according to guidelines adopted locally.

triggered. These cause problems with the conduction and rhythm of the heart and can be life-threatening. Another example is muscle contraction, which requires calcium (Ca^{2+}), sodium (Na^+), and potassium (K^+). Without the correct balance of these key electrolytes, muscle weakness or severe uncontrollable muscle contractions may occur.

Recording clinical information

It is important to obtain a full assessment and history from the patient, or the family in the case of an infant or child, and involve the health facilitator in the case of a patient with learning disabilities if there is one. This can reveal important factors affecting the patient's nutritional status. It is important to ask the patient questions about past medical history, which includes any acute or chronic illnesses (for example vomiting), any recent treatment, investigations, and medications, including prescribed drugs and over-the-counter preparations. All of this requires good communication skills; a nonjudgemental attitude towards the patient's eating habits, and accurate documentation (see Chapter 4). A number of key questions can help (see Box 6.3).

This information will assist in planning individual nutritional requirements for the patient. Those patients who are identified as being at risk of malnutrition will require a more detailed assessment. The interpretation of this data

Box 6.3 Questions to ask when taking a patient history

- Has the patient been eating a normal varied and healthy diet recently?

- How many meals does the patient eat in a day?

- What time of day does the patient eat meals?

- Who buys the food and prepares the meals?

- Does the patient have any financial constraints for buying food?

- Does the patient take any additional vitamins or supplements?

- Has the patient been 'nil by mouth' or had other dietary restrictions in place?

- Can the patient eat, swallow, digest, and absorb sufficient food to meet his or her requirements?

- Has the patient had major surgery, a chronic illness, severe infection, sepsis, cancer, or been severely burned?

- Does the patient have a physical illness that will affect the diet, for example diabetes or cardiac failure?

- Does the patient have a psychiatric condition, such as depression or an eating disorder?

- Does the patient have any specific likes or dislikes for food?

- Does the patient have any food allergies?

- Does the patient have any identified medical dietary requirements, as in diabetes, for example?

- Does the patient have any cultural, ethnic, or religious requirements?

will require judgement and setting the individual's behaviours and patterns against the clinician's values. For example—how do you judge a 'normal, varied, and healthy diet'? Remember when examining the patient's diet to take into account your own diet and BMI and consider whether your patient views you as a role model providing reliable and credible information.

Inadequate dentition for mastication (chewing) is one of the major issues associated with ill health for older adults who are in hospital or community care. This is especially the case because dental status is strongly related to age, meaning that the older the patient the more problems there will be with their teeth. As a person ages, the gums tend to recede; teeth become loose and are prone to fall out. Equally, those who wear dentures will find that they do not fit snugly when gums shrink.

When assessing a patient's ability to eat, especially in an older adult, you must first check that the patient has adequate dentition, otherwise you will have to provide a soft diet. Many patients have ill-fitting dentures and prefer not to wear them; again they will require a soft diet. If the patient has well-fitting dentures, you should ensure that they are cleaned and given to the patient to wear prior to mealtime.

Remember that young children have deciduous dentition, commonly known as 'milk teeth'. These are the first teeth, which erupt from about six months of age. Mixed dentition is present from the ages of about six (when the first milk teeth fall out) to about the age of twelve. Permanent dentition (up to 32 teeth) is usually complete by the mid-teens, although the third molars (wisdom teeth) may not appear until around the age of 21. Children can also be born with a cleft **palate** or hare lip. These will cause feeding problems and surgical intervention may be required to correct the deformity.

Dental hygiene and the appearance of an individual's teeth can have a profound effect on body image. Most people are very aware of how their teeth look; if they are in good condition and look clean and healthy. Any problems with teeth can have both painful and psychological consequences. Children may need assistance with **oral hygiene** and brushing teeth and this must be remembered.

Recording dietary information

It is also important to take an accurate account of the patient's individual diet. This is especially so if the patient is following a specific diet, perhaps because of a medical condition, such as diabetes, or for religious reasons. Information about any allergies or dislikes is particularly important, as too is information on caffeine and alcohol intake. It is important to speak to patients and listen to what they have to say about their diet so as to avoid making assumptions based on preconceived ideas about their condition or religion. Attempt to gain your knowledge and understanding based on the patient's individual preferences. Again, it may be necessary to involve the parent or guardian of a child or the health facilitator of a patient with learning disabilities.

Social information, such as the patient's job or the amount of exercise taken, can be important, since this will give some indication of how many calories are burnt generally in one day. This can help to plan for a patient's discharge or if the patient is transferring from one healthcare facility to another. Knowing who does the shopping, prepares meals, and so on, is essential so that any realistic changes can be planned. There is an issue in targeting health education at the right people: for example there is no point educating an older man on a low-fat diet, and so on, if his wife continues to cook for him in the same way that she has done for the past 50 years.

It is helpful to find out how many meals a day the patient has, where they are eaten and who prepares them. Many older adults in the community rely on meals on wheels for at least one substantial meal per day. Patients with learning disabilities may need support when preparing their meals.

Aftercare

Correct documentation in the patient clinical notes or person-centred plan is very important for continuity of care. Whatever nutritional assessment tool is used should be included in the clinical notes. If the patient is at risk, a referral should be made to members of the multidisciplinary team. This may differ, depending on the clinical environment. In some or most instances there may be a dietician, pharmacist, public health nurse, clinical nurse specialist, or community learning disability nurse for the nurse to make a referral to.

Developing your skills

It is essential to become accustomed to, and practice the skill of nutritional assessment for patients in acute care and community settings. It is also highly important that the patient is assessed and re-evaluated at appropriate times depending on the level of malnutrition. You should try and practice assessing a patient's nutritional status on your next placement. Remember that if your patient is malnourished you will need some expert help from the

qualified nursing staff and the multiprofessional team, to identify and address dietary deficiencies.

Remember that it is very important to listen to what your patients have to say. Do not assume what their diet may be. Remember that every patient is an individual and, therefore, deserves to be treated as such.

It improves confidence if you become familiar with the equipment that you are using, such as pumps. This means that you may have to ask your mentor to explain how to use it, including how to clean it afterwards. It is also necessary to know how to check that the equipment is working before use and what to do if it breaks down. Preparation of yourself and the equipment is vitally important prior to practising the skill.

Other factors to consider

Lifespan changes

Recognize that there are different dietary requirements through different ages. A growing child will have a higher metabolism and, therefore, greater energy and nutrient requirements than an older adult. This is particularly noticeable during puberty, when the child is rapidly growing and developing. It is important to ensure that teenagers receive enough energy and nutrients through their diet; however, a balance has to be struck to prevent them becoming overweight. This can be achieved by providing healthy snacks, such as fruit and vegetables, rather than sugary snacks, in between meals.

Sugary food

It is important to be able to recognize which foods are sugary and should be avoided for good dental health. It is not the amount of sugary foods that are eaten that causes tooth decay, but the number of times that the teeth are in contact with sugary foods. Therefore, limiting this to meal times only will reduce the attack on the patient's teeth. Health promotion should include encouraging nonsugary snacks in between meals.

Obesity

Obesity is a growing problem in Western society and its prevalence is increasing amongst children. Although malnutrition is not always caused by obesity, you should be aware that it is a concern. Type 1 diabetes is the most common form of diabetes in children in the UK. Of those children, who have diabetes, 90–95% of them have Type 1. This is caused by a defect in the immune system, which leads to destruction of the insulin-producing beta cells in the pancreas, so that the pancreas is unable to produce insulin. Type 2 diabetes, on the other hand, is extremely complex. There is an underlying genetic susceptibility that, when exposed to a variety of social, behavioural, and environmental factors, triggers the onset of diabetes. There has also been a strong link between childhood obesity and Type 2 diabetes.

If obesity is life-threatening then surgery may be an option, however, more commonly it is diet-controlled with encouragement to change behaviour and do more physical activity. In many cases, obesity is controlled and treated in the community care setting, and the nurse's role is to assess the patient regularly and provide advice and support.

Older people

Malnutrition is more serious among the older adult. The senses of taste and smell reduce with ageing, which can lead to a reduced appetite. Additionally, the older adult may prefer foods that are saltier or sweeter because of changes to taste buds. Added to this are dental problems and a reduced ability to chew certain foods, such as steak. Furthermore, ageing brings with it more illnesses such as **arthritis**, visual, and hearing problems, which can have an affect on how the older adult can shop for and prepare food. A nutritional assessment tool called the Mini Nutritional Assessment (MNA®) (Guigoz *et al.* 1994) has been specifically developed for the older adult.

It is, therefore, important as a student to be aware that the nutritional requirements of older adults may be more challenging. The nurse's role is to ensure that these are met. Remember that although a balanced diet with reduced fat and sugar intake is important in the older adult, it is also important to recognize that some older adults have poor appetites, and, therefore, a balance has to be made.

Metabolism decreases with age and so, too, does physical activity. However, although the energy requirement decreases with age, the actual nutrient requirement remains the same. In some cases, the older adult has an increased requirement for specific nutrients. For example, although physical activity is the best way of preventing osteoporosis, this may not be possible for older adults and, therefore, it is important to ensure that they are receiving the correct amount of calcium in their diet. Also the older adult may lack exposure to the sun and, therefore, have less opportunity to synthesize vitamin D which is essential for the absorption of calcium.

Ethical issues

There are many legal and ethical issues under debate in relation to withdrawing or withholding nutritional support for patients who can no longer feed themselves and whose medical condition offers no hope of improvement, for example in patients with severe brain damage or in a persistent vegetative state. To explore this in more detail, there are examples and detailed debates in most nursing ethics textbooks.

Religious and ethical beliefs

Remember that religious and ethical beliefs will influence the patient's food intake. Religious beliefs can affect not only food choices but also preparation and cooking methods. Various religions also have dietary restrictions. Some groups, such as Hindus and some Rastafarians, completely omit meat, while others restrict specific types of meat or animal products. Muslims and Jews, for example, do not consume pork and pork products, among other foods, while shellfish is avoided by Rastafarians.

Veganism
A vegan is someone seeking a lifestyle free from animal products for the benefit of people, animals, and the environment. A vegan, therefore, eats a plant-based diet free from all animal products, including milk, eggs, and honey.

Hinduism

Devout Hindus believe that all of God's creatures are worthy of respect and compassion, regardless of whether they are human beings or animals. Therefore, Hinduism encourages vegetarianism and avoiding eating any animal meat or flesh. However, not all Hindus choose to practice vegetarianism, and they may choose varying degrees of strictness. Some Hindus don't eat beef and pork, which are strictly prohibited in the Hindu diet code, but do eat other meats.

Rastafarianism

Rastafarians believe that food should be natural, or pure, and from the earth. Therefore, they avoid food that is chemically modified or contains artificial additives. Some also avoid added salt in foods. In strict interpretations, foods that have been produced using chemicals such as pesticides and fertilizer are not considered edible. Like many other religions, Rasta prohibits the eating of pork. Some Rastas also avoid eating shellfish because, in common with pigs, they are considered to be scavengers.

Islam

For a Muslim to eat food, it must be halal, meaning lawful. A Muslim should not drink alcohol, eat or drink blood or its by-products, or pork, and cannot eat the meat of other animals, such as chicken, beef, and lamb, without special preparation. The majority of Muslims consider fish and shellfish (including crabs, lobsters, shrimp, crayfish, and all nonpoisonous molluscs) to be halal. For meat to be considered halal, it must be slaughtered by a Muslim who pronounces the Name of Allah before killing the animal by cutting its throat, and the animal is then bled to death.

Judaism

Food must be what is termed kosher (meaning 'fit') for a Jew to be able to eat it. Kosher land animals have cloven hoofs and chew their cud (therefore, cows and most herbivores can be kosher, but pigs and all carnivores are not kosher). All birds are kosher, except for birds of prey. Kosher marine life must have fins and scales and may not be scavengers. Additionally, meat and dairy products may not be mixed, and traditional kosher Jewish homes will have separate dishes, cookware, and utensils for meat and dairy products.

6.2 **Assisting patients with eating and drinking**

Definition

You will come across many patients who require assistance with eating and drinking. Feeding, therefore, is when you have to provide the food and nourishment for patients who are unable to do this themselves. Nutrition is defined as the act or process of nourishing or being nourished. Food, as you are aware, is essential to the growth, **sustenance**, maintenance, and operation of the body.

On admission, the patient's nutritional needs are assessed using the appropriate assessment tool (see Section 6.1). This assessment will give the nurse the information required to ensure that the individual's nutritional needs are met. The challenges of feeding can vary from patient to patient.

Factors affecting the need for assistance to eat and drink include:

- Acute illness
- Chronic illness
- Physical disability
- Mental health issues, for example, depression
- Terminal illness
- Dentition
- Socio-economic status, which may affect quality of food choices

It is important that a multidisciplinary approach is taken to ensure that appropriate nutritional needs are met with the chosen feeding strategy. Medical staff will be aware of any additional dietary requirements from blood samples taken. The dietician my be involved if the body mass index (BMI) indicates that the patient is under- or overweight.

When to assist a patient with eating and drinking

It is only necessary to assist in feeding an adult or child if all other options for maintaining self-care have been tried and are unsuccessful. There are patients who need to be fed, but encouraging independence is important. Therefore, the assessment of nutrition is vitally important.

Patients with **dementia**

You may encounter patients with dementia on many of your clinical placements. The behavioural, **emotional**, and physical changes that take place as dementia progresses can all have an impact on a person's eating habits and on their intake of food and drink.

Eating and drinking difficulties for patients with dementia are very common. Many of these difficulties are a result of behavioural problems, such as craving food or needing cues to start eating. Nurses in this specialist setting are competent to deal with these behavioural difficulties and the student nurse can learn from this. A small number of patients may need to be referred to specialist nurses for eating or drinking difficulties.

In some states in the USA, it is more common to use percutaneous endoscopic gastrostomy (PEG) feeding for older people with an eating disorder. However, in the UK, PEGs are not routinely available to people with dementia. Heavy reliance is placed on a thorough assessment and appropriate strategies to assist with eating, rather than resorting to **invasive** techniques at an early stage, as many simple tasks can improve the patient's eating and drinking habits. In different circumstances, PEGs are used for individuals who have chronic **dysphagia** because of a stroke, multiple sclerosis, or muscular dystrophy.

Assessing a patient's feeding needs

The patient's needs will be assessed on first contact with the healthcare worker, and care will be planned, implemented, evaluated, and reassessed continually. The activities-of-living framework provides a good way of gaining information to assess the patient's overall needs. However, there are different nursing models that can be used for this purpose: you should be aware of what is used in the area you are working in.

Mealtimes can be an ideal time for assessment. Observe the assistance required from staff as well as the person's ability to eat and drink without help. Food assessment charts may be used over a three-day period to assess the patient's intake (see **Fig. 6.5**). This can then help to provide a guide to the dietary requirements that are not being met.

Whilst the food assessment is carried out, it is important for the nurse to assess the patient's ability to eat and drink. This is achieved from the information given on first contact with the patient and also from observation of the patient.

Procedures: Assisting a patient with eating and drinking

It is important, socially and psychologically, that all patients are out of bed for their meals unless this would cause concern or make their condition or illness worse. If this is the case, then this will be documented in their care plan and rationale provided.

The dining area should be away from the main ward or living area. If possible, the patient should be seated at a table with other patients to maintain the social aspect of eating. Sitting at a table with others can promote a sense of well-being. Be aware, however, that some patients' eating habits can be off-putting for other patients. Some patients who have swallowing difficulties may cough or gag on their food, and this can be distressing to others sitting at the table.

Key point: When it is not possible for the patient to sit with others at the table then the nurse should ensure that the reasons for this are explained to the patient. It may be that there are no dining facilities in that particular area. Another reason may be that the patient's condition merits that he or she stays at the bedside.

Preparation

The nurse should always ensure that the patient's needs are attended to prior to mealtimes:

- The patient may want to dress for meals, so ensure that this is attended to if possible

Assessment of the patient's feeding skills

EQUIPMENT
- Food assessment chart
- Appropriate cutlery
- Correct seating
- Adequate fluids
- Pen

Step		Rationale
1	Gain patient consent.	To gain cooperation.
2	Ask if patient is on any special diet due to his or her condition.	To ensure the appropriate diet is ordered and supplied to the patient.
3	Ask if the patient uses any special cutlery or table equipment.	To ensure independence and prevent embarrassment to the patient.
4	Ask if the patient would prefer a relative or carer to assist where needed.	To prevent embarrassment and promote familiarity for the patient.
5	Ask if the patient would like protective clothing.	To prevent spillage to clothes if appropriate.
6	Inform the patient of the documentation being used.	To include patient in process.
7	Complete documentation.	To ensure accurate assessment.

- Ensure that the patient has been offered toileting and hand washing facilities
- If it isn't possible to have a separate dining area, remove unpleasant and off-putting sights and sounds from the environment (such as **commodes**) to enhance the patient's appetite

It is necessary to ensure that the patient has the correct setting for meal times. It is also important to provide napkins. A member of staff should be nearby to provide assistance when needed.

Equipment

There are a number of utensils that can assist the patient in maintaining self-care when eating and drinking. A selection is shown in **Fig. 6.6**.

Grip cutlery

This is lightweight, soft, and contoured. These stainless steel utensils feature handles designed for hands with limited grasping ability. The handles have a soft, rubbery, nonslip surface. They are also dishwasher safe.

```
┌──────────────────────────────────────────────────────────────┐
│  PATIENT ID LABEL                    PATIENT WEIGHT ............ │
│                                      PATIENT HEIGHT ............ │
│                                      PATIENT BMI ............... │
│  WARD ...................                                        │
│                   Date        Date         Date                 │
│                   Day 1       Day 2        Day 3                 │
│  Breakfast                                                      │
│                                                                │
│  Mid morning                                                   │
│                                                                │
│  Lunch                                                         │
│                                                                │
│  Mid afternoon                                                 │
│                                                                │
│  Dinner                                                        │
│                                                                │
│  Other snacks                                                  │
│                                                                │
│  Comments                                                      │
└──────────────────────────────────────────────────────────────┘
```

Figure 6.5 Food assessment chart

Utensil holder

This is comfortable and fully adjustable to meet the user's particular condition and hand size (see **Fig. 6.7**). It is ideal for children and adults with little or no hand strength. It holds eating utensils, toothbrushes, or other small items.

Clothes protector

This is made of wipe-clean vinyl and has a bib. It offers clothing protection during mealtime, so that you can focus on the food rather than being careful. A continuous bottom cuff handily catches spilled food particles and liquids.

Drinking cup with spout

These are generally clear plastic feeding cups with a lid and spout. The spout is fairly wide, making it ideal for semi-solid and puréed food. See the example in Figure 6.8.

Plate guard

The plate guard is made of plastic and snaps around most normal-sized plates. One part is left open to allow the patient to gain access to the food, but the guard prevents accidental spillage of food. The plate guard provides a surface against which the person can push a fork or spoon to help pick up food.

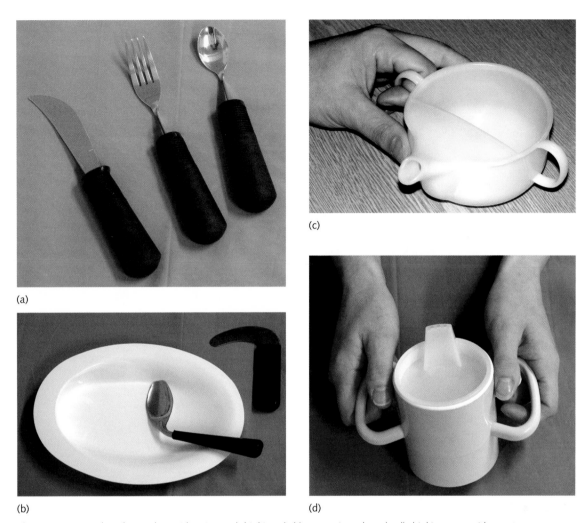

(a)

(b)

(c)

(d)

Figure 6.6 Examples of utensils to aid eating and drinking: (a,b) easy-grip cutlery, (c, d) drinking cups with spouts

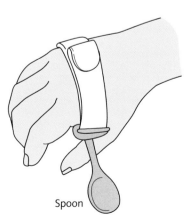

Spoon

Figure 6.7 Utensil holder

Feeding a patient who requires minimal assistance

Step	Rationale
1 Cleanse hands prior to assisting.	To prevent cross-infection.
2 Explain procedure to the patient.	To gain informed consent.
3 Ensure correct seating or positioning next to patient.	To ensure best position for eating.
4 Ensure that patient independence is promoted at all times and only assist where needed.	To prevent embarrassment to the patient and promote well-being.
5 Ensure that appropriate cutlery is used.	To aid the patient and promote independence where possible.
6 Offer mouth care or brushing teeth to the patient prior to eating (refer to Chapters 8 and 12).	To freshen the mouth before eating.
7 Ensure that adequate fluid is available at the table.	To allow opportunity for patient to refresh their mouth during eating.
8 Check that the temperature of the food is correct; neither too cold nor too hot.	To prevent scalding or burning of the mouth and unpleasant food if wrong temperature.
9 Sit down beside the patient.	To relax the patient.
10 Give adequate time between mouthfuls.	To ensure that the patient is not rushed or stressed by the procedure.
11 Always inform the patient of what you are doing and when you are doing it.	To ensure the patient is aware at all times of procedure and can ask questions as needed.
12 Cleanse hands after assisting.	To prevent cross-infection.
13 Ensure that documentation is completed.	To ensure that patient records are kept up to date and also to ensure that information is available to ensure complete and accurate assessment.

Feeding a patient who requires maximum assistance

Step	Rationale
1 Cleanse hands prior to assisting.	To prevent cross-infection.
2 Explain procedure to the patient.	To gain informed consent.
3 Ensure privacy.	To provide a comfortable relaxed setting.
4 Ensure correct seating or positioning next to patient.	To ensure best position for assisting with feeding.
5 Provide napkin or protective clothing.	To ensure that clothes or sleepwear are protected.
6 Offer mouth care or brushing teeth to the patient prior to eating (refer to Chapters 8 and 12)	To freshen the mouth before eating.
7 Ensure that the patient's meal is ready to be served and at the correct temperature.	To ensure that the patient is prepared for the meal and reduce delays that might cause tiredness.
8 Ensure that the patient or client is sitting upright in bed or chair.	To ensure best positioning to aid swallowing.
9 Ensure that appropriate cutlery is used.	To aid the patient and promote independence where possible.
10 Ensure that adequate fluid is available at the table.	To allow opportunity for patient to refresh their mouth during eating.
11 Ensure that the plate guard is in position and in front of the patient.	To aid the patient and prevent the food from spilling off the plate.
12 Offer to cut the patient's food into bite-sized pieces.	This will make it easier for the patient to manipulate food.
13 Offer to put the pieces of food into the patient's mouth.	To aid the patient, if the patient is unable to do so.
14 Give adequate time between mouthfuls.	To ensure that the patient has adequate time to chew and swallow the food.

	Step	Rationale
15	Offer fluids to the patient between mouthfuls (see Fig. 6.8).	To ensure that the patient's palate is cleansed and also to provide hydration.
16	Always inform the patient of what you are doing and when you are doing it.	To ensure that the patient is aware at all times of procedure and can ask questions as needed.
17	Monitor how well the patient is eating and if there are any problems.	To identify any problems that may result in chewing or swallowing.
18	Provide the patient with a mouthwash or facilities for cleansing the teeth on completion of meal.	To cleanse the mouth and promote good dentition.
19	Cleanse hands after assisting.	To prevent cross-infection.
20	Ensure that documentation is completed.	To ensure that patient records are kept up to date and also to ensure that information is available to ensure complete and accurate assessment.

Feeding a patient who is visually impaired

	Step	Rationale
1	Cleanse hands prior to assisting.	To prevent cross-infection.
2	Explain procedure to the patient.	To gain informed consent.
3	Ensure privacy.	To provide a comfortable, relaxed setting.
4	Ensure correct seating or positioning next to patient.	To ensure best position for eating.
5	Have patient sit upright in bed or chair.	To ensure best position adopted for swallowing and for comfort.
6	Ensure that the patient is aware of surrounding area and the position of the table.	This will provide the patient with more information, to visualize the position of the food.
7	Offer mouth care or brushing teeth to the patient prior to eating (refer to Chapters 8 and 12).	To freshen the mouth before eating.
8	Assess the need for plate guards or special cutlery.	This will help to prevent the food from slipping from the plate and will aid independence.

continued

9	Ensure that the patient has detailed information on the position of the plate and details of where the food is on the plate.	To aid the patient and promote independence where possible.
10	Continually provide information to the patient.	This will provide continual reassurance and guidance to the patient.
11	Give adequate time between mouthfuls.	To ensure that the patient has adequate time for chewing and swallowing.
12	Always inform the patient of what you are doing and when you are doing it.	To ensure that the patient is aware at all times of procedure and can ask questions as needed.
13	Cleanse hands after assisting.	To prevent cross-infection.
14	Ensure that documentation is completed.	To ensure that patient records are kept up to date and also to ensure that information is available to ensure complete and accurate assessment.

Bottle-feeding an infant

Step		Rationale
1	Cleanse hands prior to assisting with the procedure.	To reduce the risks of cross-infection.
2	Explain the procedure to the infant and the relative or carer.	To relax the infant. To gain informed consent.
3	Ask whether the relative or carer would like to participate with the procedure.	This will ensure that the child is more familiar with the procedure and help the relative or carer to feel more included.
4	An unprepared bottle must be sterilized, along with teats, according to local policy. This can be done by steam, microwave sterilizer or sterilizing solution.	To prevent spread of infection.
5	If using formula, follow the guidelines on the package for making up a feed. Use cooled boiled water. Double check this with a registered nurse.	To ensure accuracy of strength of feed.
6	Measure the milk powder with the scoop provided. Use a knife to level off the scoop, but avoid packing the powder down. Add this to the water in the bottle. Put the teat and cover on and then shake well. Don't be tempted to add extra scoops of formula powder as this can make the baby ill.	To make up an infant bottle using formula milk correctly.

7	Provide a relaxed seating area within a communal setting if possible.	This will provide social interaction for the infant and enhance his or her social skills.
8	Sit with the infant in your arms, introduce the teat into the baby's mouth and let the baby suck.	
9	Hold the bottle in such a way that the teat and the neck are filled with the formula.	To prevent the infant sucking in air.
10	When the baby stops sucking sit the baby up and gently pat or rub its back.	This may help to loosen any wind (although this tends only to be done in the UK).
11	Offer the bottle again to see if the baby wishes to feed further. Do not force the infant to finish the whole bottle.	To satisfy the baby.
12	Cleanse hands after cleaning or storing the bottle.	To prevent cross-infection.
13	Document infant's intake on fluid balance or food assessment chart, as appropriate.	This will provide a detailed account of the infant's dietary intake for that mealtime.

Feeding an infant or child

Step		Rationale
1	Cleanse hands prior to assisting with procedure.	To reduce the risks of cross-infection.
2	Explain the procedure to the patient and the relative or carer.	To gain informed consent.
3	Ask whether the relative or carer wishes to participate with the procedure.	This will ensure that the child is more familiar with the procedure and help the relative or carer to feel more included.
4	Offer mouth care or brushing teeth to the patient prior to eating (refer to Chapters 8 and 12).	To freshen the mouth before eating.
5	Provide a relaxed seating area in a communal setting if possible.	This will provide social interaction for the child and enhance his or her social skills.
6	Ensure that the child is given a choice of what is available on the menu.	To offer something that the child will like.
7	Ensure that special cutlery or equipment is available, if needed.	This will ensure that the child will be as independent as possible.
8	Assist with cutting the food into small portions.	This will ensure that the food is in more manageable pieces.

continued

9 Provide fluid.	This will ensure that the mouth is cleansed and that hydration is provided.
10 Offer mouth care or brushing teeth to the patient after eating (refer to Chapters 8 and 12).	To freshen the mouth after eating.
11 Cleanse hands after assisting.	To prevent cross-infection.
12 Document their intake on fluid balance or food assessment chart, as required.	This will provide a detailed account of the child's dietary intake for that mealtime.
13 Ensure that all information is documented in clinical notes.	This will provide a resource for all members of the multi-disciplinary team.

Aftercare

It is very important that the patient's intake and output is accurately documented in the fluid balance chart. Liquid foods, such as soups and puddings, should be entered, together with the quantities of tea, milk, or any other drink that accompanied the meal. It is important to be aware of the patient's general appetite and condition and any illnesses. This should be taken into consideration when assessing the patient's fluid intake and output. Some patients may be on a fluid restriction diet and you should be aware of this and try and ensure that it is adhered to.

A patient who has difficulty with swallowing may require additional fluids through an alternative route, for example **intravenous**ly, to supplement hydration.

Developing your skills

It is essential that you become accustomed to the requirements of a feeding assessment and develop skills in its practice. This complements the skills in providing assistance depending on the outcome of the assessment process. These skills are needed in many different care environments, including acute care and community settings. It is also important that the patient is assessed and re-evaluated at appropriate times depending on the patient's illness, recovery rate, or deterioration. Try to practice the skill of assessing a patient's feeding capability on your next placement.

Remember that if the patient has numerous problems, you will need some expert help from the qualified nursing staff and the multiprofessional team to address these deficiencies.

Remember to take into consideration the speed at which the patient eats. Too often, nurses try to rush patients when eating because they are too focused on their workload. Do not pressurize patients: let them take their own time. Also make sure that you communicate with the patient in a way that they understand.

Make sure that the correct equipment is chosen to help the patient. Getting this right can make the task of eating much easier for the patient.

Other factors to consider

The clinical assessment may reveal that the patient has many factors that contribute to decreased oral intake. Medical conditions, such as stroke, are a common example. The patient may experience dexterity problems that make food preparation difficult and prevent adequate cutting, and manipulation of food on the plate. The patient may also have swallowing difficulties. Any of these may affect the patient's nutritional intake. The patient, in this example, will be required to have a swallowing assessment carried out. The speech and language therapist (SALT) should be contacted (this usually requires a doctor's referral) to assess the patient.

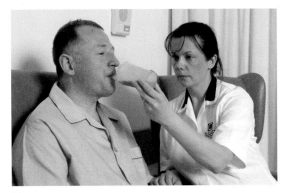

(a)

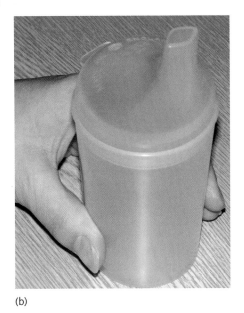

(b)

Figure 6.8 (a) Assisting a patient with drinking (b) a typical drinking cup to assist the patient

Following the assessment a suitable diet may be selected. In some situations, particularly where there is a risk of choking or **aspiration** of food into the lungs, it is necessary for the patient to have nil by mouth (NBM), until further assessments have taken place at specific intervals. Furthermore, liquid nutritional supplements are widely available in hospital and community settings.

Speech and language therapy assessment is not restricted to the adult patient. Many children with feeding difficulties and those with complex needs will require this assessment, which may lead to alternative feeding strategies for the child.

When a patient with learning disabilities is admitted to hospital it is important to refer to his or her person-centred plan or health action plan. It is also important to involve the health facilitator if there is one.

6.3 **Providing special diets**

Definition

Special diets are adaptations in people's usual eating habits for a particular purpose. The use of a special diet can be related to the prevention and treatment of disease or to achieve a general improvement in physical and mental health. Special diets can promote weight loss in obesity and may be an important part of a patient's treatment, if this is a requirement prior to surgery.

A particular diet may also be significant for religious or cultural reasons, or may be prompted by an individual's system of beliefs and values, such as is the case with vegans and vegetarians, see Section 6.1.

In the case of people who are moderately to severely overweight, there are substantial health benefits from a diet aiming to achieve a weight-loss of 10–20 lbs (4.5–9.1 kg). This can result in reduced levels of cholesterol in the blood and the lowering of blood pressure. This type of diet can also help other weight-related health problems, such as diabetes and heart disease.

Background

A healthy diet is described as one that is able to provide all of the calories and nutrients needed by the body for optimal performance, at the same time ensuring that neither nutritional deficiencies nor excesses occur. Recommended daily amount (RDA) guidelines were originally set in 1979 by the Department of Health, but have been adjusted since then in line with ongoing research (NHS Quality Improvement Scotland 2003). They are now referred to as dietary reference values (DRV) and can be different for different people. Patients who are unwell may require extra nutrients and vitamins above the DRVs, depending on what their body lacks. There are also variations with age and sex. As an example, it is recommended that the daily fat intake is 95 g for men and 70 g for women. The saturated fat intake should be no more than 30 g for men and 20 g for women.

There are common diets that patients are advised to take, depending on their condition, any investigations being carried out, and any special nutritional requirements. Hospitals provide menu-specific items for those patients on special diets. For children, there are special diets for conditions such as cystic fibrosis, diabetes, and coeliac disease.

Clear liquid diet

A clear liquid diet is often given for a short period following surgery, to give the gastrointestinal tract a rest. The diet consists of water, clear juices, broth (clear fluid), and tea.

Full liquid diet

The full liquid diet is given after surgery as a move from clear liquids to a normal diet. This diet includes all the foods on a clear liquid diet, with the addition of dairy products, such as milk, yoghurt, custard, and smooth cream soups.

Diabetic diet (normal healthy diet)

The diabetic diet principally is a normal healthy diet and is low in sugar and fat. The diet is designed to keep blood glucose (sugar) levels under control. The patient can select a meal from the normal menu, however only *sugar-free* items will be given.

Low-sodium diet

The low-sodium diet is given to patients who have conditions, such as high blood pressure, pneumonia, kidney disease, and, in certain circumstances, to people who retain water (known as oedema). A low-sodium diet may help the body get rid of excess fluids. Patients often report a lack of flavour in food with this diet.

When to provide a special diet

The nurse should assess the patient's nutritional needs on first contact with the patient. Special diets may be needed in the case of:

- Lung disease
- Heart disease
- Alcohol and drug addiction
- Cancer
- Osteoporosis
- Inflammatory bowel disease
- Renal disease
- Allergies
- Wound and ulcer management

An example may be if someone has osteoporosis. Osteoporosis is a condition where the bones, particularly those of the spine and hips, become thin and weak and break easily. As part of the treatment plan patients can be given supplements of calcium. Including more calcium in the diet can help improve the bone density and, therefore, the bones will be less likely to break.

Assessment of the patient's need for a special diet

Step	Rationale
1 Cleanse your hands prior to procedure.	To ensure no risk of cross-infection.
2 Inform the patient of procedure.	To gain informed consent.
3 Record the patient's weight.	To calculate the BMI.
4 Record the patient's height.	To calculate the BMI.
5 Record the patient's BMI.	This will give us a recording that may indicate whether the patient has special dietary needs.

continued

6	Obtain a full medical history.	This will provide information on the patient's past and present medical conditions and if the condition requires a special diet.
7	Obtain of list of present medications.	This will provide information on the patient's current therapy and provide information on any allergies or interactions.
8	Complete a nutritional risk assessment.	This will provide information on skin type, identify recent weight loss or gain, identify chronic conditions, and provide a score that may be used to indicate further referral needs.
9	Refer to dietician. For children, there are specialist paediatric dieticians. You will also find dieticians working in the community setting.	To ensure that nutritional needs are met and to ensure that correct and adequate information is provided to the patient, nurse, and relative or carer.
10	Consider referral to speech and language therapist.	This will provide a formal assessment if there are any doubts regarding the patient's swallowing ability.
11	Consider referral to occupational therapist.	This will ensure that any additional special feeding aids are available to the patient.
12	Cleanse hands after the procedure.	To prevent cross-infection.
13	Document all information using the correct assessment tools.	This will ensure that patient care is planned to suit the individual's specific needs.
14	Document all information in the clinical notes.	To ensure that all members of the multidisciplinary team are kept up to date with all information available.

Aftercare

Recording information correctly in the patient clinical notes or person-centred plan is very important. The nutritional assessment tool used to assess the patient should be specified in the clinical notes. If the patient requires a special diet, a referral should be made to members of the multidisciplinary team. This may differ, depending on the clinical environment. In some or most instances, the nurse may need to refer to a dietician, pharmacist, public health nurse, clinical nurse specialist, or community learning disability team.

Developing your skills

It is essential that you become accustomed to and practice assessing patients for special diets. You will use this skill for patients in acute care and community settings. It is also highly important that the patient is assessed and re-evaluated at appropriate times, depending on the level of malnutrition. You should try and practice assessing a patient who requires a special diet on your next placement. Remember that if a patient is malnourished, you will need some expert help from the qualified nursing staff and the multiprofessional team to address dietary deficiencies fully. It is also important that you learn about the illness and any underlying medical conditions that the patient has, to understand the requirements of the diet.

Other factors to consider

Many patients will be on a special diet not because of a medical condition, but because of ethical, spiritual, or personal reasons. It is important to learn about these diets and become accustomed to what the patient can and cannot eat. See Section 6.1.

Student nurses will be involved in assisting patients to choose their diet from the hospital menu and, therefore, it will help the patient if you know what they can and cannot eat. In some instances, the nurse provides the patient's meal on a tray served at the bedside or at a table. In some hospitals and wards, healthcare assistants or catering staff serve meals. If this is the case, it is important to monitor what the patient is eating, ensuring that each patient receives the correct meal and is actually eating it. A danger is that meal trays can be left at the patient's bedside and removed later without them actually eating anything. This can be for a variety of reasons: the meal may be unappetizing, or the patient may be unable to eat the meal unaided, may be unable to reach the meal, or may simply be unable to open the packets or containers. It is important, therefore, to check food intake after every meal.

6.4 Caring for a patient suffering from vomiting or nausea

Definition

Vomiting is when the contents of the stomach are forced up through the oesophagus and out of the mouth or nose. Nausea is the feeling of having the urge to vomit.

Nausea is described as being unpleasant and a wave-like sensation at the back of the throat and the stomach. Nausea can occur without vomiting and vomiting can occur without the preceding nausea, although this is less usual. Nausea can occur more often than vomiting. If left untreated nausea can lead to the patient having a reduced appetite or **anorexia** (loss of appetite).

It is important to collect and measure the amount of vomit expelled to help determine the patient's fluid loss, which can sometimes be considerable and, in severe cases, can lead to dehydration.

Background

The expulsion of contents from the stomach happens when there is a strong downward contraction of the diaphragm and the abdominal muscles tighten while the stomach is relaxed and the sphincter (muscle) is open. Therefore, the contents of the stomach are sent up and out of the mouth or nose (Haughney 2004).

The control of vomiting involves four areas (shown in **Fig. 6.9**):

1   The vomiting centre in the medulla oblongata (part of the brainstem), where the vomiting reflex is initiated.
2   The chemoreceptor trigger zone (CTZ) in the area of the fourth ventricle of the brain acts as the entry point for vomiting stimuli. The CTZ is outside the blood–brain barrier and, therefore, responds to stimuli from either the cerebral spinal fluid (CSF) or the blood.
3   The vestibular apparatus (balance from the middle ear).
4   The gastrointestinal tract neurotransmitters.

Vomiting is a complex response. The vomiting centre in the medulla oblongata in the brain responds to stimuli from the gastrointestinal tract, other organs, the cerebral cortex, the vestibular apparatus (balance) and the chemoreceptor trigger zone (CTZ), and even severe unpleasant sights, odours (smells), and pain. The vomiting centre can have different levels of stimulus in different individuals. Some people vomit readily and with little effort at the least stimulus. Other people rarely vomit even with severe stimuli.

Causes of nausea and vomiting

The nurse should try and find out the most likely cause for the nausea and vomiting prior to administering any prescribed **anti-emetic** drugs (Butler and Courtenay 2002). Nausea and vomiting are very common and can occur for a number of reasons. These include:

- Alcoholism
- Brain tumours
- Bulimia and self-induced vomiting
- **Chemotherapy** in cancer patients
- Constipation (common)
- Food allergies
- Food poisoning
- Medication (especially chemotherapy and **anaesthetic** medications); this is common

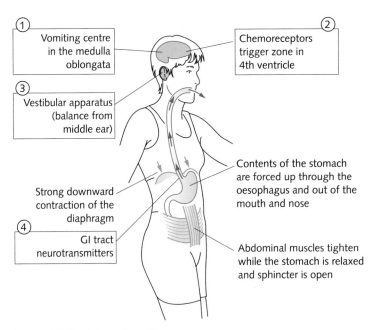

Figure 6.9 Physiology of vomiting

- Morning sickness during pregnancy
- Migraine headaches
- Motion or seasickness
- Pain; this is common
- Viral infections

Key point: Nausea and vomiting are extremely common when patients are receiving chemotherapy treatment.

There are additional possible causes in infants:

- Pyloric stenosis (constriction of the outlet from the stomach)
- Milk intolerance
- Gastroenteritis
- Overfeeding
- Intestinal obstruction
- Accidental drug or poison ingestion

Effects of nausea and vomiting

If vomiting continues and is poorly controlled, it can lead to a number of health problems. Patients can become reluctant to eat anything, because this leads to nausea or vomiting and, therefore, they can lose their appetite. This can lead to food aversion, or anorexia, which can become so extreme that the patient has severe weight loss.

Dehydration can also develop through excessive vomiting. This is a condition in which the body contains an insufficient volume of water for normal functioning. This can be caused by a variety of situations, such as prolonged physical activity without consuming adequate water, especially in a hot or humid environment. The combination of severe diarrhoea and vomiting can be particularly problematic and life-threatening, as it can lead to electrolyte imbalance. The most serious electrolyte disturbances involve abnormalities in the levels of sodium, potassium, or calcium. For example, an extremely low potassium or calcium level can lead to heart-rhythm disturbances and death. A very low sodium level can cause confusion and convulsions.

In post-operative patients, abdominal wound **dehiscence** (the wound bursting open) is an extremely distressing complication of excessive post-operative vomiting. This is caused because the large muscles in the abdomen contract strongly during vomiting and can pull on the wound that is trying to heal. To prevent this, you can advise the patient to hold the wound and abdomen when vomiting.

Lastly, a serious and potentially fatal health problem is caused by the aspiration of vomit. This is a common problem for the semi-conscious, sedated, or anaesthetized patient who vomits. Rather than being expelled through

Assessment of nausea and vomiting

If a patient is acutely unwell, it is important to carry out a thorough assessment to determine the cause prior to providing any medication. A number of questions can be used in the assessment, such as:

1   How long has the nausea or vomiting lasted?

2   Is the nausea constant?

3   Does the nausea always lead to vomiting?

4   Do you get vomiting without nausea?

5   When do you get the symptoms?

6   Is there a specific trigger for the symptoms?

7   Have you tried anything to reduce the symptoms?

8   What type of vomit is it—projectile, amount, colour, content, odour?

the mouth, the contents of the stomach could enter the lungs because of a suppressed cough reflex. This is serious and life-threatening, and explains why many patients, except in very urgent cases, are always fasted before receiving an anaesthetic.

Aftercare

Ensure that the amount of vomit is recorded on the fluid balance chart. Documenting information correctly in the patient clinical notes is very important. It is also important to recognize if there is an identifiable trigger that can be treated, to reduce or stop the symptoms of nausea and vomiting.

Some consideration should be given to the administration of medicines for patients suffering from nausea and vomiting. The patient's prescription chart should be checked to see if an anti-emetic (anti-sickness drug) has been prescribed, and under what circumstances it may be administered. If the patient is not prescribed an anti-emetic and continues to suffer from nausea and vomiting, then medical staff should consult to decide if it is appropriate to prescribe one. If a drug is prescribed, the student, along with a trained member of nursing staff should administer the drug through an appropriate route. Choosing the correct route to administer a drug to patients who are vomiting is a major decision, as the oral route becomes so unreliable. Medications prescribed for oral administration normally need to be changed, and medical and pharmacy staff should be consulted. Assured routes of drug administration for actively vomiting patients may be for example, the **buccal** route (oral mucous membrane or **sublingual**) or **intramuscular** injection. However, the intravenous route is preferred for children who already have a cannula *in situ,* to prevent further pain and discomfort.

Caring for a patient who is vomiting and alert

Step		Rationale
1	Ensure privacy	To prevent embarrassment and maintain dignity.
2	Temporarily limit the patient's food intake.	To prevent further vomiting.
3	Put on disposable gloves.	To prevent contamination of self.
4	Ensure that the patient's airway is being maintained.	To ensure adequate oxygenation.
5	Provide the patient with a disposable sick bowl; or the toilet or some form of receptacle that can be easily cleaned if in a community setting.	To collect vomit in a disposable container.
6	Assist patient to sit up and lean forwards.	To maintain the airway and assist in expelling the contents of the stomach.
7	Support and comfort the patient while vomiting.	To reduce embarrassment and self-consciousness.
8	When sick bowl is full replace with a fresh sick bowl (or empty down the toilet if in a community setting).	To collect vomit in a disposable container.
9	When patient has finished vomiting, remove the bowl.	To remove any vomit away from the patient.
10	Measure the amount of vomit.	To record fluid loss accurately.
11	Dispose of the sick bowl and vomit in the macerator (or according to policy).	To dispose of the vomit.
12	Provide the patient with a damp cloth to wash face and freshen up.	To freshen up face and hands.
13	Provide patient with a mouthwash or drink of water.	To rinse vomit from mouth.
14	If vomit is on bedclothes or patient's clothes, change these.	To clean clothes and bed clothes.
15	Dispose of gloves and wash hands.	To follow infection control policy and prevent contamination.

| 16 | Inform trained nursing or medical staff that the patient has vomited. | To communicate to a trained nurse or doctor for further treatment. |
| 17 | Note that the patient has vomited in the clinical record. | To provide accurate documentation. |

Key point: An infant or a child who is vomiting may find this particularly distressing especially if they have never experienced vomiting before. The child may have little understanding of what is happening and will need to be comforted. The child's parent, family, or carer may find this distressing to witness and will also need to be comforted.

Caring for a patient with impaired consciousness who is vomiting

Step		Rationale
1	Ensure privacy.	To prevent embarrassment and maintain dignity.
2	Call for help.	You will not be able to deal with this on your own.
3	Put on disposable gloves.	To prevent contamination to self.
4	Turn patient onto side using manual handling guidelines.	To prevent aspiration of vomit.
5	Ensure that the patient's airway is maintained (this means that the patient is breathing more than eight breaths per minute).	To ensure adequate oxygenation.
6	Place sick bowl under side of face to collect any vomit, or allow vomit to go onto the floor or bed.	To collect vomit in a disposable container.
7	When patient has finished vomiting, remove the bowl.	To remove any vomit away from the patient.
8	Measure the amount of vomit.	To record fluid loss accurately.
9	Dispose of the sick bowl and vomit in the macerator (or according to policy).	To dispose of the vomit.
10	Suction any food debris left in the mouth (this is an advanced skill).	To clear the airway (this must be carried out by a senior student or trained staff).
11	Provide oral hygiene (see Chapters 8 and 12).	To clean the mouth of any vomit.

continued

12	Wash the patient's face.	To clean any residual vomit from the patient's face.
13	Dispose of gloves and wash hands.	To follow infection control policy and prevent contamination.
14	Inform trained nursing or medical staff that the patient has vomited.	To communicate to a trained nurse or doctor for further treatment.
15	Record that the patient has vomited in the clinical record.	To provide accurate documentation.

Developing your skills

It is essential that you become accustomed to and practice caring for a patient who has nausea and vomiting, in acute care and community settings. It is also highly important that patients are assessed and re-evaluated at appropriate times depending on their changing symptoms. It is important to understand the causes *of nausea and vomiting* in order to provide nursing care for the patient.

Other factors to consider

In all patients, exhaustion is a problem due to the expenditure of energy and strong contractions of muscles used in vomiting. Therefore, the student should try and provide the patient with as much rest as possible once the vomiting has stopped.

There are alternative treatment options for nausea and vomiting. Knowing these can help in alleviating the patient's symptoms. Common alternative therapies are:

- Aromatherapy scents
- Acupressure
- Acupuncture
- Nerve stimulation
- Music

Nausea and vomiting can interfere with normal nutrition, reducing fluid intake and causing dehydration. The nurse must remember this and be alert to this happening. It is important to check the patient's electrolyte levels (urea and electrolyte blood test). It is important that you are able to recognize abnormal levels and report them to nursing or medical staff. Once an abnormality is recognized, the correct action for returning the urea or electrolyte levels to normal can be discussed.

6.5 **Monitoring fluid balance**

Definition

Fluid balance refers to the regulation of fluid quantities in the body, with the amount of fluid taken into the body normally equalling the amount of fluid lost from the body. Fluid balance is one of the body's vital homeostatic mechanisms.

Many illnesses can cause problems with the balance of fluid within the body; therefore, monitoring fluid balance is an important skill for a nurse to perform. The balance of water in the body is important and the nurse will need to recognize if a patient is becoming dehydrated, either by not drinking enough, or by losing too much fluid. Additionally, the patient should not take in too much fluid through drink or other means, and should also be able to pass out a normal amount of fluid through the kidneys.

Background

Body fluid is located in two types of locations or 'compartments'. Most body water is located inside cells; this is called intracellular fluid. The remaining fluid forms the extracellular compartment. This extracellular fluid is divided into interstitial fluid (fluid that is in the tissue space between and around the cells) and intravascular fluid (the watery plasma, or serum, of the blood) (Docherty and Foudy 2006).

The body uses three interrelated control mechanisms to maintain fluid balance (Docherty and Coote 2006).

1 The brain, where antidiuretic hormone (ADH) is produced in the posterior pituitary and causes water to be retained by the body.

2 The kidneys, where more than a million nephrons in each kidney perform a vital role in controlling fluid excretion, and where the hormone renin is produced and secreted into the blood.

3 The adrenal glands, where aldosterone is produced and works with renin and angiotensin in the blood to control the pressure of blood flowing to the kidneys and, in turn, the amount of water excreted in the urine.

These hormonal control mechanisms play an important role in fluid balance. Antidiuretic hormone is produced in response to decreased circulating blood volume and increased serum **osmolarity**. This means that if the body becomes dehydrated (there is too little fluid) then there is an increase in secretion of this hormone, which causes the kidneys to conserve water by reducing urine output. The patient can show signs of this by producing dark concentrated urine.

Conversely, when the body has excess fluid and there is a reduction in the secretion of this hormone, the result is an increase in urine production by the kidneys, and the urine is lighter in colour.

Also if the patient has a low blood pressure (hypotension) then there will be less blood flow through the kidneys and, therefore, less urine is produced. This happens because the juxtaglomerular cells in the kidney recognize the reduced blood flow and secrete renin into the bloodstream. A complex process takes place, involving the liver and lungs, and results in renin converting angiotensin I to angiotensin II. This is a strong **vasoconstrictor** (tightens blood vessels) and, therefore, causes the blood pressure to increase.

Fluid can be lost normally from the body in a number of ways:

- Through the skin, as perspiration
- In the urine and faeces
- Through vomiting
- Through breathing

Fluid loss through sites where the loss is not measurable and usually goes unnoticed is known as insensible loss. For example fluid loss through breathing is impossible to measure and can only be estimated.

Fluid is taken into the body by:

- Food (for example an apple is 90% water)

- Metabolism of food (carbohydrates are broken down in the body for energy, producing water as a by-product)
- Drinking

Total body water (TBW) is about 65–70% of the body weight in men and 55–60% of body weight in young women: there is a difference because women, on average, have a greater proportion of body fat than men. The average urine output for an adult is 1.5 litres a day. You lose almost an additional litre of water a day through breathing, sweating, and bowel movements, as mentioned previously. Food usually accounts for 20% of your total fluid intake, so if you drink 2 litres of water or other beverages a day (a little more than eight tumblers or glasses), and have a normal diet, you will typically replace the lost fluids.

Illness can affect the fluid balance of the body. For example, someone who is very breathless will lose more fluid through breathing. Similarly, someone with a high body temperature will lose more body fluid through sweating. It is easy to imagine that vomiting and diarrhoea can both quickly lead to acute and possibly life-threatening dehydration. Hormonal problems affecting ADH, aldosterone, and renin production can have major effects on the body's ability to maintain fluid balance. Sometimes, treatment can have serious consequences too: for example, during surgery, patients may lose fluid but not have the ability to replace this naturally through drinking because of altered consciousness, risk of vomiting, and so on. It is, therefore, necessary to recognize some of these situations and be alert to the effects that they can have on a patient's fluid balance.

Key point: When the body retains too much fluid, the patient is said to have a *positive balance* (fluid gain is greater than fluid loss). This can cause the patient's weight to increase. When the body loses too much fluid the patient is said to have a *negative balance* (fluid loss is greater than fluid gain). This can cause the patient's weight to decrease.

When to monitor a patient's fluid balance

Common drugs, such as caffeine and alcohol, both suppress the secretion of ADH; therefore, the kidneys reabsorb less water and this leads to an increase in urine output. Illnesses can produce much more complicated effects. Patients are at risk of fluid loss due to vomiting, diarrhoea, and haemorrhage (blood loss). There are also some conditions that cause the body to retain fluids, such as **heart failure**. Additionally, some patients, such as stroke patients, surgical patients fasting for theatre, and unconscious patients, may have problems with eating and drinking and, therefore, have difficulty in maintaining adequate hydration. Failure to maintain an accurate fluid balance for a patient can have serious consequences. Patients who have an imbalance in fluid are unable to oxygenate vital organs in the body efficiently or transport waste products to be excreted.

Procedures

When assessing fluid intake, the aim is to gain information on the amount, time, and type of fluid consumed by the patient. This information can be recorded on a fluid balance chart. Any loss of fluid can also be recorded on the same chart; this can be from urine, vomit, diarrhoea, and so on. This allows the appropriate amount of fluid intake and output for the patient to be checked. A healthy adult should drink 1.5 to 2 litres of fluid in 24 hours. However, this will vary depending on the patient's condition and illness. In addition to this, it is important to use other observation signs to assess the patient's hydration. Dehydration may be indicated by dry lips, a loss of elasticity in the skin, and low blood pressure (Shepherd 2001).

The amounts of fluid intake and output are normally calculated daily. The chart can start at midnight, 6 a.m., or 8 a.m., and is calculated at the same time each day. A combination of the fluid balance chart and daily weight measurement is used for stable patients. If the patient is unstable, then hourly fluid input and output recording is carried out.

Assessing hydration

Assessing an individual's state of hydration can be carried out in a number of ways. It is important to recognize some of the clinical features that can be presented; these are shown in **Table 6.1** and **Fig. 6.10**.

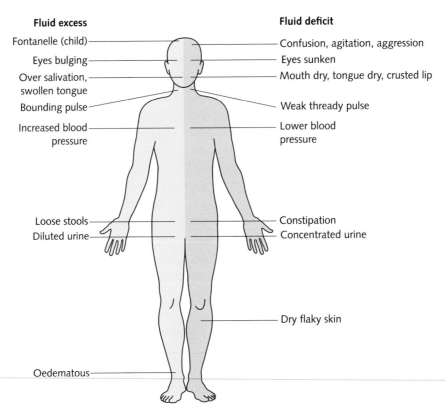

Fluid excess

Fontanelle (child)
Eyes bulging
Over salivation, swollen tongue
Bounding pulse
Increased blood pressure

Loose stools
Diluted urine

Oedematous

Fluid deficit

Confusion, agitation, aggression
Eyes sunken
Mouth dry, tongue dry, crusted lip
Weak thready pulse
Lower blood pressure

Constipation
Concentrated urine

Dry flaky skin

Figure 6.10 Dehydration versus fluid overload

Recording fluid intake

Key point: Fluid intake must include all fluids that the patient takes into the body. This includes all liquids, any ice, liquid foods, such as soup and ice cream, any intravenous infusions and any fluids administered through feeding tubes.

Step   Rationale

	Step	Rationale
1	Identify whether the patient should have a fluid balance chart	To identify whether the patient is at risk of over- or under-hydration.
2	Explain the purpose of keeping a fluid balance chart to the patient.	To keep the patient informed.
3	Measure all fluid intake including oral, intravenous, medications, and tube feeding. Orally taken fluids include milk on cereals, soup, and ice cream.	To gauge fluid intake accurately.
5	Record the time and amount of fluids taken in the appropriate space on the chart.	To maintain an accurate chart.
6	Record all forms of fluid intake over the 24-hour period.	To record all fluid intake.
7	Add together all fluid intake for the 24-hour period.	To calculate fluid balance between intake and output.
8	Check the addition so that an error is not made.	To recheck fluid intake and prevent error.
9	Notify the charge nurse of any imbalance.	To ensure that any possible imbalance in fluid intake and output is communicated to a trained member of staff.

Recording fluid output

Key point: Fluid output must include all fluids that the patient passes out of the body. This includes all liquids (urine, vomit), as well as diarrhoea, which will contain a large volume of fluid, and any volume from **drains** such as after surgery.

Step	Rationale
1 Identify whether the patient should have a fluid balance chart.	To identify whether the patient is at risk of over- or under-hydration.
2 Explain the purpose of keeping a fluid balance chart to the patient.	To keep the patient informed.
3 Measure all fluid output including vomit, urine, bowel movements, drains.	To gauge fluid output accurately.
4 Record the time and amount of fluids in the appropriate space on the chart.	To maintain an accurate chart.
5 Record all forms of fluid output over the 24-hour period.	To record all fluid output.
6 Add together all fluid output for the 24-hour period.	To calculate fluid balance between intake and output.
7 Check the addition so that an error is not made.	To recheck fluid output and prevent error.
8 Notify the charge nurse of any imbalance.	To ensure that any possible imbalance in fluid intake and output is communicated to a trained member of staff.

Aftercare

Recording information correctly in the patient clinical notes is very important. All too often a patient's fluid balance chart has not been kept up to date and, therefore, does not provide necessary information. It is important to be vigilant in completing the fluid balance chart (see **Fig. 6.11** for an example). Remember after every mealtime to record fluid intake. Be sure to make a record if the patient loses any fluid by any means, such as normal **micturition** (passing urine) or in abnormal ways such as blood loss and vomiting.

Developing your skills

It is essential that you practice completing a fluid balance chart for patients in acute care and the community setting. It is very important to complete the fluid balance chart throughout the day. This is best done after mealtimes and regular intervals. The fluid balance chart should not be left until the end of the day to complete. It is also highly important that patients are assessed and re-evaluated at appropriate times, depending on their level of hydration and their illnesses, to decide whether they should still be monitored using a fluid balance chart and have this observed.

Table 6.1 Clinical features indicating fluid excess or deficit

Body site	Fluid excess	Fluid deficit
Head and neck		
Fontanelles (child)	Bulging	Sunken
Eyes	Bulging	Sunken
Mouth	Over-salivation, swollen tongue	Dry, shrunken tongue, dry crusted lips, dry mouth, thirst
Trunk and abdomen		
Weight	Weight gain	Weight loss
Bowel function	Loose stools	Constipation
Respiration	Crackles in lung bases, increased respiratory rate	Raised respiratory rate
Kidney function	Diluted urine, increased urine output	Concentrated urine, reduced urine output
Skin	Oedematous	Dry and tight
Sacrum	Oedematous	
Extremities		
Blood pressure	Increased blood pressure, but may be hypotensive if in cardiac failure	Lower blood pressure
Pulse	Bounding pulse, increase in pulse rate	Weak, thready pulse, increase in pulse rate
Legs	Oedematous	Dry flaky skin
Cognitive		
Behaviour		Confusion, agitation, aggression

Other factors to consider

Many factors can affect fluid balance. It is important to remember that such things as age, acute or chronic illness, and psychological, cultural, and environmental factors can affect an individual's fluid balance.

You should become familiar with the volumes of fluid contained in the drinking vessels used in the clinical areas: this includes cups, glasses, mugs, and so on. Juice cartons and cans have the volume written on them.

time	Fluid Intake			Fluid Output		
	oral	IV/SC	Other	Urine	Vomit	Other
0100						
0200						
0300						
0400						
0500						
0600						
0700						
0800						
0900						
1000						
1100						
1200						
1300						
1400						
1500						
1600						
1700						
1800						
1900						
2000						
2100						
2200						
2300						
2400						
total						

PATIENT ID LABEL

WARD ... ...

DATE ... ...

Previous day input ... ...

Previous day output ... ...

Total input ... ...   **Total output** ... ...

Figure 6.11 Fluid balance chart

 Scenarios

Consider what you should do in the following situations, then turn to the end of the section to check your answers.

Further scenarios are available at

🌐 **www.oxfordtextbooks.co.uk/orc/docherty/**

 Scenario 1

You are a student on placement in a care home and a patient, a Miss Brown, is being transferred from acute care. She is a 90-year-old woman who has had a recent stroke that has left her paralysed down the right side. She has been in acute hospital care for three months. Although she has had extensive rehabilitation, she remains bed-bound. As part of your admission assessment, you must carry out a nutritional assessment. This involves finding out Miss Brown's height and weight. Miss Brown does not weigh the same as when she was first admitted to hospital.

How can the height and weight of a patient who is in bed be measured?

What other assessment measures can be made to tell if Miss Brown has gained or lost weight?

How will the fact that Miss Brown has had a stroke affect her eating capabilities?

 Scenario 2

You are a student on clinical placement with a health visitor. You are attending a baby clinic, where mothers bring their children to have their development assessed regularly. One of the common assessments carried out at these clinics is the baby's weight. You are asked to assist in recording the weights of children under 3 years old. How should you do this?

Scenario 3

You are a student nurse working in a learning disability placement, where children attend daily, sometimes for respite and at other times for treatment, education, and support for the families. A child attending has special needs; he is autistic and has developed dietary problems. Food has become a source of fear or revulsion and he will not try anything new. How are you going to ensure that he is provided with a balanced diet that meets his daily requirements?

 Scenario 4

You are working in a care home and assisting with the care of an elderly gentleman, a Mr Patel, who is 82 years old. He has dementia and tends to wander about the home. He has recently been transferred to the home. Before his transfer, he lived at home with his elderly wife who cared for him and prepared all his meals. They ate together at a table for every meal and she ensured that he had a balanced nutritional diet. On assessment to the care home he has a normal BMI and his nutritional assessment did not alert the nursing staff to any problems. As a student nurse, you notice that he has not had an assessment carried out for a number of weeks and decide to make an assessment again, for practice. You notice that he is now underweight with a BMI of less that 18.5. Why do you think this may be happening and what can be done about it?

Website

🌐 **www.oxfordtextbooks.co.uk/orc/docherty/**

You may find it helpful to work through our short online quiz and interactive scenarios intended to help you to develop and apply the skills in this chapter.

References

BAPEN (2003). *Malnutrition Universal Screening Tool: 'MUST'*. British Association for Parenteral and Enteral Nutrition, Redditch.

Butler M and Courtenay M (2002). Anti-emetics. *Nursing Times,* **98**, 48. www.nursingtimes.net/ntclinical/antiemetics.html

Corkins MR, Lewis P, Cruse W, Gupta S, and Fitzgerald J (2002). Accuracy of infant admission lengths. *Paediatrics,* **109**(6), 1108–11.

Docherty B and Coote S (2006). Fluid-balance monitoring as part of track and trigger. *Nursing Times,* **102**(45), 28–9.

Docherty B and Foudy C (2006). Homeostasis—part 4: fluid balance. *Nursing Times,* **102**, 22. www.nursingtimes.net/ntclinical/homeostasis__part_4_fluid_balance.html.

Guigoz Y, Velles B, and Garry PJ (1994). Mini nutritional assessment: a practical assessment tool for grading the nutritional state of elderly patients. *Facts and Research in Gerontology,* **4**(suppl. 2). 15–59. Mini nutritional assessment tool available at www.nestlenutrition.co.uk/Healthcare/gb/pages/rtnnpublications.aspx.

Haughney A (2004). Nausea and vomiting in end-stage cancer. *American Journal of Nursing,* **104**(11), 40–8.

Johnstone C, Farley A, and Hendry C (2006a). Nurses' role in nutritional assessment screening—part one of a two-part series. *Nursing Times,* **102**(49), 28–9.

Johnstone C, Farley A, and Hendry C (2006b). Nurses' role in nutritional assessment and screening (part 2). *Nursing Times,* **102**(50), 28–9.

Kondrup J, Allison SP, Elia M, Vellas B, and Plauth M (2002). ESPEN Guidelines for nutrition screening. *Clinical Nutrition,* **22**(4), 415–21.

NHS Quality Improvement Scotland (2003). *Food, Fluid and Nutritional Care Standards.* NHS Quality Improvement Scotland, Edinburgh.

NICE (2006). *Nutrition Support in Adults.* NICE, London. http://guidance.nice.org.uk/CG32/guidance/pdf/English.

NMPDU (2002). *Nutrition Assessment and Referral in the Care of Adult Patients in Hospital. Best Practice Statement.* NMPDU, Edinburgh.

Shepherd M. (2001). Assessing fluid balance. *Nursing Times.* **97**(6), 11. www.nursingtimes.net/ntclinical/assessing_fluid_balance.html

Todorvic V, Russell C, Stratton R, Ward J, and Elia M (2003). *The 'MUST' Explanatory Booklet: a Guide to the Malnutrition Universal Screening Tool.* BAPEN, Redditch. www.bapen.org.uk/pdfs/must/must_explan.pdf.

Useful further reading and websites

BAPEN (2003). *Malnutrition Universal Screening Tool: 'MUST'*. British Association for Parenteral and Enteral Nutrition, Redditch.

The MUST was developed by the Malnutrition Advisory Group (MAG) of BAPEN and first produced in November 2003. The MUST has been validated for use in the hospital, community, and care settings, and its evidence base is contained in the MUST report. An explanatory booklet on MUST is also available for use in training and implementation. Copies of both the report and booklet are available from the BAPEN Office.

Gilbert R (2006). Fluid intake and bladder and bowel function. *Nursing Times*, **102**(12), 55–6.

Holmes S (2003). Undernutrition in hospital patients. *Nursing Standard*. **17**(19), 45–52.

Khair J and Morton L (2000). Nutritional assessment and screening in children. *Nursing Times*, **96**, 2.

Mamaril ME, Windle PE, and Burkard JF (2006). Prevention and management of postoperative nausea and vomiting: a look at complementary techniques. *Journal of PeriAnesthesia Nursing*, **21**(6), 404–10.

This article deals specifically with nausea and vomiting after surgery and will be useful when attending a surgical placement.

MENCAP (2007). *Death by Indifference*. MENCAP, London. www.mencap.org.uk/document.asp?id=284.

This is a large document; however, you can save it onto your computer rather than printing it. It provides insight and guidance on caring for patients with learning disabilities.

Noble KA (2006). Stop spinning world: postoperative nausea and vomiting. *Journal of PeriAnesthesia Nursing*, **21**(6), 431–5.

This article deals specifically with nausea and vomiting after surgery and will be useful when attending a surgical placement.

Reid J, Robb E, Stone D, *et al.* (2004). Improving the monitoring and assessment of fluid balance. *Nursing Times*, **100**(20), 36–9.

This article deals specifically with fluid balance and will provide you with more detailed information.

Sandlin D (2006). Alternative treatment options for postoperative nausea and vomiting. *Journal of PeriAnesthesia Nursing*, **21**(6), 436–38.

This article deals with alternative therapies to drug treatment for nausea and vomiting.

British Association for Parenteral and Enteral Nutrition. www.Bapen.org.uk/.

British Heart Foundation. www.bhf.org.uk.

British Nutrition Foundation. www.nutrition.org.uk/home.asp?siteId=43&sectionId=s.

Food Standards Agency. *Height/Weight Chart*. www.eatwell.gov.uk/healthydiet/healthyweight/heightweightchart/.

Food Standards Agency. *Healthy Weight*. www.eatwell.gov.uk/asksam/healthydiet/healthyweightq/.

Healthier Scotland. *Take Life On, One Step at a Time*. www.takelifeon.co.uk/.

National Institute for Clinical Excellence. http://guidance.nice.org.uk/CG32/quickrefguide/pdf/English.

Royal College of Nursing. www.rcn.org.uk/newsevents/campaigns/nutritionnow/tools_and_resources/nutritional_assessment.

Check 🌐 **www.oxfordtextbooks.co.uk/orc/docherty/** for changes and new developments. Updated research, guidelines, or equipment will be added every four months.

 Answers to scenarios

 Scenario 1

There are a number of ways to estimate Miss Brown's weight when she is in bed.

- Self-reported height and weight. Ask Miss Brown: she may know. Patients' self-declared heights and weights are generally realistic and reliable. However, since Miss Brown has been ill for a while, and an inpatient, she may not accurately know her weight or height

For height:

- Measure the length of Miss Brown's forearm and use a conversion table
- Measure Miss Brown's knee height and use a conversion table
- Measure Miss Brown's demispan (from the sternal notch—the top of sternum—to between the middle

and ring finger of the right hand) and use a conversion table

For weight:

- Look at Miss Brown's clothes and jewellery: are they loose fitting?
- Sitting scales can be used. Miss Brown can be transferred onto them using a hoist
- Measure Miss Brown's mid-upper arm circumference (MUAC)
- Measure a skin fold thickness, such as Miss Brown's triceps skin fold thickness (TSF)
- Measure Miss Brown's mid-arm muscle circumference (MAMC)
- Measure Miss Brown's waist–hip ratio (WHR)

The 'MUST' assessment tool explains these procedures for assessing nutrition if the patient cannot be weighed, or the patient's height cannot be measured.

A stroke can affect a patient in many ways, related to eating and drinking, and on different levels. Some patients may never be able to eat or drink naturally again and will require more advanced feeding techniques such as nasogastric tube or PEG tube feeding. Some patients are not affected at all. It is essential, when a stroke occurs, that a full and proper assessment is conducted.

 Scenario 2

Weighing scales will be different for different ages of children. The type of scales used will depend on the infant or child's age, size, and general condition. Infants and toddlers under three years should be weighed naked, or with very little clothing on. The child should be placed centrally on the scales and the reading should be taken in kilograms.

The weight should be recorded in the infant's medical notes and on a centile chart.

A single weighing of an infant is not generally helpful; infants are generally weighed frequently, to chart the progress of their development and weight gain according to age. This can be compared with previous weights and their clinical history.

 Scenario 3

It is important to involve others, as appropriate, such as parents, classroom teachers, dietician, psychologist, and GP to try to get a picture of the pattern of causality of the child's fear and revulsion for food. For example, from a physical perspective it might be that the child is unwell. However, the fear or revulsion is attributed to the autism (a classic case of diagnostic overshadowing). It might be that some form of behaviour therapy could be beneficial, but this would have to be based, of course, on a **holistic** assessment. Any goals (SMART or otherwise) should be child-centred.

Creating a daily menu card can help in a number of ways. The menu can help children to organize and make sense of the day, in whatever setting they are in. The menu can form part of a food diary to record, over a period of time, the range of foods a child will eat.

The menu is a good tool to use to increase the intake of different foods. The menu can reinforce a child's love of structure and routine, which makes it difficult for the child to ignore written instructions. A child may ignore a verbal instruction, but a verbal instruction combined with symbols as a visual display may be more effective. The menu can be used for many reward systems, for example, just licking the food, biting the food, or chewing a food item.

 Scenario 4

Malnutrition can be very common for patients who have dementia. Mr Patel was used to sitting at home at a table with a regular routine that his wife maintained. In the care home, he tends to wander and possibly no one is checking that he is sitting at the table until he finishes his meals. Providing Mr Patel with a regular routine of sitting at a table and ensuring that he finishes his meals, by taking him back to the table if he wanders, may be enough to help him regain weight. However, expert advice from a dietician could help in the short term to replace the weight that Mr Patel has lost.

7 Eliminating

MARY BALLENTYNE AND VALERIE NESS

Introduction

This chapter provides students with the fundamental skills of assessing and helping patients with elimination problems. Elimination is a basic human process, essential to life, which concerns itself with the excretion of waste from the bladder (urine) and evacuation of waste products from the bowel (faeces). The ability to control these processes is called continence. The maintenance of continence depends on many physiological factors, which will be discussed in this chapter. Problems with these processes affect other activities and can have devastating physical and psychological effects. Many of these problems can begin in childhood before the physiological processes have matured, for example, bedwetting (enuresis) and faecal soiling (encopresis), or can affect those with physical or learning disabilities.

This chapter will discuss the physiology of elimination, the assessment of the patient with elimination problems, including the collection of specimens, and the management of some of these problems, including aiding patients to eliminate and the care of urinary catheters. The skills discussed in this chapter should be dealt with sensitively as they may cause embarrassment to patients, given that they are activities normally undertaken in private.

Learning outcomes

These outcomes relate to numbers 9, 10, and 26 of the NMC's Essential Skill Clusters and specifically to Care Domains 2 and 3 of the NMC's Standards of Proficiency for Pre-registration Nursing (outcomes to be achieved for entry to branch).

On reading the chapter and associated web pages and undertaking supervised activities, the student will be able to:

- Understand the physiology of the bladder and bowel
- Select appropriate equipment for the care of the patient's bladder and bowel needs
- Perform the skills necessary to assist patients to maintain normal elimination
- Document the patient's bladder and bowel output accurately
- Recognize deviations from normal intake and output

Prior knowledge

To perform the clinical skills in this chapter it is important that you have knowledge and understanding of the following anatomy and physiology. This can be obtained from a number of reference books.

- The urinary system, consisting of the kidneys, ureters, bladder, and urethra
- Regulation of the balance of acid–base balance, fluid, and electrolytes
- The digestive system, consisting of the mouth to the anus including the mouth pharynx, oesophagus, stomach, small intestine, and large intestine

Background

Normal bladder function

The bladder and lower urinary tract have two main functions: the storage and expulsion of urine. From a physiological perspective, urinary continence is defined as control of the **detrusor** muscle, competence of the urethral sphincter mechanism, and the anatomic integrity of the urinary tract, so that urine exits the system only during voluntary urination (Gray 2006).

The anatomical structures involved in both the storage and expulsion of urine are:

- The bladder and bladder neck
- The urethra and urethral sphincter mechanism
- The pelvic floor

The bladder

The bladder (see **Fig. 7.1**) is a hollow muscular organ, which lies in the pelvis behind the symphysis pubis. In adults, as the bladder fills it expands upwards and is palpable in the lower abdominal cavity. Alpha and beta receptors are found in the bladder wall. These facilitate the stimulation and **contraction**, as well as the inhibition and relaxation of, smooth muscle. The bladder, therefore, stores and coordinates the emptying of urine (Yeung 2001).

The bladder has the ability to stretch and distend to enable it to fill, when, in adults, the urge to pass urine occurs. A full adult bladder can contain 300–400 ml. The child's bladder will accommodate 50–200 ml of urine and, as the child's urinary system matures, the ability to store more urine develops. Patterns of urinary elimination depend on many things, such as the amount of fluid consumed, an intact central nervous system, *the amount of fluid loss through perspiration*, circadian rhythm, opportunities to **void**, and personal habits. It is considered that the individual may void 6–9 times in 24 hours (Abrams *et al.* 2002) (**Figure 7.2** explains the micturition cycle which governs urinary continence.).

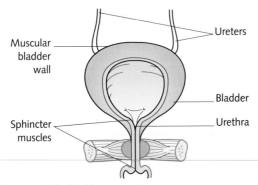

Muscular bladder wall

Sphincter muscles

Ureters

Bladder

Urethra

Figure 7.1 The bladder

Introduction to urinary dysfunction

Urinary incontinence is defined as a sign or symptom; not a condition or disease (Abrams *et al.* 2002). It is also defined as the involuntary leakage of urine, which may be demonstrated **objectively** (Abrams *et al.* 2002).

Types of urinary incontinence

Imbalance between bladder and urethral pressures may result in urinary incontinence. Depending on the particular balance of these forces, individuals may experience one or two types of urinary dysfunction: overactive bladder (OAB) or urge urinary incontinence (UUI), stress urinary incontinence (SUI), overflow, or mixed urinary incontinence (MUI) (see **Table 7.1**).

Prevalence of urinary incontinence

Urinary incontinence is a common condition affecting both men and women. In the UK, up to 20% of women living at home and up to 70% of patients in continuing care are affected. The Department of Health (2000) report the prevalence of this condition in relation to people's age: they note that 1 in 14 women aged between 15 and 44 years experiences urinary incontinence, likewise 1 in 33 men will also experience urinary incontinence. However, the incidence of urinary incontinence in the elderly population is proportionately greater, as the prevalence of this condition increases with age. Furthermore, these figures increase dramatically if a person is in an institutional setting.

Recent research observed that both nursing staff and older patients did not see urinary incontinence as a treatable condition (Horrocks *et al.* 2004; Shaw *et al.* 2001). The prevalence by type and age has been well established (Hunskaar *et al.* 2004; Nitti 2001; Perry 2002; Royal College of Physicians 1995; Thomas *et al.* 1980).

Predisposing risk factors leading to elimination problems

There are many risk factors for urinary problems. Stress urinary incontinence, that is, leakage of urine on coughing,

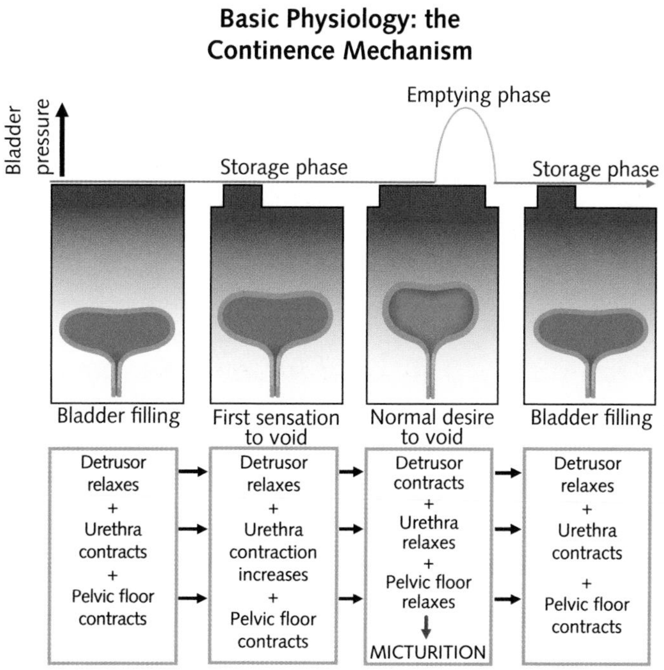

**Basic Physiology: the
Continence Mechanism**

Figure 7.2 The micturition cycle. Viktrup L. International Journal of Clinical Practice 2002; **56 (9)**: 694–700. © Wiley Blackwell 2008.

laughing, and sneezing is considered the most prevalent type of incontinence in women over 25 years of age (McGrother *et al.* 2001). This leakage can range from dampness to flooding. In the UK, this type of urinary incontinence is reported in 41% of women with urinary incontinence. Other studies report that a further 30% of women have combined stress and urge symptoms (the compelling sensation to void urine).

The next most prevalent type of urinary dysfunction with incontinence is described as the overactive bladder. Pregnancy and childbirth, with the traumatic and pressure effects in the region of the lower pelvis, are strongly associated with urinary dysfunction with increased risk after four or more births (Foldspang *et al.* 1999; Viktrup 2002). There are lower urinary tract symptoms (LUTS), which are referred to as storage or voiding problems (frequency, incontinence, terminal dribbling, **dysuria**, and so on).

Menopause is also considered a risk factor, although there is scant evidence to support this (Abrams and Artibani 2004).

Having both stress and overactive bladder symptoms is termed 'mixed urinary incontinence' and can account for symptoms that occur within an older age group. Other recognized risk factors include weight gain and constipation, which result in significant problems for the pelvic floor muscles (Bump and Norton 1998; Cardozo *et al.* 2000; Moller *et al.* 2000; Parazzini *et al.* 2000).

In the adult male, the prevalence of incontinence increases with age. The increasing risk of prostate enlargement as the male ages is a common predisposing factor. Males can also have the symptoms of an overactive bladder. However, the major prevalence of urinary problems in the population is in the frail elderly and those suffering from long-term conditions, such as multiple sclerosis, stroke disease, and those who are physically disabled (Viktrup 2002).

Psychological issues associated with urinary problems

Patients affected by urinary problems report it as bothersome. This is not surprising, as urinary symptoms can interrupt an individual's lifestyle or limit their social activities. This can be particularly disturbing for young and

Table 7.1 Types of urinary incontinence

Type	Signs	Causes	Treatment	Outcome
Stress urinary incontinence (SUI)	Leakage of urine on coughing, laughing, sneezing. Leakage can be damp to flooded.	Weak bladder neck sphincter	Individual pelvic floor training regime; biofeedback; lifestyle changes, such as weight loss, prevention of constipation, fluid advice, **oestrogen** replacement; surgery where indicated.	Prevention of leakage on exertion, strengthen pelvic floor muscles, improve quality of life.
Urge UI (OAB)	Involuntary leakage accompanied or immediately preceded by urgency: frequency, **nocturia**, urge incontinence	Urinary tract infection, central nervous disorder, anxiety, restricted fluid intake, secondary to prostatic enlargement	Lifestyle strategies: advise on fluid intake, decrease all irritants, such as caffeine and coffee, but aim for a good fluid volume of 2 litres per day; exclude or treat urinary tract infection; bladder retraining: individual programme for 12 weeks; teach individual pelvic floor muscle exercise (PFME) programme: antimuscarinic drug therapy	Reduce number of visits to the toilet, reduce leakage episodes, increase bladder capacity, improve quality of life, and gain confidence.
Obstructive (for example benign prostatic hypertrophy [BPH])	Frequency, urgency, hesitancy, nocturnal, poor stream, intermittent flow, incomplete emptying, and urinary tract infection, secondary to symptoms	Enlarged prostate in men, stricture formation or, in the female, severe pelvic organ prolapse	Depends on watchful waiting and prostate assessment. Medication; surgery; catheterization; stricture therapy	To relieve obstruction, to complete bladder emptying, improve symptoms and protect the upper tracts
Neurogenic underactivity	Incomplete emptying or retention; urinary tract infections; frequency; urge; dribbling	Diabetic neuropathy; any central nervous disorder	Intermittent self-catheterization (first choice); suprapubic catheterization; indwelling urethral catheter; medication; voiding techniques	To relieve symptoms, allow bladder to empty sufficiently, reduce number of urinary tract infections and protect the upper tracts

Table 7.1 (*Continued*)

Functional incontinence	May be the result of poor dexterity, immobility, confusion, or urinary tract infection, with no aetiology within the bladder	Poor attention to toileting by care staff, confusional state, environment; acute illness	Attention to good toileting programmes; address contributing factors leading to functional incontinence; assess and exclude urinary tract infection or constipation; plan programme towards the individual; document and be aware of client's toileting needs and habits	Express bladder needs in a safe and comfortable environment, promote continence, maintain dignity

middle-aged people who still maintain an active lifestyle. Because of the fear of urinary leakage and odour, individuals may limit or avoid social or sexual relationships. It is without doubt that urinary problems significantly decrease the overall quality of life (Lekan-Rutledge 2004).

The **social stigma**, embarrassment, and taboos of urinary dysfunction are prevalent in today's society. It is, therefore, essential that nurses treat people with sensitivity, tact, and confidence. Many people can be successfully treated for their urinary problems despite their anxiety at coming forwards for help. However, nurses need to be aware of how they approach the person with urinary problems, be able to perform an assessment of the patient's bladder needs, and, therefore, plan appropriate care (Brittain *et al.* 2001).

It is also important to remember that there can be functional causes of urinary incontinence. Conducting an accurate assessment of the patient's bladder and bowel status will assist in the determination of appropriate strategies to help improve the patient's continence level.

Through careful and detailed assessment, the nurse can hopefully exclude some of the following, which may contribute to the patient's continence status:

- Inability to reach the toilet owing to poor mobility or **arthritis**
- Poor eyesight may hinder the patient from going to the toilet
- Poor lighting in the toilet area and lack of privacy
- Confusional states where the patent is unable to recognize signals from the bladder, or recognize the toilet

- Medications may also predispose the patient to becoming incontinent

These can also be remembered with the acronym DIAPPERS (Fonda *et al.* 1999):

- Delirium
- Infection
- Atrophic vaginitis
- Pharmaceuticals
- Physiological disorders
- Endocrine disorders
- Restricted mobility
- Stool impaction

These variables are often reversible and so the identification and management of these factors may improve the patient's continence status.

Normal bowel function

A clear understanding of normal and abnormal bowel function is necessary in the care of patient's bowel evacuation needs.

The digestive system is involved in four basic processes: ingestion, digestion, absorption, and **defecation**. With regards to bowel management, the part of the digestive system we need to focus on is the working of the large bowel. The contents of the small bowel are mainly fluid (a large amount of water may be absorbed here). Water continues to be absorbed from the large bowel and the contents gradually solidify.

When faeces enter the rectum their presence is detected by **sensory** nerve endings in the muscle around the rectum. This results in the feeling of rectal fullness and the desire to go to the toilet. Defecation involves the relaxation of two sphincters; the internal anal sphincter (under autonomic control) and the external anal sphincter (under both autonomic and voluntary control). A volume of about 150 ml of faeces causes autonomic relaxation of the internal anal sphincter. Faeces then enter the anal canal. Its sensitive nerve endings relay messages to the brain, which are interpreted as urgency—similar to the way the bladder works.

When it is convenient to defecate, the external sphincter also relaxes. A **reflex** action from the spinal cord will initiate defecation. In adults, this can be inhibited by the cerebral cortex when it is inconvenient to defecate: this is a learned process. The stool is then expelled by rectal contraction. The position of the patient's body is also important, as gravity and abdominal effort (forcing **expiration** against a closed glottis) aids expulsion. Unless the stool is hard (because of constipation) only a small amount of abdominal effort is required to propel the stool through the anal canal.

Bowel habits and common complaints

An individual's s bowel habits are influenced by diet, fluid intake, lifestyle factors, and mental state. The average adult will have one brown, soft, and cylindrical bowel motion per day, of about 100–150 g of faeces. Changes in bowel habits and colour, consistency, and shape can be a sign that there is a problem. Common problems are outlined in **Table 7.2**.

Table 7.2 Common bowel complaints

Type of complaint	Manifestation	Causes
Faecal incontinence, Group 1	Have faecal incontinence but intact anal function.	Cerebrovascular accidents, diarrhoea, faecal impaction.
Faecal incontinence, Group 2	Have faecal incontinence and compromised anal sphincter function.	Congenital abnormality or obstetric trauma.
Diarrhoea	Faeces contain excess water and the frequency of elimination is greater.	Infection, medications, inflammatory bowel conditions, stress, tumours, malabsorption conditions. Can also occur in patients who are constipated, because of faecal overloading.
Constipation	Faeces are hard stools, defecation is less frequent than normal for the patient, owing to a problem with colonic propulsion or rectal evacuation, there may be other abdominal and general symptoms.	Often caused by poor low-fibre diet (treat by increasing fibre intake to 35 g per day), also medications, organic disorders, for example, **thyroid**, tumours; poor fluid intake—increased intake or ignoring the 'call to stool', that is, the natural sensation to empty the bowel (this can lead to problems, such as overstretching the rectum or megacolon; this may be habitual or because of depression, confusion, or **dementia**.
Alternating constipation and diarrhoea	As for constipation and diarrhoea.	Can be a sign of irritable bowel syndrome (IBS) or a partial obstruction that could be caused by cancer.

7.1 **Assessment of elimination**

Definition

Before the nurse can assist the patient with elimination problems, it is important that the individual's continence status is determined. This can be a sensitive and embarrassing process for the patient and it is important that the nurse deals with this sensitively and ensures that the patient is treated with confidence and dignity. The nurse must remember that although incontinence is a common condition, it still evokes embarrassment and individuals have difficulty expressing how the problem affects them.

Nurses need to remember when caring for patients with elimination problems, to use the necessary key skills. These skills are in listening, comforting, and allowing patients to discuss and explain their symptoms and feelings regarding their condition. It is also important that the nurse has the underpinning knowledge in order to plan the most appropriate pathway of care for the patient. These essential elements in the process of continence assessment allow the nurse to understand the patient's expectations of treatment.

General approaches to assessment of elimination

When considering the patient with elimination needs we need to consider the approach that is most appropriate for the individual. To determine urinary or bowel problems, it is best to use a structured list of questions; cluster or trigger questions; an **integrated care pathway**; or an individualized continence tool. Whatever form the elimination assessment takes, the nurse must remember at all times that this is a sensitive subject for many patients, as it carries a degree of stigma and social taboo and must be treated with the greatest respect.

The approach to conducting a continence assessment varies according to the patient, local policies, procedures, and nursing styles. Assessments can vary from taking a single patient's history on a one-to-one basis, to adopting a 'patient group' approach, which is sometimes preferred by some continence teams. It may also involve the use of an observational tool if the patient is confused or has a learning disability and cannot give a verbal history.

Subjective data should be collected and should include the patient's **perceptions** of their symptoms and indications of how the problem has changed their lifestyle, or coping strategies. The objective data are where the nurse observes (for example, perineal examination or observation of leakage of urine on coughing), listens (using **active listening** skills and utilizing clinical judgement when interpreting history) and measures (flow rates, urine output, pelvic floor examination, use of quality-of-life scales and symptom scores, frequency–volume charts).

Caution should be exercised when using lay terminology to describe elimination processes and products. Whereas it is generally good advice to speak to patients at their level of understanding, you could inadvertently cause offence by using lay terminology when discussing urine, faeces, **micturition**, and defecation. Be sensitive to this and err on the side of caution.

However, the core components of the assessment should include a symptom profile (urge, urgency, nocturia, frequency) a quality-of-life questionnaire as a marker of patient expectations to treatment, dipstick urinalysis, a frequency–volume chart covering at least three days, MSSU, post-void **residual** tests, and, in women, genitalia examination.

In assessing bowel function and stools, the pattern of defecation and any changes to this, stool colour, shape, and consistency should be assessed. The Bristol Stool Chart (see **Fig. 7.3**) is a very common tool used in many areas to help with accurate and consistent recording. A bowel and food diary may also be used (see **Fig. 7.4**).

When to perform an assessment of a patient's elimination needs

The assessment of a patient's elimination needs should be undertaken as part of a **holistic** assessment. These assessments often highlight problems that patients have perhaps never mentioned to anyone before. An essential part of the initial management of urinary problems is a thorough assessment to establish causes and to identify complex cases or serious conditions.

Assessment of continence status

Step	Rationale
1 Find a private area in which to carry out the assessment and explain the reason for the assessment.	Some questions may cause embarrassment and so the patient's bedside may not be appropriate.
2 Begin the assessment with some key trigger questions, such as: **How long have you had the problem and when did it begin? If you leak urine, is this leakage small, moderate, or large? Do you go to the toilet often and, if so, how often? Do you get up to go to the toilet at night and if so how many times? Do you wear pads to protect your clothes? Do you leak on the way to the toilet?**	To gain insight into the patient's elimination status and perceived incontinence problem, providing a good baseline from which to commence any planned treatments and review successful outcomes.
3 Assess the other influencing factors in relation to elimination:	
Patient's ability to move,	For example, can patient use a commode, lift on to a bed pan?
Condition of patient's skin,	Are there red or broken areas?
Dependence, independence,	Does patient need assistance with clothing?
Frequency and amount of urine passed,	As a part of continence assessment or to detect abnormalities.
Appearance of urine, urinalysis,	To detect abnormalities.
Frequency, consistency, appearance of stools.	To detect abnormalities.
Consider the factors affecting the patient's elimination, that is: Biological: muscle tone or damage, neurological disorders, mobility, **Medication that could affect urinary function (see Box 7.1),** Psychological: altered cognitive state (for example, dementia), emotional state, attitude, and behaviour, **Sociocultural: cultural and religious practices,** Environmental: access to toilet, home, and hospital environment **Politico-economic: diet, money, access to services**	To ensure that a holistic assessment of the patient is completed.

4	Ask the questions in an unhurried manner and use appropriate terminology and language.	To ensure understanding, to allow time for the patient to answer and reduce anxiety.
5	You may need to consult with the patient's carer in some instances.	Certain patients, for example, children, those with learning disabilities, or mental health problems may have difficulty answering questions (ensure that you have **consent** to involve the carer).
6	Refer to appropriate specialist service if a more thorough assessment is required.	There are many specialist investigations that can be carried out if the patient has problems with the maintenance of their continence.

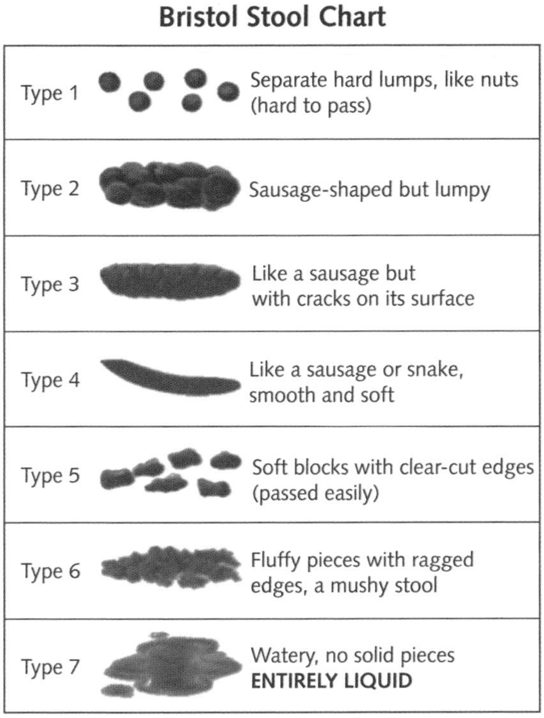

Bristol Stool Chart

Figure 7.3 Bristol stool chart. Reproduced by kind permission of Dr K W Heaton, Reader in Medicine at the University of Bristol. © 2000 Norgine Pharmaceuticals Ltd.

Aftercare

The assessment should be documented in the nursing notes. If a thorough, specialized assessment is required, the patient should be referred to the appropriate health professional, such as the continence nurse specialist. Part of this assessment may include bladder diaries or frequency volume charts and a bladder scan.

Bladder diaries or frequency volume charts

Bladder diaries are recommended by NIHCE (2007) and SIGN (2004) as one of the tools in the assessing of urinary problems. Both bladder diaries and frequency–volume charts are good ways to review *micturition* patterns of the patient. In some cases, the patient may be encouraged to keep and fill out their own diary, particularly if attending on an outpatient basis. If a patient is unable to complete these, a carer may be able to, provided the patient has consented to do so (for example, in a nursing home or residential care environment).

Patients are encouraged to maintain the diary for three consecutive days, including one working and one leisure day (NIHCE 2007). Ideally, the patient should document the number of trips to the toilet and the volumes voided in each 24-hour period. Additionally, the patient should also write the number of leakage episodes and the amount of fluid consumed. From bladder diaries, the nurse can ascertain the amount the patient voids per micturition episode, revealing a large or small capacity bladder, the infrequency or frequency of voids and pattern, the number of trips to the toilet during the night, the number of incontinent episodes and whether these are associated with anything such as movement, exercise, coughing, or urgency.

Bladder scan

This is carried out to exclude *urinary residual problems*. The ICS (Abrams *et al.* 2002) consider that a residual measurement post void is anything over 150 ml. However, the nurse undertaking the bladder scan must

DIET & BOWEL DIARY	WEEK COMMENCING:_____

Please record all you eat and drink each day including times. Also fill in each time you have a bowel action, whether in the toilet, a bowel accident or leakage. Include in this section if you need to change a pad or pants.

FOOD AND DRINK (and time)	BOWEL ACTION (and time)
<u>Monday</u>	
<u>Tuesday</u>	
<u>Wednesday</u>	
<u>Thursday</u>	
<u>Friday</u>	
<u>Saturday</u>	
<u>Sunday</u>	

Figure 7.4 Bowel and food diary

be competent in the procedure (see **Fig. 7.5**) and at interpreting the scan. Detecting whether the patient has a residue of urine is important as the presence of a large residual volume may mimic other characteristics of other types of urinary problems, such as stress urinary incontinence. A large residual volume may also be the cause of recurring urinary tract infections and clinically suggests that the patient has difficulty in emptying the bladder fully.

Developing your skills

It is important to remember that the assessment process is an ongoing process. The patient's elimination needs should not be looked at in isolation as they will affect many of the other activities of living.

Other factors to consider

Nurses also need to be aware that certain medications may contribute to elimination problems. During the history-taking process, it is important to find out what medications the patient is taking and to determine whether the bladder dysfunction could be a direct consequence of medication, whether prescribed or not.

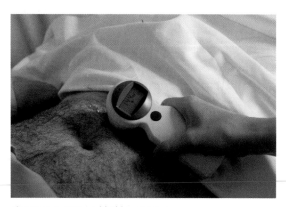

Figure 7.5 Using a bladder scanner

7.2 **Collection and analysis of urine specimens**

Definition

The analysis of urine is an important part of the general elimination assessment process. This 'urinalysis' can provide the nurse with important information about the patient's health, for example, diabetes, renal, urological or liver conditions, infection, and hydration and can screen for abnormal substances that can alert staff to organize further investigations. Other tests can also be carried out, for example, pregnancy testing (by the detection of hormonal changes).

Background

Urine is approximately 95% water, in which are dissolved several substances or waste products, including nitrogenous waste, electrolytes, toxins, pigments, hormones, and other abnormal substances, such as blood, glucose, albumin, or calculi (small stones). This urine is excreted by the kidneys. The kidneys maintain **homeostasis** by regulating the water, electrolyte, and acid-base content of the body. They do this by varying the amount of water and electrolytes leaving the body in the urine.

Three main processes are involved in the excretion of waste products: glomerular filtration, tubular reabsorption, and tubular secretion. The blood plasma is processed to form urine. The urine is then excreted through the ureters, the urinary bladder, and the urethra to the outside of the body (see **Fig. 7.6**).

The volume of urine excreted over a 24-hour period is considered to be 1200 ml, on average. An output of less than 400 ml per day is considered abnormal and may result from low fluid intake, excess fluid loss, or kidney dysfunction (**oliguria** <0.5 (ml/kg)/hr). An output of greater than 3000 ml per day is considered excessive and may result from high fluid intake, diuretic medication, or any metabolic endocrine disease (Abrams *et al.* 2002). If the patient has nocturnal **polyuria**, a referral to a GP may be sought to exclude the diagnosis of a cardiac condition (Abrams *et al.* 2002). Further information about fluid balance can be found in Chapter 6.

Box 7.1 Medications that can affect urinary function	
Drug	Side effect
Antidepressants, antipsychotic, sedatives, **hypnotics**	Sedation, retention (overflow)
Diuretics	Frequency, urgency (OAB)
Caffeine	Frequency, urgency (OAB)
Anticholinergics	Retention (overflow)
Alcohol	Sedation, frequency (OAB)
Narcotics	Retention, constipation, sedation (OAB and overflow)
Alpha-adrenergic blockers	Decreased urethral tone (stress incontinence)
Alpha-adrenergic agonists	Increased urethral tone, retention (overflow)
Beta-adrenergic agonists	Inhibited detrusor function, retention (overflow)
Calcium channel blockers	Retention (overflow)
ACE inhibitors	Cough (stress incontinence)

When to collect and analyse urine specimens

Collection of a urine sample and analysis, by observation or urinalysis, is performed as part of the general assessment process both in acute and community settings.

A midstream specimen of urine (MSSU) is required if a urinary tract infection is suspected. This sample is sent to bacteriology for culture and sensitivity testing, to detect any abnormal microorganisms.

Sometimes a 24-hour urine collection will be requested. This procedure measures the components of urine or the concentration of these components over a 24-hour period and can, therefore, be used to assess kidney function.

Much of the literature suggests using the first void of the day, where possible, as a urine sample, because it contains the highest bacterial count (Dougherty and

The kidney

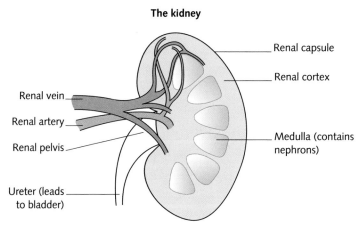

Figure 7.6 The kidney

Lister 2008; Wilson 2005); however, some authors disagree with this; there is **urinary stasis** within the bladder in the morning (Nicholls 1997). An early-morning urine sample for acid and alcohol-fast bacilli testing (AAFB for tuberculosis, TB) must be the first urination of day, and is usually collected for three days in a row. Whenever the sample is taken, it is important that subsequent samples are taken at the same time of the day to allow comparison. Specimens can also be taken directly from catheters; this is discussed later in this chapter.

Procedure: Obtaining a midstream sample of urine (MSSU)

Collecting an MSSU from a child

It may be difficult to obtain an MSSU from a child. It may be easier if the child sits on the toilet seat facing the back of the toilet. This allows the nurse or parent to stand behind the child and collect the specimen in the container. A clean potty specimen may be taken if the child is trained, or adhesive bags can be used for those who are not toilet trained. These bags are attached to the infant and removed straight after urination, so that a specimen can be collected. For example:

- Application of a sterile paediatric urine collection pouch for children who cannot pass urine on request
- Insertion of a Euron collection pad into the child's nappy and withdrawing urine using the equipment provided in the pack

Developing your skills

A wide variety of reagent strips is available for urinalysis testing, so when you are on your clinical placement ask your mentor about them and read the manufacturer's instructions. Also, different collection bottles and labels are used in different clinical environments, for example, a culture of a urine specimen often requires a different container; again, discuss these with your mentor and read the local procedure manual.

Obtaining a midstream sample of urine (MSSU)

Step		Rationale
1	Draw curtains round bed area or close room door.	To ensure patient privacy.
2	Explain the procedure and reason for the sample being taken and obtain consent.	To obtain informed consent and cooperation.
3	Ask patient to clean the genital areas with simple unperfumed soap and water. The patient may need some assistance with this: if so disposable gloves and apron should be worn for your protection.	To prevent contamination and false readings.
4	If the patient is able to urinate, ask the patient to pass urine into the toilet then catch the middle section of the stream in the container (15–25 ml), then pass the remaining urine into the toilet.	This is to ensure that the urine collected is representative of the urine actually in the bladder, uncontaminated by urethral organisms.
5	Collect urine in a single-use sterile container.	To prevent contamination.
6	The patient or nurse should ensure that the specimen container does not touch the patient's genital area and that the inside of the container is not touched by the patient's fingers.	To prevent contamination.
7	Screw the lid securely back onto the container.	To prevent spillage or contamination.
8	If you have been assisting, then remove disposable gloves, apron, and wash hands.	To reduce spread of infection and maintain personal hygiene.
9	Allow the patient hand-washing facilities	
10	Transfer specimen into sterile specimen container immediately and label container with the patient's details.	To prevent contamination and to ensure that sample is correctly identified.
11	Ensure container lid is secure.	To prevent spillage in transit.

continued

12	Fill in the microbiology form with patient details. It is important to check details with patient to ensure they are correct.	To ensure correct patient information is supplied.
13	Give as much detail as possible, including symptoms and current diagnosis.	Helps the laboratory analyse the results.
14	Send the sample to the laboratory as soon after collection as possible for microscopy, culture, and sensitivity (MC&S). If not collected immediately then refrigerate.	Light and room temperature affect the analysis of results, for example, increase microorganisms, change the **pH**, break down bilirubin and urobilogen, increase bacterial growth.
15	Record in nursing notes specimen obtained.	To ensure that the test is not carried out again by mistake.

Procedure: Assessing a urine sample

Observe the characteristics of the urine sample, as shown below

Observation	Interpretation
Colour	
Light yellow (straw colour)	Normal
Dark yellow	**Dehydration**
Bright red or red-brown	May signify blood in the urine (haematuria)
Brown-green or strong yellow	May signify bilirubin (an indication of liver or gallbladder problems)
Some foods or drugs also influence the colour	
Clarity	
Cloudiness or debris	May signify **pus**, protein, or white blood cells (owing to infection, urinary stasis, or kidney stones)
Odour	
'Fishy' smell	May be a sign of infection or suggest that the sample has been waiting too long for collection
'Pear-drop or **acetone**' smell	May suggest that ketones (produced during the metabolism of fat) are present
Foods and medications can produce certain smells	

Obtaining and testing a urine specimen for urinalysis

▶ Step   Rationale

	Step	Rationale
1	Explain the procedure and obtain informed consent. In children, use appropriate terminology.	To obtain informed consent and cooperation.
2	Assess patient's ability to carry out the task.	To allow assistance to be given if required.
3	Explain carefully how the specimen is obtained.	To ensure patient cooperation.
4	Assistance or supervision may be required (if so wear disposable gloves and apron).	To prevent contamination and reduce spread of infection.
5	Ensure that genital area is cleansed using plain water and dried with a towel.	To prevent contamination.
6	Once client begins urinary stream, the initial portion should be allowed to escape.	This initial stream flushes the urethral orifice and **meatus** of **resident bacteria**. The specimen is collected from the midstream.
7	Prior to urine testing, check the expiry date of the reagent strips and ensure that the container has not been left open. Using disposable gloves, dip the test strip into the urine, ensuring that all the test pads are wet with urine.	To ensure accurate results.
8	Withdraw the strip, wiping along rim of container to remove excess urine.	To prevent droplets of urine falling from test strip.
9	Wait for the time recommended by manufacturer.	To ensure accurate results.
10	Compare the test strip (see Fig. 7.7) with the label on the side of the test strip container (see Table 7.3 for common tests and values).	Must be the same container as the test strip to ensure accurate results.
11	Document results and dispose of waste correctly in yellow clinical waste bag.	To keep a record and to follow policy.
12	Report any abnormalities to appropriate nurse.	
13	Remove disposable gloves and apron and wash hands at end of procedure.	To prevent contamination.

Obtaining a 24-hour urine collection

Step		Rationale
1	Explain the procedure and obtain informed consent. In children, use appropriate terminology.	To obtain informed consent and cooperation.
2	Assess patient's ability to carry out the task.	To allow assistance to be given if required.
3	Give the patient a urine collection container, labelled with the patient's details (full name and hospital number). The patient may need more than one container.	To allow the patient to collect the urine and to ensure that the correct details are given.
4	Sometimes the container will contain a small amount of acid; therefore, care must be taken.	This acts as a preservative. Acids can be corrosive.
5	Ask the patient to empty his or her bladder prior to commencing the collection and record the time.	To allow patient and staff to know the exact time that the collection started.
6	Ask the patient to collect all the urine passed in the next 24 hours in the container. The patient should not pass urine directly into the container—another container, such as a clean jug, should be used, and the contents transferred.	To collect a 24-hour sample. To prevent contamination.
7	Ensure that the lid is always securely fitted after collection.	To prevent spillage.
8	The patient may need to keep the container refrigerated throughout the collection.	To preserve the urine specimen.
9	End the collection exactly 24 hours after beginning by getting the patient to urinate and adding this sample to the container.	To ensure accurate collection.

Aftercare

Once obtained, the MSSU specimen should be placed in the specimen fridge for transporting to the laboratory. If collected in a red-topped bottle, the specimen can be stored at room temperature until taken to the laboratory.

It is important to document that an MSSU has been taken and when. This prevents another test being done unnecessarily.

It is also important that you know what urinalysis findings mean, so that you can report any abnormalities.

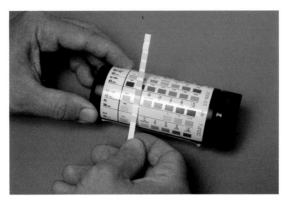

Figure 7.7 Urine reagent strips

Table 7.3 Urinalysis findings

Test	Normal values	Common causes of changes
Glucose	Not normally present in urine.	Raised blood glucose (diabetics or those on glucose infusion); pregnancy; renal conditions
Bilirubin	Not normally present in urine.	Liver damage (paracetamol overdose, hepatitis, bile tract obstruction, for example, gallstones)
Ketones	These are produced by the breakdown of fatty acids.	Fasting (especially with fever and vomiting), diabetic ketoacidosis
Specific gravity	Tests the concentration and diluting power of the kidneys. Normal values vary depending on fluid balance, usually between 1.000 and 1.030.	High—dehydration, renal failure Low—high fluid intake, diabetes insipidus, renal failure
Blood pH	This is not normally present. A false positive test may result if patient is menstruating. 4.5–8.0	Haematuria—kidney or urinary tract disorders, Haemoglobinura—sickle cell disease crisis Low—diabetes, starvation, reduced potassium High—stale urine, alkalaemia if caused by vomiting, UTI
Protein	This is best tested in the morning. Normal urine has a low level of albumin.	UTI, renal conditions, fever, **heart failure**, pre-eclampsia
Urobilinogen	Small amount is normally present.	High—red blood cell disorders Low—biliary tract obstruction
Nitrate	Not normally found in urine. Best tested using the first morning specimen.	UTI with nitrate-producing organisms
Leucocytes	Not normally present in urine.	Urinary tract infection

7.3 **Collecting and analysing stool specimens**

Definition

The number of times that people pass stools (faeces) in a day and the colour and consistency of them varies dependent on many factors such as diet, lifestyle, and mental state. Faeces consist of 30–50 g of solids (cellulose, epithelial cells, bacteria, salts, and a brown pigment) and 70–100 g of water. The smell is caused by bacterial decomposition.

Assessment of a patient's normal elimination habits will allow any changes to be identified. Stool specimens can be sent for analysis to detect microorganisms, such as intestinal pathogens or other parasites, if there is a suspicion of a gastrointestinal infection. The main types of microbiological test are antibody-antigen tests (which detect viruses), examination for parasites and their eggs under the microscope, and routine cultures. Stool samples can also be sent to detect **occult haematuria** (hidden blood), either in the laboratory or with a faecal occult blood (FOB) testing kit in the clinical environment if there is a suspicion of bleeding. Stool samples can also be used to measure faecal fat and elastase content.

When to collect a stool specimen

A stool specimen is often requested when there is a change in bowel habit or there are visible changes in a patient's stool. The specimen will be sent to the laboratory and analysis, such as microscopic examination, chemical testing, and microbiological testing, will be carried out. Often a culture test will be used to detect and identify **pathogenic** bacteria.

Collecting a stool specimen

Key point: Single specimens are usually requested if there is a suspicion of infection. These are sent off to the laboratory for culture and sensitivity to detect microorganisms. Multiple samples at later times (consecutive) are often requested if there is a suspicion of fat or blood in the stools.

Step   Rationale

	Step	Rationale
1	Explain reasons for sample being taken and obtain informed consent.	To ensure informed consent and cooperation.
2	Ask patient to perform procedure in a locked toilet cubicle.	To ensure privacy.
3	Ask patient to clean the genital areas with soap and water.	To prevent contamination.
4	Collect faeces in a single-use clinically clean bedpan.	To prevent contamination and false readings.
5	Wash hands and put on nonsterile gloves and apron.	To comply with **universal precautions**.
6	Observe stool for consistency and colour and note findings.	To identify any obvious abnormalities.

7	Unscrew the top of the sample container without contamination.	To prevent contamination.
8	Collect a sample of stool using the spoon incorporated in the lid of container.	This remains attached to the lid do not remove.
9	Screw the lid securely back onto the container.	To prevent spillage or contamination.
10	Dispose of remaining faecal matter immediately into macerator.	To dispose of the remaining stool.
11	Remove gloves and apron and wash hands.	To prevent any contamination. Hands can become contaminated when removing gloves.
12	Label the specimen pot with all the patient's details.	To prevent misidentification.

Observations of stool specimens

- If the stool appears black and tarry (melaena), this indicates bleeding from the upper gastrointestinal tract, for example, oesophageal varices or bleeding duodenal or peptic ulcer
- If the stool is more maroon in colour, this often indicates bleeding from the lower gastrointestinal tract, for example, inflammatory bowel disease or malignancy (cancer)
- Fresh blood in the stools usually indicates haemorrhoids or diverticular disease but could also indicate the previous conditions

When to test for faecal occult blood (FOB)

If there is suspicion of bleeding but no blood can be seen in the stools, the faecal occult blood test should be carried

Testing for faecal occult blood (FOB)

Step		Rationale
1	Explain reasons for sample being taken and obtain informed consent.	To ensure informed consent and cooperation.

continued

2	Follow procedure for collecting a stool sample until the step involving the sample container.	
3	Obtain the FOB testing kit.	To obtain the correct equipment.
4	Using a scraper, take a small sample of the faeces and smear it on to the piece of card from the testing kit (the instructions on the kit will tell you what to do).	To prepare the sample for testing.
5	Drop the chemical (from the bottle provided) on to the sample.	To start the reaction.
6	If there is a change in colour after adding the chemical, there is blood present.	This is how the test is observed.
7	Dispose of remaining faecal matter immediately into macerator.	To comply with health and safety procedure.
8	Remove gloves and apron and wash hands.	To prevent any contamination. Hands can become contaminated when removing gloves.
9	Document findings in patient's notes.	To keep correct records.

out. A positive result can indicate one of the previously mentioned conditions; in this case, further investigations should be carried out.

Faecal occult blood testing can also be used as a screening tool to detect early bowel cancer. However, it should be noted that a positive result does not mean that the patient has cancer. Further investigations would be offered to find the cause of the bleeding.

When testing for FOB, it may be that more than one test is required, often at two or three separate times or days. This will allow for gastrointestinal bleeding disorders to be detected; sometimes bleeding occurs at different times of the day.

Aftercare

Ensure that you detail in the patient's notes that a specimen has been collected and sent for analysis. This prevents any additional samples being collected unnecessarily. Document any findings as appropriate.

Developing your skills

Familiarize yourself with the FOB testing kit that is used in your area and read the manufacturer's instructions. Different specimen bottles and labels are used in different clinical environments. Discuss these with your mentor and read the local procedure manual.

7.4 **Aiding patients to urinate or defecate**

Definition

In some cases the patient may be unable to use the toilet due to illness or immobility and will have to be provided with a bedpan, commode (**Fig. 7.9**), or urinal. Again, the nurse must exercise tact and sensitivity as the patient may find using these aids highly embarrassing.

There are both male and female urinals. The female urinal, often referred to as a 'slipper' comes in various types and tends to either sit under the thighs or between the thighs, tucked under the perineum. They can be formed as shallow dishes or deeper jugs, often with mouldings and sometimes with detachable drainage bag containers.

There are two types of bedpan—disposable and plastic. Disposable bedpans are single-use only and need to be put in plastic holders (see **Fig. 7.8**). They are then destroyed, usually in a mechanical bedpan disposer that macerates them to pulp. The plastic bedpans are usually sterilized after each use in a sterilizing machine, according to the manufacturer's instruction.

When to assist a patient to urinate or defecate

When a patient requests to either urinate or defecate it is essential that the nurse responds immediately and in an approachable way. Failure to do so can cause patients distress and they may change their behaviour accordingly, that is, limit their fluid intake to reduce the number of times they will need the toilet. This can lead to incontinence, retention, infection, and constipation as well as patient distress. At all times, the patient should be screened to ensure privacy and dignity.

Assisting the patient to use a bedpan

Step	Rationale
1 Explain the procedure and gain patient's consent.	To gain informed consent and patient compliance.
2 Assess patient's moving and handling needs; consider risk assessment.	To determine whether further help is required and patient's risk of falls.
3 Collect bedpan—may be a disposable bedpan in a rigid holder or nondisposable.	To prepare for procedure.
4 Cover with disposable cover.	To prevent embarrassment.
5 Draw curtains around patient's bed area or close room door.	To maintain patient privacy.
6 Put on disposable gloves and apron.	To prevent spread of infection.
7 Assist patient to adjust clothing to expose the area.	To prevent any of clothing from becoming soiled.

continued

8	Ask patient to raise bottom off the bed or assist them with this if necessary.	Ensure that correct moving and handling techniques are used.
9	If the patient wishes, it may be advisable to place a waterproof or incontinence pad underneath the patient.	To prevent any leakage or spillage onto the sheets.
10	Place bedpan on top of the pad, underneath patient, and ensure that it is safely in place.	To prevent any contamination onto the sheet.
11	Ensure the bedcovers are covering patient appropriately.	To maintain dignity.
12	If the patient is able, leave toilet paper with the patient and wait outside the curtains or room; give patient nurse call button.	To allow the patient privacy.
13	Assist patient to wipe if necessary and ask patient to lift up off bedpan and remove it.	
14	If the patient's output is being recorded, the toilet wipes should not be disposed of in the bedpan but in another receptacle.	To allow accurate output recording.
15	Allow patient to wash hands.	To maintain personal hygiene.
16	Cover bedpan with disposable cover and remove from the area.	To reduce embarrassment.
17	Ensure that patient is left in a comfortable position.	To maintain comfort and dignity.
18	Observe urine or faeces prior to disposal and measure if required.	To assess patient.
19	Dispose of bedpan as appropriate.	
20	Wash and dry holder.	To prevent spread of infection.
21	Wash and dry hands.	To prevent spread of infection.

Assisting the patient to use a commode

Step	Rationale
1 Explain the procedure and gain patient's consent.	To gain informed consent and patient compliance.
2 Assess patient's moving and handling needs; consider risk assessment.	To determine whether further help is required and if patient is at risk of falls.
3 Ensure that the commode is clean.	To reduce spread of infection.
4 Place the commode at the person's bedside and ensure that the wheels of the commode are locked. Ensure that there is a bedpan receiver in place under the commode (see Fig. 7.9).	To prevent any falls or accidents.
5 Draw curtains around patient's bed area or close room door.	To maintain patient privacy.
6 Assist the patient onto the commode. If safe, leave the patient; give the patient a nurse call button.	To maintain patient privacy.
7 Once patient has finished using the commode, assist patient to stand.	
8 Wear gloves. If patient requires assistance using toilet paper, wipe the patient's bottom using toilet paper, from front to back, followed by skin cleanser and wipe area clean.	To prevent the spread of infection from the bowel area to the urethra (this is especially important in women who have a very short urethra).
9 Ensure that you pat the skin dry after doing this.	To prevent skin breakdown.
10 Assist the patient to wash and dry hands.	To maintain personal hygiene.
11 Before removing the commode, ensure the lid is placed on top of it. Then assist the patient back to bed and pull back the screens.	To maintain patient dignity.
12 Dispose of the bedpan in the normal way in the macerator.	To reduce spread of infection.
13 The contents may need to be measured and recorded accurately in the patient's fluid balance chart.	To assess and monitor patient.

continued

Step	Rationale
14 Wash the commode.	To prevent spread of infection.
15 Wash and dry hands.	To prevent spread of infection.

Assisting the patient to use a male or female urinal

Step	Rationale
1 Explain the procedure and gain patient's consent.	To gain informed consent and patient compliance.
2 Assess patient's moving and handling needs.	To determine whether further help is required.
3 Draw curtains around patient's bed area or close room door.	To maintain patient privacy.
4 Put on gloves and apron.	To prevent spread of infection.
5 **For males:** Assist patient to stand if able. Ask him to place his penis completely in the urinal and hold it there (assist if necessary—ensure you are wearing gloves).	To assist in urination. To avoid urine spillage.
For females: Positioning of the patient depends on the type of female urinal being used and the ability of the patient. Generally, the patient should tuck the urinal into position from the front or pivot it into position under the thigh from the side or by rolling her from her side onto the pre-positioned urinal.	To position patient correctly on to the urinal to prevent spillage.
6 Leave the patient, if safe to do so, leaving a nurse-call button.	To maintain patient dignity.
7 Remove urinal and allow patient to wash hands.	To maintain patient's personal hygiene.
8 Ensure that you leave the patient in a safe and comfortable position.	To maintain patient comfort and safety.
9 Observe and measure urine if required and dispose of urinal in macerator.	To assess for abnormalities. To comply with health and safety procedures.
10 Wash and dry hands.	To prevent spread of infection.

Aftercare

Any abnormal findings should be documented in the nursing notes and passed on to the appropriate professional. Measurements should be documented on the fluid balance chart.

It is important to maintain the patients' independence and encourage them to have as much control as possible over their own elimination needs. This may involve teaching patients to be independent each time they request the toilet, orientating them to the environment, or ensuring that they have a nurse-call button. If a patient has sensations of urgency, a bed near to the toilet may be all that is required to prevent the patient from developing a continence problem.

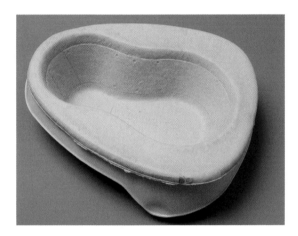

Figure 7.8 Disposable bedpan

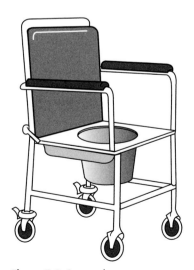

Figure 7.9 Commode

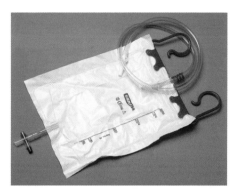

Figure 7.10 Urine drainage bag

Developing your skills

Familiarize yourself with the various aids that are used in your clinical placements and observe your experienced members of staff help patients to use these. Always remember to assess your patients prior to assisting them with their toileting needs and ensure that you maintain their dignity at all times.

Other factors to consider

With children, it may be that the parents wish to be involved. The nurse should, therefore, ensure that they know where appropriate equipment can be found. They may bring in the child's potty with them, as a familiar object can help reduce the anxiety related to a hospital visit.

As a student you may encounter cultural issues, for example, the patient may ask for a same-sex nurse. Muslim women will often not discuss their elimination habits in the presence of their husband or a male interpreter. Initial assessment of the patient should alert nursing staff to these sensitive requests and, where possible, their needs should be met.

7.5 **Catheter care**

Definition

A urinary catheter (**Fig. 7.10**) is a hollow tube that is positioned in the urethra with its end in the bladder, from where urine can be drained and collected. There will be times when a patient you are caring for may have a urinary catheter *in situ*. Nurses must ensure that the catheter

Meatal cleansing - care of bedbound patients with a urinary catherter *in situ*

▶ Step | Rationale

	Step	Rationale
1	Explain the procedure and gain patient's consent.	To gain informed consent and patient compliance.
2	Gather necessary equipment.	To prepare.
3	Draw curtains around patient's bed area or close room door.	To maintain patient privacy.
4	Position patient to allow for access and patient comfort.	For patient comfort and ease of procedure.
5	Wash your hands and put on disposable gloves and apron.	To prevent spread of infection.
6	Use a fresh cloth/wipe and soap and water to clean the area.	Studies have shown that there is no need to use antiseptic or antibacterial agents.
7	Cleanse the external urethral meatus. Clean downwards in females, away from the meatus. In males, retract the foreskin before cleansing and then replace afterwards.	To prevent spread of infection. To allow access to the meatus: replacing the foreskin will prevent a paraphimosis. To remove any discharge.
8	Clean the shaft of the catheter away from the catheter–meatus junction.	
9	Ensure that the area is dried thoroughly.	To prevent skin breakdown.
10	Ensure that the patient is left in a comfortable position.	For patient comfort and dignity.
11	Remove equipment and remove disposable gloves, apron.	To prevent spread of infection.
12	Wash hands.	To prevent spread of infection.

Emptying a catheter bag

Key point: If you are asked to empty a catheter bag and you find that there is very little urine in it, you should consult the patient's fluid balance chart to see if this is abnormal and alert the patient's nurse. It could be that the catheter is blocked or kinked, or incorrectly placed, so further assessment would need to be carried out.

Step	Rationale
1 Explain the procedure and gain patient's consent.	To gain informed consent and patient compliance.
2 Gather necessary equipment.	To prepare.
3 Draw curtains around patient's bed area or close room door.	To maintain patient privacy.
4 Wash hands and put on disposable gloves and apron.	To prevent cross-infection.
5 Clean the outlet port with an alcohol swab and allow to dry.	To prevent risk of infection.
6 Open the port and allow the urine to drain into a collecting receptacle, for example, measuring jug.	To empty the catheter bag.
7 Close port and clean again with alcohol swab.	To prevent risk of infection.
8 Reposition catheter bag.	
9 Cover the receptacle and dispose of contents in the sluice. Observe for any abnormalities and measure contents as appropriate.	To reduce contamination and to assess patient's elimination needs.
10 Remove gloves and apron.	To prevent spread of infection.
11 Wash hands.	To prevent spread of infection.

Collection of a catheter specimen of urine

Step	Rationale
1 Explain how the specimen is obtained and why it is necessary and obtain informed consent.	To gain informed consent and patient compliance.
2 Assess patient's ability to carry out the task.	To ensure compliance or to organize assistance.
3 Wash hands and wear disposable gloves.	To prevent spread of infection.
4 Clamp the drainage tubing of the urine bag and wait until sufficient urine collects to allow specimen to be collected.	Never clamp the catheter as this can damage the balloon port lumen and prevent the balloon from being deflated.
5 Swab the sampling port with 70% alcohol swab and allow to dry for 30 seconds.	To prevent contamination.
6 Insert a needle attached to a syringe into the port at a 45° angle. (Some tubes contain ports that connect directly to the syringe.)	This section is made of self-sealing material.
7 Withdraw the correct amount of urine: 15–25 ml.	The sample must be large enough for the laboratory to test.
8 Remove the needle and syringe and transfer urine to the sterile specimen pot.	
9 Dispose of sharps correctly.	To prevent sharps injury.
10 Transfer specimen into sterile specimen container immediately and label container with the patient's details.	To prevent contamination. To prevent misidentification.
11 Ensure that container lid is secure.	To prevent spillage in transit.
12 Remove gloves and apron.	To prevent spread of infection.
13 Wash hands.	To prevent spread of infection.
14 Fill in the microbiology form with patient details. It is important to check details with the patient to ensure that they are correct.	To complete request form correctly.

15	Give as much detail as possible to help the laboratory including symptoms and current diagnosis.	
16	Send the sample to the laboratory for microscopy, culture, and sensitivity tests (MC&S).	To perform the test.
17	Record in nursing notes that a specimen has been obtained.	To ensure the test is not carried out again by mistake.

is patent at all times and that every effort is made to prevent ascending infection in the catheterized patient.

The catheter is kept in place in the bladder by an inflated balloon. This prevents the catheter from accidentally slipping out of the bladder. Once the catheter has been inserted into the urinary bladder through the urethra, this balloon is inflated with sterile water.

Background

There are many clinical reasons for catheterization:

- Retention of urine
- Haemodynamic monitoring
- Post-operative care
- Post labour,
- Receiving chemotherapy drugs,
- Prostatic obstruction,
- Imaging studies of the lower urinary tract.

When to provide catheter care

Cleaning a catheter and the surrounding area should be considered as a general part of personal hygiene. If the patient is independent and can have baths or showers, then the cleansing can be done as part of the normal routine. Over-cleansing can cause irritation and increase the incidence of infection.

A catheter bag should be emptied when it becomes almost full or is heavy for the patient to carry, or it may be emptied hourly if an accurate fluid balance is required. A specimen of urine may be requested from a catheter, for reasons previously discussed in the section on urine specimen collection.

Procedures

Key point: In all procedures in relation to catheter care, infection control measures are vital as catheter infections are very common (NHS Quality Improvement Scotland 2004).

Aftercare

Any abnormalities detected during cleansing should be documented in the patient's notes. For example, was there any discharge from the catheter, or was there any leakage around the catheter? If any abnormalities are detected when emptying the catheter bag, they should also be documented and the urine should not be discarded until this information has been passed on to the appropriate nurse or doctor, as a sample may be requested.

Developing your skills

There are many different catheter bags available, in all shapes and sizes. You will become familiar with these during your placements. The drainage system should be chosen to be appropriate for the patient. Many of these are worn on the thigh, calf or, trunk and attached with belts or straps, or can be supported in a holster or a pocket sewn into normal clothing. Tube lengths, bag size, and tap designs vary, again to allow for individualized patient care. There are also bags that are more suited to day or night. Larger bags can be used at night or the patient's normal bag can be attached via the outlet tap to a night drainage bag that can hold more urine and can be supported in a holder to keep it off the ground.

Patient scenarios

Consider what you should do in the following situations, then turn to the end of the section to check your answers.

Further scenarios are available at **www. oxfordtextbooks.co.uk/orc/docherty.**

Scenario 1

Jane is 28 years old. She visits the clinic with a history of two previous urinary tract infections, the latter one resulting in admission to hospital, where she was also found to have a high residual volume. She was treated on both occasions with an **antibiotic**. She experiences pain when she has a urinary tract infection. Her medical history is unrevealing and she is not taking any medication. She describes initial hesitancy in micturition and admits that when she has a urinary tract infection she drinks three litres to distend her bladder. She also reveals that she has a problem in urinating in toilets other than her own. She goes on to reveal that when she went on holiday last year she did not need to go to the toilet for nine hours, which she says is not unusual.

1   Consider the issues that affect Jane.
2   What else do you need to know about her history?
3   Devise an action plan for Jane detailing treatment strategies. Explain your reasons.

Scenario 2

John is an 11-year-old boy, who has had surgery after breaking his leg. He is in a full-leg plaster and is unable to bear weight. You are a student nurse caring for him and he tells you that he needs to pass urine.

1   What options are available to you?
2   What will you assess in order to choose the best option for John?

Scenario 3

Craig is a 52-year-old patient on the general medical ward where you are a student. He has been admitted for investigation of central chest pain. He is normally continent at home, however, for the past two days he has had episodes of urinary incontinence.

1   What assessment would you carry out?
2   What may be the cause of these episodes?
3   What management strategies could you adopt?

Scenario 4

Mrs McDonald is 78 and has a history of early-stage dementia. You are in her home visiting her with the district nurse when her home help tells you that she has been increasingly incontinent at night (nocturnal enuresis) sometimes in bed and sometimes on the way to the toilet.

1   What would you include in your assessment?
2   What could be the cause?
3   What management strategies could you adopt?

Website

 www.oxfordtextbooks.co.uk/orc/docherty/

You may find it helpful to work through our short online quiz and interactive scenarios intended to help you to develop and apply the skills in this chapter.

References

Abrams P, Cardozo L, Fall M, et al. (2002). The standardisation of terminology of lower urinary tract function: a report from the standardisation sub committee of the ICS. *Neurourology and Urodynamics,* **21**, 167–78.

Abrams P and Artibani W (2004). *Understanding Stress Urinary Incontinence.* Ismar Healthcare, Belgium.

Brittain K, Perry S, and Williams K (2001). Triggers that prompt people with urinary symptoms to seek help. *British Journal of Nursing,* **10**(2), 74–6.

Bump R and Norton PA (1998). Epidemiology and natural history of pelvic floor dysfunction. *Obstetrics and Gynecology Clinics of North America,* **25**, 723–46.

Cardozo L, Staskin D, and Kirby M, eds (2000). *Urinary Incontinence in Primary Care.* Isis Medical Media, Oxford.

Department of Health (2000). *Good Practice in Continence Services.* The Stationery Office, London.

Dougherty L and Lister S (2008). *The Royal Marsden Hospital Manual of Clinical Nursing Procedures,* 8th edn. Blackwell, Oxford.

Foldspang A, Mommsen S, and Djurhuus JC (1999). Prevalent urinary incontinence as a correlate of pregnancy, vaginal childbirth and obstetric techniques. *American Journal of Public Health,* **89**, 209–12.

Fonda D, Benvenutti F, Castleden M, *et al.* (1999). Management of incontinence in older people. In Abrams P, Khoury S, and Wein A, eds, *Incontinence: 1st International Consultation on Incontinence,* pp. 731–73. Health Publication Ltd, Plymouth.

Horrocks S, Somerset M, Stoddart H, and Peters TJ (2004) What prevents older people from seeking treatment for urinary incontinence? A qualitative exploration of barriers to the use of community continence services. *Family Practice,* **21**(6), 686–96.

Hunskaar S, Lose G, Sykes D, and Voss S (2004). The prevalence of urinary incontinence in women in four European countries. *British Journal of Urology International,* **93**, 324–30.

Lekan-Rutledge D (2004). Urinary incontinence strategies for frail elderly women. *Urology Nurse,* **24**(4), 281–301.

Moller L, Lose G, and Jorgensen T (2000). The prevalence and bothersomeness of lower urinary tract symptoms in women 40–60 years of age. *Acta Obstetricia et Gynecologica Scandinavica,* **79**, 298–305.

McGrother CW, Shaw C, Perry SI, Dallosso HM, and Mensah FK (2001). Epidemiology (Europe). In Cardozo L and Staskin D, eds, *Textbook of Female Urology and Urogynaecology,* Chapter 3, pp. 21–34. Isis Medical Media Ltd, Hampshire UK.

NIHCE (2007). *Urinary Incontinence: The Management of Urinary Incontinence in Women.* National Institute for Health and Clinical Excellence, London.

NHS Quality Improvement Scotland (2004). *Urinary Catheterisation and Catheter Care.* NHS Quality Improvement Scotland, Edinburgh.

Nicholls C (1997). Urological investigations. In Fillingham S and Douglas J, eds, *Urological Nursing,* 2nd edn, pp. 30–56. Balliere Tindall, London.

Nitti VW (2001). *The Prevalence of Urinary Incontinence.* Department of Urology, New York University School of Medicine, New York.

Parazzini F, Collii E, Origgi G, *et al.* (2000). Risk factors for urinary incontinence in women. *European Urology,* **37**, 637–43.

Perry S (2002). Prevalence of faecal incontinence in adults aged 40 years or more living in the community. *Gut,* **50**, 480–4.

Royal College of Physicians (1995). *Incontinence: Causes, Management and Provision of Services.* Royal College of Physicians, London.

SIGN (2004). *Management of Urinary Incontinence in Primary Care.* Scottish Intercollegiate Guideline Network, Scotland.

Shaw C, Tansey R, Jackson C, Hyde C, and Allan R (2001). Barriers to help seeking in people with urinary symptoms. *Family Practice,* **18**(1), 48–52.

Thomas TM, Plymat KR, Blannin J, and Meade TW (1980). Prevalence of urinary incontinence. *British Medical Journal,* **281**(6250), 1243–5.

Viktrup L (2002). The risk of lower urinary tract symptoms five years after the first delivery. *Neurourology and Urodynamics,* **21**, 2–29.

Wilson LA (2005). Urinalysis, *Nursing Standard,* **19**(35), 51–4.

Yeung CK (2001). Pathophysiology of bladder dysfunction. In Gearheart JP, Rink RC, and Mouriquad PDE, eds, *Paediatric Urology.* WB Saunders, London, 453–69.

Useful further reading and websites

Baillie L and Arrowsmith V (2005). Meeting elimination needs. In Baillie L, ed., *Developing Practical Nursing Skills,* 2nd edn, Hodder Arnold, London.

Bonner L and Wells M (2008). *Effective Management of Bladder and Bowel Problems in Children.* Class Publishing, London.

Continence Resource Centre (2005). *Frequency Volume Chart.* NHS, Greater Glasgow and Clyde.

Dingwall L (2008). Promoting effective continence care in older people: a literature review. *British Journal of Nursing,* **17**(3), 192–7.

This is a useful article, which highlights the problems and offers solutions in managing continence in the elderly population.

ERIC (Education and Resources for Improving Childhood Continence). www.eric.org.uk.
This is a useful site with content focused on childhood incontinence.

Foxley S (2007). An overview of urinary incontinence. *British Journal of Healthcare Assistance,* **1**(1), 35–8.

Gray M (200). An update on the physiology of urinary incontinence. *Continence UK*, **1**(2).
A useful article on urinary incontinence.

Getliffe K and Dolman M (2003). *Promoting Continence: A Clinical Research Resource*, 2nd edn. Bailliere Tindall, London.
This is a useful book, which looks at all aspects of the promotion of continence.

Heaton KW (2000). *Bristol Stool Scale*. University of Bristol, Bristol.

KidsHealth. http://kidshealth.org/kid/htbw/kidneys.html.
This is an interactive website for children to discover how their kidneys and urinary tract works.

NHS Greater Glasgow and Clyde. Southern General Hospital (2007). *Protocols for Bowel Management*. NHS, Greater Glasgow and Clyde.

NHS Quality Improvement Scotland (2005). *Continence: Adults with Urinary Dysfunction*. NHSQIS, Edinburgh.

Pellatt GC (2007). Anatomy and physiology of urinary elimination. Part 1. *British Journal of Nursing*, **16**(7), 406–10.
This article gives a good summary of the anatomy and physiology of urinary elimination.

Stegall MJ (2007). Urine samples and urinalysis. *Nursing Standard*, **22**, 14–16.

Trigg E, Mohammed TA (2006). *Practices in Children's Nursing: Guidelines for Hospital and Community*, 2nd edn. Churchill Livingstone, Edinburgh.
This textbook offers guidelines for the testing of urine and catheter care in children.

Bladder and Bowel Foundation. www.bladder and bowel foundation.org.

A useful website which will inform you on all aspects of continence.

Check ⊕ **www.oxfordtextbooks.co.uk/orc/docherty/** for changes and new developments. Updated research, guidelines, or equipment will be added every four months.

Answers to scenarios

Scenario 1

1 Consider the issues that affect Jane.
- Frequent urinary tract infections with pain result in time off work and poor quality of life
- On hospital admission she was found to have a high residual volume, over 450 ml, with a spontaneous void of 100 ml
- She deliberately distends her bladder when she has an infection to try and dull the pain, causing some denervation of her bladder

2 What else do you need to know from her history?
- How many times she urinates and the amount of infrequency or frequency in 24 hours
- The number of times she has difficulty in initiating micturition in a 24-hour period
- How long she has not been able to use public toilets and whether there is a root cause to this?

3 Devise an action plan for Jane, detailing treatment strategies and why.
- Educational needs: explain normal bladder function and issues that arise when infrequent voiding occurs
- Maintain fluid volume of 2 litres per day
- Initiate regular toileting throughout the day, even if she does need feel the need to do so. Arrange a scheduled two-hourly void
- Repeat measurement of residual volume at the clinic with pre-spontaneous void if possible
- If there is still a residual volume after scheduled toileting, consider intermittent self-catheterization
- Discuss the issue of micturition difficulty and history: consider possible desensitization therapy
- Jane may require prophylactic long-term low-grade antibiotic with or without clean intermittert self-catherization (CISC).

Scenario 2

1 What options are available to you?

As John is unable to bear weight, your only options are to assist him on to a bedpan on his bed (placing a pad under the bedpan would help absorb any spillage) or to give him a urinal (he may need assistance with this).

2 What will you assess in order to choose the best option for John?

- You would assess his mobility and his dependence (can he lift himself up on to a bedpan, can he move his clothing out of the way)
- You would assess his pain and his sedation to establish whether he could be moved and assess his understanding about what was required of him (that is, whether he knows how to use a urinal)
- You would ask whether he wished his parents to help or not.

Scenario 3

1 What assessment would you carry out?

- You would assess Craig's normal elimination habits, and his ability to understand and communicate.

2 What may be the cause of these episodes?

- The unfamiliar environment may affect Craig's ability to remember where the toilet is; psychological and social factors may add to the stress of his hospital stay, which may lead to incontinent episodes
- Craig may not be able to communicate his needs

3 What management strategies could you adopt?

- Craig should be orientated to the ward environment—this may need to be done regularly rather than as a one-off. Show him where the toilet is and how it works; use the same route each time
- Speak to Craig's health facilitator, carers or next of kin to establish how he normally communicates—perhaps a signal or sign could be used. Craig may have a health action plan that can be reviewed on his admission to establish any needs
- Prompted voiding may help—that is, asking Craig if he needs the toilet at regular intervals

Scenario 4

1 What would you include in your assessment?

You would make a full assessment to determine the cause of this change in normal elimination pattern (for example, medication changes, changes to fluid intake). You could take a urinalysis in case Mrs McDonald has acquired an infection.

2 What could be the cause?

There could be a urine infection or Mrs McDonald's dementia could be worsening so that she has problems getting to the toilet.

3 What management strategies could you adopt?

- If it is an infection, antibiotics would form part of the management strategy
- If it is dementia, you would wish to promote her independence and so various strategies could be adopted, for example, timed voiding if she has home helps or carers regularly, label the toilet door, involve occupational therapy to see if aids would be helpful, give Mrs McDonald a routine, ensure that she is wearing easy to remove clothes

Personal cleansing and dressing

8

CHARLES DOCHERTY, KIRSTEEN LANG AND JOHN TIMMONS

Introduction

This chapter encompasses the fundamental nursing skills related to the activities of personal cleansing and dressing. These require specific attention because, in fit healthy individuals, they are taken for granted to the extent that it is difficult to imagine what a nurses' role might be, except, of course, when someone becomes ill, infirm, disabled, or depressed. Personal cleansing and dressing then becomes an issue and an indicator of an underlying problem that nurses can influence through the process of assessment, planning, implementing, and evaluating.

It is also an activity with a lifespan component: an elderly patient may recently have lost the ability to undertake this activity completely independently, and will need help in coming to terms with this. At the other end of the spectrum, young children may only recently have acquired skills in this area, and will need encouragement and time to practice.

Of course the activity of personal cleansing and dressing doesn't stand in isolation. You will not be able to persuade a patient who is feeling cold and shivery to enter a bath or a shower. Neither will you be able to persuade a patient to wear a heavy coat on a hot summer's day. So regulating body temperature is intimately linked with this activity.

Similarly, the activity of living 'expressing sexuality' must also be taken into consideration when assisting a patient with personal cleansing and dressing. For example, a young boy would be very upset if he was dressed as a little girl. That seems simple enough but stereotypes can be hazardous and what might be perfectly acceptable for one individual may cause great offence to another. The length of skirt, neckline, colour of clothes, and whether arms are exposed or not, may be highly significant to the individuals concerned. So things we take for granted are heavily value-laden and subject to stereotypes: accepting these without thinking can lead to poor quality care of an individual. Therefore, careful assessment is vital before any action is contemplated.

This chapter is also concerned in some detail with the care of skin and, where skin is damaged or broken, in wound care. This can be a difficult area, as wound care can be very complex, requiring specialist skills and experience that only comes through postgraduate studies. So for now we will concentrate on the principles that underpin all wound care, which can be built on in years to come.

Learning outcomes

These outcomes relate to numbers 3, 5, 8, 9, 10, 16, 22, and 25 of the NMC's Essential Skill Clusters and specifically to Care Domains 2 and 3 of the NMC's Standards of Proficiency for Pre-registration Nursing (outcomes to be achieved for entry to branch).

On reading the chapter and associated web pages and undertaking supervised activities, the student will be able to:

- Understand the complexity of skills in personal cleansing and dressing
- Apply the principles of skin care in different contexts through assessment and planning
- Perform skin care in community and hospital contexts
- Cleanse eyes

- Demonstrate oral care
- Care for the hair of bedbound patients
- Wash a patient in bed
- Shave facial hair
- Organize and plan total patient care
- Describe the principles of aseptic techniques
- Care for wounds, and remove sutures, staples and clips
- Understand the legal and professional issues around personal care and touch

Prior knowledge

To use the clinical skills in this chapter, it is important that you have related knowledge and understanding obtainable from a large range of reference books that specialize in the sciences associated with nursing, particularly biology and physiology.

Skin   It is recommended that you revise your knowledge of the anatomy and physiology of the skin.

Eye   It is recommended that you understand the basics of the anatomy and physiology of the eye. It is not necessary to understand the complexity of vision, but you should be able to name and understand the relationships between the structures surrounding the eye.

Mouth   You will need to know the basic anatomy and physiology of the structures in the oral cavity, to be able to make a simple assessment with an external light source.

Background

Skin

The skin is the largest organ of the body and is the boundary between our internal and external environments. As such, it has many functions including defence against infection, protecting internal organs against damage from external pressure, shearing forces and harmful radiation. It also has more subtle functions, such as temperature regulation, and excretion. Section 3.1 provides further

detail on the structure and function of the skin. More subtle still are the effects that skin colour, skin health, and disfigurement can have sociologically and psychologically.

Remember that 'the skin' includes its appendages, such as hair and nails. Knowing how these grow and the factors that influence their appearance in health and disease is very useful when it comes to assessing your patient. An experienced nurse can often identify a health problem in an individual by examining the skin. Similarly, natural differences in skin colour create added complexity when assessing the skin: for example, a blueish colour (cyanosis) that is readily identifiable in fair-skinned people is more difficult to detect in people of Afro-Caribbean origin. It is also important to note the normal biology of the skin, and to understand that it is usual for bacteria to live on the skin, and that these play an important defensive role against the more harmful, or pathogenic, microorganisms that live in the environment. Additionally, the process of repair and healing of the skin should be revised.

Perceptions of physical contact and skin exposure

In this multicultural world in which we live, it is important to recognize that what we take for granted as the norm might cause offence to another. Cultural differences in body contact, touch, skin exposure, and the significance of using the left hand for one thing and the right for another, is very important when we come to assist patients in personal cleansing and dressing activities. Naturally, with an awareness of local culture, you will be expected to respect sensitivities that you know that people might have.

Uninvited touch may be considered assault in certain situations, and this is a potential risk when students undertake personal care without permission. This relates to vulnerable patients with learning disabilities; those with mental health problems; and elderly adults and children. Similarly, if you are caring for someone from a different culture from your own then it is your responsibility to familiarize yourself with the norms and beliefs of that person's culture and religion, to avoid offence. Some patients have specific needs in terms of washing before prayer, covering their hair, using one hand for toileting and the other for eating. The sex of the carer may be an issue, too. There is too much potentially relevant information to be included here, so find out by asking: find out by searching the Internet, but don't find out by trial and error.

Assessment of personal cleansing and dressing needs

The assessment of a patient in relation to personal cleansing and dressing is multifactorial, requiring a **holistic** approach in the context of patients' individual circumstances. Most nursing models facilitate this approach; however, the following can be relevant:

- The patient's level of dependency on others
- Age and age-related health problems
- Cultural factors, such as religion
- Personality and sensitivity
- Dignity and privacy
- Disability
- Moving and handling capabilities and limitations
- Lifestyle or home circumstances, such as home heating and dampness
- Compliance or concordance and understanding
- Elimination norms and continence
- Eating and drinking and dietary preferences (dentition and oral care)
- Links to maintaining a safe environment (internal and infection control)
- Temperature control and clothing choices

8.1 **Skin care**

Definition

Caring for the skin involves grooming, nail care, washing, and bathing, and relieving pressure to avoid skin damage. Some of these aspects of skin care are covered elsewhere in this chapter; pressure care is explained in detail in Chapter 3. This section will confine itself to the principles of skin cleansing and washing. It is important to remove dirt, sweat, and excess oil produced by **sebaceous glands** in the skin, which can result in body odour and skin breakdown if left to accumulate. It is also vitally important to remove any urine or faeces from the skin, as these can alter skin **pH** and reduce its effectiveness as a barrier to infection.

These skills also have **therapeutic** value in building a trusting relationship, which is particularly important in children, people with learning disabilities, and those with mental health problems.

When to provide skin care for a patient

Skin cleansing is a common need that all people have, but being able to satisfy this need at the appropriate time and sufficiently often can be thwarted by health problems that reduce functionality and impair the individual's ability to undertake this important activity. If, however, a skin cleansing regime is chosen inappropriately, perhaps too frequently, this can cause alterations in skin pH, destruction of the normal **skin flora**, and skin irritation, breakdown, and infection. Assessment and evaluation of skin cleansing practices are essential to discuss the frequency and nature of skin care with the patient, and to respect individual patient choices.

Assessment of individual patients' needs

It is vital to make an assessment of the patient's skin, noting blemishes, pressure damage, variations in normal coloration, redness (**erythema**), inflammation, swelling, dryness, and any breaks in the skin's integrity. Skin conditions, such as **psoriasis** and **dermatitis**, are important to note: these ought to be drawn to the attention of medical staff if their location is not readily visible, and if the patient has omitted to mention them.

Most patients are perfectly capable of meeting their own needs in relation to normal skin care; however, certain circumstances can arise to make professional nursing intervention essential. The patient's mobility and continence will have a marked effect on the condition of the skin in particular areas, such as the buttocks and sacral area, where pressure and excoriation can combine with toxic chemicals in urine and faeces to create a very high risk of pressure-sore development and skin breakdown. Inappropriate skin cleansing can contribute to this problem (Cooper *et al.* 2006).

Most tools designed to assess pressure-sore vulnerability, such as the Waterlow Scale, combine risk factors for mobility, continence, and the state of general health to give a holistic measure of risk. Assessment of the patient's skin should be made regularly as it can change so rapidly, especially in the acutely ill or in individuals who suddenly develop problems with mobility and continence.

Caring for the whole patient requiring skin care is essential as patients may be embarrassed, and great efforts are required to make this procedure dignified and pleasant for the patient.

Aftercare

- The patient should be left comfortable and repositioned. Where frequent repositioning is required, a position chart is useful
- Clean bedsheets, pulled taut to avoid wrinkles and pressure points will help to keep the skin clean and healthy and free from pressure sores. Any observed changes to the patient's condition should be recorded
- Where lotions or creams are prescribed, enter details in the drug administration chart, according to the policy on administration of medicines
- Tidy the area and safely dispose of any soiled materials and wet linen. Return any patient's belongings to locker; ensuring that wet soap is allowed to dry, and that damp towels are allowed to air

Developing your skills

The intention should be to encourage the patient to be self-caring in this activity. Setting realistic goals and developing a progressive plan of care with the patient, under the supervision of your mentor, can help coordinate care and achieve longer-term goals.

Other factors to consider

The patient's nutritional status will have an important influence on skin care. If the patient is emaciated, dehydrated, and lacking in **subcutaneous** fat, extra care needs to be taken to avoid damage to the skin through shearing forces while washing and applying creams or lotions. Conversely, if the patient is overweight, greater care needs to be taken in removing soap or cleanser and thoroughly drying between skin folds, between buttocks, and so on.

The patient's general state of health should be considered, too, and sometimes it is as appropriate to bathe and sponge a patient for comfort reasons, as it is for personal cleansing reasons. If a patient has **pyrexia** (Chapter 9), it may be necessary to change sweaty bedclothes and sponge the patient down several times per day. Care needs to be taken in this situation not to use too much cleanser: plain water may be preferred, to avoid denuding the skin of essential oils.

Where incontinence is a problem, requiring frequent skin care in a confined area of the body, it is important to protect the skin after each wash, otherwise the skin will become dry and prone to breakdown.

Key point: Skin care is unique to individual patients and requires their involvement in choices and in giving consent.

8.2 **Showering or bathing a patient**

Definition

Caring for patients' skin also involves washing the skin by means of a shower, bath, or assisted wash in bed. The nurse must assess the patient and involve the patient in deciding which means of washing is the most desirable and appropriate. All patients should be encouraged to participate in showering or bathing as much as is possible, with the nurse encouraging their independence, whilst maintaining the patient's safety.

While washing a patient, the nurse can also assess the condition of the patient's skin and to identify changes in the skin.

When to shower or bathe a patient

Showering or bathing is necessary when a patient requires assistance. It is assumed that the patient is conscious

Skin care

Step	Rationale
1 Cleanse hands.	To avoid the risk of cross-infection.
2 Wear apron , gloves.	Contact with patients' skin can cause 'normal' skin flora and **commensals** to be exchanged between patient and nurse. Some of these microorganisms can be problematic; therefore, gloves serve as protection for both patient and nurse.
3 Gain patient's **consent**, incorporating choices and preferences.	This respects patients' autonomy. It is important to have full cooperation, since touching a patient in sensitive areas can have social and psychological significance. Consent to touch an individual in your care is necessary. Unexpectedly touching a patient can cause offence and can, in some situations, be considered as assault and have legal ramifications.
4 Provide privacy.	People can be embarrassed at having to expose skin that is normally kept covered, particularly the elderly, teenagers, and some religious groups, such as Muslims. Involving family members in patient care is considered a good idea in general but caution needs to be exercised when skin exposure and the intimacies of personal cleansing are required: it may be that an individual would rather this be performed by a professional carer than a family member.
5 Assess the patient's needs for skin care.	Patients have individual needs for skin care, however, all patients will need a review of skin care products and cleansing regime to ensure that best practice is followed (for example, avoidance of strongly perfumed soaps and moisturizers).
6 Negotiate the practice of skin care with the patient or the patient's family: provide explanations and rationale.	Patients will have preferences for skin care products and practices and inappropriate habits associated with their use will need to be unlearned. Some skin care regimes may be medically prescribed and, therefore, should not be subject to substantial change without medical referral.

continued

7	**Select appropriate equipment.**	In hospital, patients should be provided with their own basin, kept at their bedside, for cross-infection purposes. This may be lined with a disposable polythene film for single-use bathing. Comfortably warm water should be used for skin cleansing. Towels should be cleaned regularly, and allowed to dry and air between use. Traditional facecloths should be discouraged because they tend to remain wet and can harbour pathogenic microorganisms. Soiled bedlinen should be disposed of in accordance with local infection control policy.
8	**Prepare the patient for examination and skin care.**	Psychological preparation is needed to enable the patient to feel comfortable when exposing skin. Expose only those parts of the body to be examined at any one time (see Fig. 8.1).
9	**Observe the condition of the skin.**	Is it dry or flaky? Moist or oedematous? Are there any breaks? Any rashes? Any discolouration? Bruising?
10	**Select soap, cleanser, or emollient cleanser.**	The patient's own toiletries should be selected, but it needs to be appropriate. It may be opportune to use this occasion to educate on the most suitable cleanser for the patient's skin type.
11	**Rinse.**	Ensure that all traces of cleanser are removed from the skin by rinsing with clean water prior to drying. Some skin cleansers contain a barrier preparation which should not be removed by rinsing.
12	**Dry.**	Ensure that all areas of the body are properly dry, paying particular attention to areas where opportunistic fungal growth can be problematic, such as between toes, buttocks, and groin area, under breasts, and axillae.
13	**Apply lotion or cream; this should be smoothed not rubbed.**	In addition to skin cleansing, moisturizers may need to be applied to keep skin in good condition. Where appropriate, lotions and creams should be applied with the smoothing movement of a gloved hand moving in the direction of skin hair. Do not rub, as this can cause damage to structures beneath the skin.

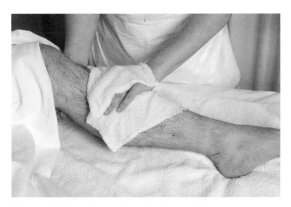

Figure 8.1 Exposing only one leg for washing

(otherwise a bed bath would be required), and may be able to complete some parts of the skill with minimal assistance or independently.

Reasons for showering or bathing:

- Cleanse skin
- Easing pain or discomfort
- Therapeutic, for skin conditions
- Relaxation

Concern for the patient's safety should be paramount at all times and the nurse should assess whether the patient's safety is likely to be compromised. There may be instances where it is not appropriate to assist the patient to take a bath or shower:

- Where the patient's consciousness is altered
- Impaired mental status, for example, the patient is confused or disorientated
- Impaired mobility; appropriate equipment and knowledge of how to use it should be available before considering showering or bathing this group of patients. The patient's environment should also be assessed to ascertain whether adequate space and facilities are available

Special considerations

Medical equipment

The patient may have attached equipment or devices, such as **intravenous** drips, central lines, and nasogastric feeding tubes. These should, ideally, be disconnected before bathing the patient, but there may be cases when it is not safe or appropriate to do so, such as with an insulin infusion. The student should always seek the advice of a more senior member of the nursing team to assess whether equipment should be disconnected or not. If lines and equipment have to be disconnected, this should only be done under supervision by a more senior member of the nursing team or medical staff.

Procedure: Showering or bathing the semi-independent patient

Points to consider:

- Patients may prefer a family member to assist with bathing. In particular, children may prefer a parent or guardian. This should be arranged, if appropriate
- Patients' own cleansing equipment needs to be considered for appropriateness, as highly perfumed and traditional soaps could cause irritation and dryness

Preparation

Discussion with the patient

Explain the procedure to the patient and ask if patient has any preferences, for example:

- Shower or bath? The patient may have a preference or may not wish to wash at all
- How much assistance is required? The patient may require assistance with fundamentals such as mobilizing. Also, the patient may be independent at home, but desires assistance in the hospital environment for reassurance
- Own equipment, for example, towel, skin cleansers, shampoo, and so on

Cultural and religious considerations

The nurse should be aware that the patient may feel embarrassed and vulnerable and should be sensitive to cultural and religious considerations when bathing a patient. A patient's beliefs should never be assumed and the nurse should discover the patient's preferences in the assessment stage.

Showering or bathing the semi-independent patient

EQUIPMENT

- Cleanser
- Disposable cloths or wipes
- Towels
- Change of clothing
- Gloves
- Apron

Key point: The nurse should be aware of changes to a patient's skin condition and should report any such changes to senior nursing staff or medical staff in addition to documenting them in the patient's nursing notes. These changes may be caused by a variety of factors, such as infection, disease processes, pressure damage, allergies, or side effects from drugs or **topical** therapies.

Step	Rationale
1 Prepare shower or bath area: the area should be adequately cleansed according to local infection control policies and procedures.	To prevent cross-infection and transmission of infection.
2 Cleanse hands prior to the procedure, put on gloves and apron.	To prevent cross-infection.
3 Explain procedure to the patient.	To facilitate informed consent.
4 Gain patient's consent and incorporate choices and preferences.	To gain cooperation and respect autonomy.
5 Ensure privacy—curtains, door closed with displayed engaged sign.	To prevent embarrassment and maintain patient dignity.
6 Ensure access to the patient does not pose any physical risk to nurse or patient.	To protect nurse and patient from injury.
7 Collect all equipment and have ready in shower or bathroom.	To ensure smooth procedure and prevent need to leave patient alone.
8 Shower: run water to reach desired temperature, checking temperature of water on back of forearm. Bath: run water to desired depth and check temperature on back of forearm.	To assess correct temperature to ensure patient's comfort and safety. To assess correct temperature to ensure patient's comfort and safety.
9 Assist patient to the shower or bathroom using appropriate moving and handling techniques or equipment.	To ensure safe and comfortable movement of the patient.

10	Assist patient to wash, using cleanser and cloths. Patient may wish to be left to wash independently. If safe, explain how to use the emergency call system, to alert for help.	To facilitate independence, whilst maintaining patient safety.
11	When patient has finished assist patient to exit the shower or bath using appropriate moving and handling techniques and equipment.	To ensure safe and comfortable movement of the patient.
12	Assist the patient to dry, taking particular care to dry adequately between skin folds.	To achieve dry skin for patient's comfort and to reduce risk of infection.
13	Apply emollient to skin, ensuring correct amount is used.	To moisturize skin without causing excessive dryness or moisture.
14	When patient has finished, assist to exit shower or bathroom, using appropriate moving and handling techniques/equipment.	To ensure safe and comfortable movement of the patient.

Aftercare

The shower or bathing area should be cleaned according to local infection control or cleaning policies. The nurse should take adequate precautions to protect themselves from risk of cross-infection and any caustic cleaning materials, according to local decontamination guidelines. Any laundry should be contained for cleaning; soiled laundry should be wrapped and cleaned according to local policies.

The nurse should continue to assess the condition of the patient's skin, applying more emollients or creams as indicated and reporting any changes to a more senior member of nursing or medical staff. Any changes and emollients applied should also be documented in the patient's nursing documentation.

Other factors to consider

Effects of soap on skin

Soap can have a drying effect on skin, which can increase the risk of skin breakdown, making it more susceptible to infection. Soap-free cleansers, which have a pH closer to the skin's pH, are recommended to help minimize skin dryness. This should particularly be considered with patients who have existing dry skin (Ersser *et al.* 2007).

The ageing process

As skin ages, it loses its strength and elasticity, therefore, extra care should be taken when bathing elderly patients, as their skin can be more fragile and susceptible to damage from **friction** and shearing forces.

Infants and children

It may be appropriate to bathe a young infant in a baby bath. Local policies and protocols should be followed regarding procedure and cleansing products.

Effects of medication or therapies

There are many drugs and treatment regimes that can have implications and effects on a patient's skin. Patients undergoing radiation therapy, for example, can develop reactions such as redness, itching and dryness. Oral and topical drug therapies can also cause skin reactions. It is vital that the nurse is aware what therapies their patients are receiving and their possible effects in skin appearance and integrity.

Urinary and faecal incontinence

The bacteria in urine and faeces coupled with exposure of the skin to excessive moisture can compromise skin integrity. Specialized emollient cleansers are available for the purpose of cleaning these patients' skin.

8.3 **Washing a patient in bed**

Definition

This activity, known alternatively as a 'bed bath' or 'blanket bath' is reserved for the most **dependent** of patients, who simply cannot mobilize to a more appropriate area, such as bathroom or shower for washing, or whose condition requires them to rest and, therefore, not get out of bed to wash. This will, therefore, involve washing the whole of the patient in bed and attending to all other care requirements. It does not mean to say that the patient is helpless: far from it. You should approach washing a patient in bed from the perspective that this is an opportunity to engage with the patient and make a detailed assessment of the patient's mobility, strength, capability, skin condition, mental state, and mood. On the other hand, the patient may be extremely weak, sedated, unconscious, or dying with limited capacity to participate.

When to give a bed bath

Reasons for bed-bathing:

- Cleanse skin
- Ease discomfort
- Therapeutic for skin conditions
- Relaxation or rest

Procedure
Preparation

The room should be comfortably warm, draught free, and private. In an open ward area, screens should be closed. The time of day should suit the patient and not intrude on visiting, or expected medical activity such as the ward round, blood sampling, or procedures such as X-rays or scans. Make sure that the patient's condition is stable and the patient feels comfortable about the procedure at the scheduled time. Some medical conditions can be made worse by washing, as cooling the skin has a physiological effect—for example, **heart failure** and **hypertension** can be exacerbated by **peripheral vasoconstriction** (caused by skin cooling): so make sure that this planned nursing activity is consistent with the patient's overall plan of care.

Before beginning, assess exactly what you'll need. The patient ought to have his or her own towel, skin cleansers, and toiletries. Prepare a trolley with everything you require, such as basin, water, towels, and any linen that you think may need to be changed.

You don't need written consent but approval from the patient is necessary. Sometimes patients are reluctant and may require reassurance that the procedure will be as quick and efficient as possible and that their dignity and privacy will be maintained throughout, to ease any embarrassment; this may be acute for some, particularly teenagers and younger adults.

Aftercare

Dispose of any used material appropriately. Clean and dry the basin and return the patient's equipment in locker. Ensure that patient's towel, if used, is left in a position where it can dry, or leave it with used night attire for the patient's relatives for collection at visiting time.

Washing a patient in bed

EQUIPMENT

- Cleanser
- Disposable cloths or wipes
- Towels
- Basin
- Change of clothing
- Gloves
- Apron

▶ Step

Rationale

	Step	Rationale
1	**Explain the need for the procedure, reassure and gain consent, incorporating patient choices and preferences.**	To ease embarrassment, gain patient's cooperation, and respect autonomy.
2	**Prepare all necessary equipment in advance.**	To facilitate the efficient performance of the procedure and prevent unnecessary exposure of the patient midway through the procedure.
3	**Cleanse hands, put on gloves and apron.**	To prevent cross-infection.
4	**Ensure privacy: curtains and door closed with displayed engaged sign (if available).**	To prevent embarrassment and maintain patient dignity.
5	**Ensure that help is available from another member of the ward team to assist with mobilizing (if required).**	To prevent undue stress on the patient and to maintain patient safety.
6	**Ensure that there is sufficient room to arrange basin, cleanser, towel, in a safe and orderly fashion on a stable work surface.**	To prevent accidental water spillage.
7	**Assist patient out of their night attire. Loosen bed-clothes and remove excess blankets, leaving the patient sufficiently covered.**	To maintain dignity and body temperature for the duration of the procedure.
8	**Position waterproof/protective materials strategically around the patient (such as water-absorbent pads) if necessary, repositioning as required (see Fig. 8.2).**	To prevent saturation of bed-linen.
9	**Dependent on patient's condition: hand-hot water (no hotter than 45° C) should be used. Slightly cooler water may be more appropriate if the patient is febrile (has a fever).**	This temperature is comfortably warm when applied to patient's skin and will prevent shivering and loss of body heat. Cool (tepid) water applied to the skin may assist in maintaining body temperature within the normal range.

continued

10	Consider patient's preferences for soap, cleanser, toiletries, or other products.	To maintain patient's dignity and choice and to facilitate the expression of patient's sexuality.
11	Apply soap or cleanser sparingly and rinse thoroughly.	To avoid skin drying and irritation. Pay particular attention to skin folds and ensure that all traces of soap and moisture are removed. Particular areas for attention: beneath breasts, between toes, and axillae.
12	Change water regularly.	To avoid build up of soap or cleanser in bathing water and to maintain correct water temperature.
13	Take a systematic approach, washing, rinsing and drying as you go. Begin with the patient's hands, then face and neck, then arms, axillae, the front of the upper body, legs and feet, then perineum/groin. Change water before turning patient onto their side and finishing with upper body, buttocks and anal region. Expose only those areas necessary for washing.	To avoid unnecessary moving and handling; to maintain dignity and privacy and to avoid unnecessary spread of microorganisms from areas of high concentration (such as the anal region) to areas of low concentration (such as the face).
14	Immerse hands, and if possible, feet in water when washing these parts (see Fig. 8.3).	To promote comfort and relaxation.
15	Use disposable materials as required.	To avoid the risk of cross-contamination.
16	Involve the patient in the procedure: particularly washing of face, and the perineal/groin area, and in repositioning.	To maintain independence, to avoid undue embarrassment.
17	Ensure effective drying, especially between toes; cleft of the buttocks, axillae, and perineum.	To prevent skin excoriation and creating a niche for microorganisms that cause thrush, athletes foot, and so on.
18	Pat dry rather than rub dry.	To prevent shearing forces causing skin damage.
19	Apply emollient to the skin, as appropriate, ensuring correct amount is used.	To moisturize the skin without causing excessive dryness or moisture.
20	When bathing is complete, change any linen as required and remake bed, assist patient into fresh night-attire, and leave in a comfortable position.	To promote comfort, rest, and relaxation.

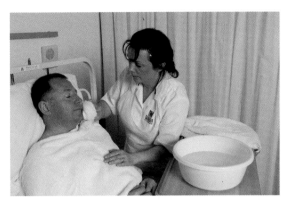

Figure 8.2 Position of protective materials for bed bath

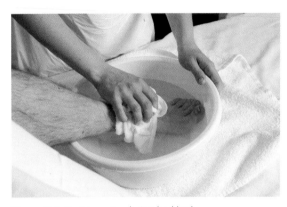

Figure 8.3 Feet in water during bed bath

Developing your skills

Update the patient's documentation to reflect the care performed. With your mentor, consider whether any aspect of the care plan could be reviewed in light of your experience in performing this activity with your patient.

Other factors to consider

This skill can be complicated by the presence of intravenous devices, urinary catheters, and surgical wounds, as well as levels of patient dependency. A bed bath often comes in combination with other skills such as shaving, hair washing, wound dressing, and so on, greatly increasing the complexity of the intervention.

8.4 **Shaving**

Definition

A patient may also need or wish to be shaved. Some patients may wish their facial hair to be shaved, and some may wish hair elsewhere on their body to be shaved. Shaving my also be required prior to an operative procedure to that particular area.

Shaving can be achieved using either a manual or electric razor. The procedure described here will be that for using a single-bladed disposable razor.

When to shave a patient

Reasons for shaving:

- Shaving of facial hair
- Shaving of body hair for cosmetic reasons
- Shaving of pre-operative sites

The frequency of shaving required will be determined by both the patient's preference and the rate at which the hair grows. The rate at which an individual's hair grows varies; for facial hair some patients may need to be shaved daily, whereas others may need to be shaved less often. The patient's appearance should be assessed and the patient consulted, if able, regarding the frequency of shaving required.

Pre-operative shaving

Some patients may need shaving of hair prior to surgery in that area of the body. There is, however, no conclusive evidence either to support or the purpose of shaving, with regards to post-operative infection rates (Tanner *et al.* 2006).

Shaving an area prior to surgery may also be deemed necessary to aid access or visibility to the site.

When not to shave a patient

Some patients may not wish their facial hair to be shaved: they may simply like having a beard or moustache, and some may have cultural or religious beliefs that require them to have their facial hair unshaved. Some patients may also be apprehensive of someone else shaving them, as there is the potential to be cut, and patients may not wish a stranger to carry out this task. As with all procedures, the patient's preferences should be respected at all times.

Risk of bleeding

It should be considered that there is a risk of causing a break to the patient's skin during shaving and if the patient's **blood clotting** is impaired it should be considered whether or not to shave the patient at all.

Alternative intervention

Removal of hair can be achieved by use of **depilatory creams**, lotions or foams. These products should be considered in the same way as any topical therapy, and may require consultation and approval by medical staff before their use.

Procedure

Preparation

Patients should always be consulted prior to shaving. If this is not possible, due to illness or another communication problem, it may be appropriate to ask the family or next of kin.

- Disposable razor
- Shaving foam, cream, or emollient
- Apron
- Gloves
- Other equipment, for example, towel, skin cleansers, shampoo, and so on

Key point: Patients may be taking medications, or have a disease process that affects clotting. The nurse taking care of the patient should be aware of such factors and consider these prior to shaving patients.

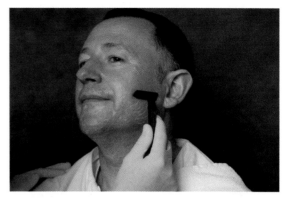

Figure 8.4 Shaving stroke direction

Aftercare

The nurse should assess the skin that has been shaved. Pressure should be applied to any bleeding areas with a clean gauze swab to aid haemostasis. Bleeding that appears excessive or continues for a prolonged period should be reported to a more senior member of nursing or medical staff, and recorded in nursing documentation. The razor should be disposed of in a **sharps** container as per local protocols.

Razors should also not be left in the close proximity of more vulnerable patients, for example children, the visually impaired and those with a history of self-harm issues. Irrespective of the client group, razors should not be left lying where the nurse, patient, or someone else could be harmed on the exposed blade.

It should be documented when the patient has been shaved, what type of razor has been used, and any foams or emollients that have been applied to the skin. This is particularly important if the patient's skin shows any localized irritation that may be linked to the razor and/or any cleansers or moisturizers used.

Other factors to consider

Other types of razors

The patient may have his or her own razor or an electric razor and these can be used provided they pose no risk to the patient and comply with policies and protocols. For example, an electric razor used in an inpatient area should be checked for safety as per the area policy before use.

Shaving facial hair

Step	Rationale
1 Explain the procedure to the patient.	To facilitate informed consent.
2 Gain patient consent.	To gain cooperation.
3 Cleanse hands prior to the procedure, put on gloves and apron.	To prevent cross-infection.
4 Ensure privacy: curtains, door closed with displayed engaged sign.	To prevent embarrassment and maintain patient dignity.
5 Ensure that access to the patient does not pose any physical risk to nurse or patient.	To protect nurse and patient from injury.
6 Collect all equipment and have ready to patient's vicinity.	To ensure smooth procedure by minimizing interruptions to collect equipment.
7 Fill bowl or basin with warm water and check temperature on own forearm.	To ensure patient's comfort and safety.
8 Wet area and apply shaving cleanser.	To assist smooth movement of razor over patient's face, contributing to patient's comfort.
9 Shave patient using slow, short strokes, following hair growth (see Fig. 8.4).	To maintain patient comfort and reduce risk of causing abrasions. Also to reduce risk of development of in-grown hairs.
10 Once completed, wash residual cleanser from patient's face.	To remove excess cleanser, which may contribute to dryness of skin.
11 Dry patient's skin with a clean dry towel.	To ensure that skin is dry, for patient comfort and prevention of excess drying from environment.

8.5 **Hair care**

Definition

For the purposes of this book, hair care will be restricted to caring for a patient's hair when the patient is unable to meet this need independently. This may be in an acute or continuing care setting.

When to care for a patient's hair

This skill may be required in a situation where an individual is admitted to hospital following trauma or an accident and is unable to care for his or her own hair. Settings include intensive care units, acute surgical wards, spinal injury units, and neurology units.

There is another group of patients who require assistance with hair care: the long-term ill, bedbound, and incapacitated patients. Ideally, hair should be washed in the bath or shower but for some patients this is not possible. In addition, some patients with scalp conditions, such as eczema and psoriasis, may be prescribed a specific medicated shampoo. Follow the rules for administration of medicines in this instance.

Breathlessness

The breathless patient may not tolerate more than two or three minutes lying completely flat; therefore, this procedure would need to be assessed for suitability for this patient.

Aftercare

Return patient's belongings—shampoo, hair dryer, comb, brush—to their place in the locker.

Update nursing documentation to reflect the care carried out. If medicated shampoo has been administered as prescribed, record this according to policy.

If in consultation with your mentor and your patient it is considered that professional hair care is required, this can often be facilitated for the patient, at their own expense.

Other factors to consider

Head lice

An itchy, flaky scalp may be indicative of dandruff or something a little more sinister, such as head lice. Be aware of this possibility in all patients, and seek expert help from your mentor in identifying and treating this condition. Tact and diplomacy will be required, as having an **infestation** carries with it a degree of **social stigma**.

8.6 **Eye care**

Definition

Eye care describes the cleansing and care of the structures surrounding the eye, the eyelids, and the eyelashes. Simple eye care is aimed at facilitating normal physiological processes, to enhance these when these are reduced or compromised through age, and to improve cleanliness and comfort of the skin and structures surrounding the eye. Eye care may also be required as a comfort measure to soothe the eye or to precede the instillation of eye drops or eye ointment.

Background

Eye

The eye is a complex structure, but for the purposes of eye care, you don't need to understand the mechanics of vision. It is, however, useful to be able to name the main structures of the eye (see **Fig. 8.5**) and its surroundings, and to understand basics such as how the eyes move, where tears come from, and why it is that our noses run when we cry.

Tears have an **antimicrobial** action: any infection of the surface of the eye itself is controlled and limited by the constant flow of tears being produced, washing over the eye, and draining into the **naso-lachrymal duct**. Normally

Hair care

EQUIPMENT

- Waterproof pads or drawsheet and polythene lining
- Shampoo and conditioner of patient's choice
- Hair dryer
- Head and shoulder tray
- Jug with warm water for rinsing
- Large bucket to collect water

Step	Rationale
1 Explain the need for the procedure, reassure, and gain consent. Incorporate patient choices and preferences.	To gain the patient's cooperation and to respect autonomy.
2 Gather the equipment, including any prescribed shampoo.	To ensure that the procedure is enacted as efficiently as possible in as short a timescale as possible; to prevent chilling of patient.
3 Position the patient correctly.	To make sure that water does not escape from the tray and saturate bedlinen.
4 Test water temperature: it should feel warm to touch.	Too warm can scald the patient: too cold will make the procedure unnecessarily unpleasant.
5 Wet hair, apply shampoo, and massage into scalp for two or three minutes (follow product guidelines and instructions).	To ensure an even application of shampoo to the scalp area.
6 Rinse hair, massaging the scalp, and removing all trace of shampoo.	To ensure that scalp dryness and irritation does not result from soap residue.
7 Repeat if necessary.	To ensure thorough cleansing.
8 Apply conditioner, if required, massaging into scalp and throughout the length of the hair.	To prevent over-dryness of the hair and scalp.
9 Rinse thoroughly.	To avoid accumulation of conditioner in hair and scalp.
10 Remove tray, all wet and damp linen, and bucket.	To minimize hazard from water and potential spillage. Potential electrical hazard in the presence of hairdryer.
11 Wrap patient's head in towel.	To begin the drying process and to prevent water running down patient's neck and back.

continued

12	Reposition patient upright if possible and dry hair with hairdryer, noting patient preference for style, and so on.	For comfort, self-image, and expressing sexuality.
13	Remove equipment from the environment.	To avoid health and safety risks.

this goes unnoticed by the individual, but when tear production is increased as part of an emotional response, or when there is irritation of the eye, or when the naso-lachrymal duct is blocked, tears can overflow and run down the skin of the face.

When **pus** is formed through bacterial action on the surface of the eye, sometimes this cannot pass through the naso-lachrymal duct and overflows onto the lower eyelid, where it can dry out and cause encrustation and discomfort.

When eye care is required

Simple eye care may need to be repeated several times daily, and should be timed to precede the administration of any local eye medication, such as ointment and drops.

Semi-conscious patients will require particular attention, as their eyes are prone to drying and infection if they are unable to blink effectively or to completely close their eyes.

Elderly people may have diminished tear production and drooping eyelids, leading to problems with dry or weepy eyes.

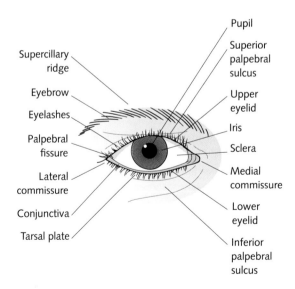

Figure 8.5 External structures of the eye

Eye care

EQUIPMENT
- Gallipot
- Swabs
- Disposable towel
- Gloves
- Disposal bag
- Sterile solution (normal saline)

▶ Step   Rationale

	Step	Rationale
1	**Cleanse hands.**	To prevent cross-infection.
2	**Explain the procedure to the patient.**	To facilitate informed consent: full cooperation is required from the patient for this procedure to be carried out successfully.
3	**Ensure privacy.**	To prevent any embarrassment and to maintain patient dignity.
4	**Prepare sterile equipment: gallipot, swabs and disposable towel (see Fig. 8.6).**	Equipment needs to be sterile to prevent cross-infection. In community settings, gallipots may be washed in warm soapy water, dried with paper towels and reused.
5	**Nontouch technique: consider the possibility of wearing gloves.**	Gloves may be appropriate if the patient's eyes are heavily contaminated or there is a risk of introducing infection. Balance this risk against the extra dexterity that is needed when wearing gloves.
6	**Pour prescribed solution into gallipot.**	This may be antiseptic or antibacterial or simply normal saline (0.9% sodium chloride solution).
7	**Prepare patient and environment.**	The patient should be seated or sitting upright in bed, with head inclined at a slight backwards angle. The area should be well lit to allow maximum observation of the eye. The towel should be draped around the neck to catch any spillage.
8	**Ask the patient to close the eyes.**	This will prevent any solution accidentally entering the eye; it will also minimize the risk of the swab touching the conjunctiva or cornea—very sensitive areas painful to touch and easy to damage.
9	**Begin with the uninfected eye or the eye least affected.**	To prevent transmission of infection to the healthier eye.

continued

10	Moisten the swab in the solution.	Too much solution will cause excessive fluid to run down the patient's face.
11	Applying gentle pressure, swab from the inner aspect of the eye (canthus) outwards, starting with the lower eyelid (see Fig. 8.7).	This will gently remove any debris.
12	Use one swab per sweep.	To prevent introducing infection from one part of the eye to another.
13	Continue procedure until debris is completely removed from the lower eyelid, then repeat for the upper eyelid.	A systematic approach will ensure efficient and effective performance.
14	On completion, ensure that the patient is comfortable and that all used equipment is disposed of properly.	To remove potential biological hazards in the environment.

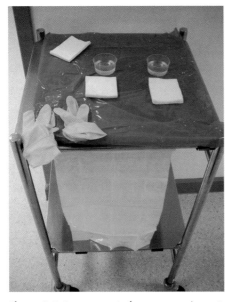

Figure 8.6 Arrangement of eye care equipment

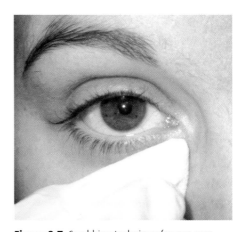

Figure 8.7 Swabbing technique for eye care

Assessment of the eye

- Pain in and around the eye, redness, blurred vision, grittiness, stickiness, and excessive tear production may all be signs of infection and need to be reported to a medical practitioner for treatment, usually with antibiotic ointment or drops
- Severe pain inside the eye may indicate an emergency situation, such as glaucoma, where pressure builds up within the eyeball itself

- Excessively dry eyes may also be accompanied by some of these symptoms, but not as severely. Dry eyes can normally be treated with over-the-counter preparations at pharmacies, with proprietary lubricants, or artificial tears
- It is important to note from the person's history whether he or she wears glasses, uses contact lenses, or has had recent surgery, such as cataract removal, as these could have a bearing on future care

Aftercare

Record the procedure in the patient's notes, documenting any findings, being specific regarding the right or left eye. Anything untoward, for example, pain during the procedure, should be notified to medical staff.

The patient should be taught self-care in this procedure, particularly if it is a recurring need.

Other factors to consider

A swab of any discharge may be required prior to performing eye care. This will be sent to the bacteriology department for analysis that will inform the prescription of any antibiotic drops or ointments.

8.7 **Mouth care**

Definition

Mouth care in this chapter includes the process of brushing teeth and caring for dentures. More detailed mouth care is covered in Chapter 12.

Good oral care involves the removal of **plaque**, the stimulation of **saliva** and the avoidance of conditions leading to the drying of the tongue and **mucosa**, tissue cracking, and fissuring.

Oral care describes the measures that can be taken to help patients to maintain the cleanliness of their teeth or dentures and to encourage a moist tongue and mucosa through the stimulation of saliva, or through artificial means.

Background

Mouth

The mouth is complex, containing a number of important structures (see **Fig. 8.8**) and performing vital functions. It is essential to two physiological systems—the digestive system and the respiratory system. Clearly, if something is seriously wrong, for example excessive swelling or inflammation, or infection developed in this part of our anatomy, it could be life-threatening. In terms of everyday health,

though, the mouth is taken for granted but serves a number of different purposes: we laugh, smile, speak, kiss, eat, drink, or smoke using our mouths and they, therefore, serve more than a physiological function; they are essential for psychological and social well-being.

Much effort is applied to maintaining health in this region from early childhood until old age: an examination of the mouth can tell a lot about a person's respiratory status, state of hydration, standards of personal hygiene,

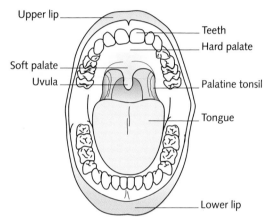

Figure 8.8 The structure of the mouth

and whether the person smokes or not. Dental care is an important aspect of healthcare that is quite often considered a separate entity; however, examining the mouth can reveal indications of diseases in other parts of the body, even cancer. Accessing a patient's dental records is often difficult, though, as these tend to remain in the dental practice. Asking a patient about his or her dental health may be the only reliable means of getting information about things like dentures, toothache, dental sensitivity, and any special tooth-care requirements. Where communication barriers are present, such information is difficult to convey, therefore, dental problems will be indicated in different ways, such as loss of appetite, aversion to very hot or very cold drinks, and so on.

The mouth contains many millions of different types of bacteria and other microorganisms, which take advantage of the ready supply of nutrients, oxygen, warmth, and moisture. Often, these accumulate in a translucent grey or white sticky film called 'plaque' covering teeth and gums. The natural defences of the body allow these potentially pathogenic microorganisms to be held in check. However, at times of ill health, and through eating patterns involving too much sugar, particularly sucrose, or through drinking too many acidic carbonated drinks, this balance may tilt in favour of the microorganisms and cause infections of **salivary glands**, ulceration of the mucosa, tooth decay and toothache. In patients who are unable to express themselves verbally, or who suffer confusion or **dementia**, toothache can be particularly distressing. In caring for such patients, always be alert to pain being a possible cause of restlessness, loss of appetite, and inability to sleep. One study demonstrated that as many as 60% of patients with dementia in nursing homes had dental pain, so it is a very common occurrence (Chalmers and Pearson 2005).

When mouth care is required

Adults

Oral hygiene is indicated when the patient is dehydrated or has limited oral intake of either fluids or food: chewing normally **stimulates** the flow of saliva. It is also indicated in patients who are unable to chew properly, as in some patients suffering a stroke or those affected by a neuromuscular problem affecting the face; in those patients who are nauseated or who have recently vomited, those prescribed certain drugs that have a drying effect on oral mucosa, and in those suffering dementia.

Any patient who is bedbound, who cannot move to a sink, who has a mobility or dexterity problem, or who has altered consciousness will need assistance with oral hygiene, but the extent of assistance that is required will need to be carefully determined by assessing and discussing with the patient.

Children

Oral hygiene is indicated in children who are too young to have mastered the intricacies of tooth cleansing. Toddlers are vulnerable to developing caries, particularly if sweets and fruit juices are a regular feature of their diet, especially if consumed between meals. The constant slurping of such drinks means that the teeth are under constant attack. As part of the dental care of children, it is important to emphasize to parents the harm that seemingly innocuous practices can inflict. If sweets are to be given to children, perhaps immediately following a meal is the best time, shortly followed by toothbrushing.

The practice of brushing teeth, with a small-headed, soft toothbrush should commence as soon as teeth appear, using a little fluoridated toothpaste. Parental supervision and encouragement is required in preschool years and into early school years, until the child is able to appreciate its importance and is autonomous in this regard. Six-monthly dental check-ups are important to monitor the loss of primary teeth and the emergence of permanent teeth, dealing with any orthodontic issues as they arise. **Fissure sealant** is an important dental treatment that can reduce the incidence of **dental caries** if applied at the right time. Dental care may be complicated by the use of orthodontic braces and children will need coaching and encouragement to care for these properly.

Assessment of the patient's mouth condition

If available, use an oral assessment tool to assist in guiding the assessment process.

- While visually examining the mouth, note any dentures, bridges, veneers, dental caries, loose, or broken teeth. Also look for redness, swelling, ulceration, and bleeding
- The colour of the tongue and its smoothness should also be noted
- Look for any food remnants lodged between gums and cheeks, and trapped between teeth. Sometimes a drink of plain water or a mouth rinse is sufficient to deal with this problem
- Take note of any strange smells from the patient's breath: a foul, fetid smell may indicate a lack of oral hygiene and tooth decay; a smell of **acetone** (pear drops) may indicate diabetes or extreme malnourishment; alcohol may be detected on the patient's breath, as may cigarette smoke

Brushing a patient's teeth

EQUIPMENT

- Patient's own toothbrush (or equivalent), toothpaste, floss, denture cleaning materials. The size of toothbrush should be appropriate to the individual
- A small torch may be required
- Prepare some plain, tepid water for rinsing
- Prepare a receptacle (disposable bowl) to collect expelled mouth-rinse
- Tissues

Step	Rationale
1 Wash hands.	To protect the patient from cross-infection.
2 Wear gloves.	To protect yourself from contamination from oral secretions and possible infection.
3 Explain and gain consent, incorporating patient choices and preferences.	This is an **invasive** procedure and potentially hazardous to the nurse if full cooperation is not gained from the patient. A full explanation is required.
4 Provide privacy.	Most people are sensitive to the fact that they have dentures and are reluctant to clean these in public.
5 Gather materials.	Being organized will allow the patient to feel comfortable that the nurse is confident and competent at the procedure.
6 Prepare patient. Position patient upright where possible, in a good light. Where the patient's condition prohibits this position, the patient should adopt a position on their side.	To provide good visualization. To prevent **aspiration** of toothpaste or rinsing fluid. The procedure is otherwise the same.
7 Drape towel around the patient's shoulders.	To absorb any spillages.
8 Inspect the mouth.	To identify any collections of food, any areas of mucosa and tongue that may be ulcerated and painful. Remember to look at the **palate**, as sometimes food can be trapped here, adhering to the roof of the mouth. A small torch is useful.

continued

9	**Provide the patient with their toothbrush, prepared with a pea-sized amount of toothpaste.**	The effort and coordination involved in putting toothpaste on the brush may be too much for some patients. Too much toothpaste may irritate the patient's mucosa. If this occurs even with a small amount of toothpaste, try changing brands to a less highly flavoured variety.
10	**If necessary, assist the patient to manipulate the toothbrush and move it in such a way as to achieve a cleansing motion (see Fig. 8.9). Use a teddy or doll to demonstrate the movements required to a child.**	The fronts and backs of teeth can be cleaned by gently moving the brush to and fro, along the gum margins. An up and down movement of the brush, from the gums to the tips of the crowns and back, will clean the front and back surfaces. A back and forth movement on the tops of the teeth will clean biting surfaces. If the tongue is coated, but not painful, a gentle brushing will help remove excessive build up of secretions and plaque.
11	**Assist the patient to expel used toothpaste and food particles into disposable bowl: finish with a rinse of tepid water and offer tissues to dry lips.**	The mouth should feel fresh and all visible trace of toothpaste should be removed.
12	**If appropriate, apply lip balm, and if prescribed, apply medication such as acyclovir for herpes simplex if present.**	Lips can dry and crack if the patient is dehydrated; some prescribed medications can have the same effect. Herpes simplex infections of the lips can be dormant until activated through stress.

Aftercare

Leave the patient comfortably positioned if in bed, removing towel and replacing any used materials belonging to the patient. Make written notes of any findings regarding dental health, and the needs of the patient for mouth care. Inform the nurse in charge of any issues or concerns; recommend updating the patient's care plan if the frequency and nature of planned care will not meet the patient's needs.

The patient should be encouraged and facilitated to make the transition from dependence to independence in this recurrent need, if possible.

Other factors to consider

Where dentition is poor, or teeth are painful, a better quality of life can be achieved for the patient by calling on the services of a dental surgeon. Occasionally this needs to be done as an emergency in acute care settings, but more often than not it is required routinely in continuing care.

Children have particular needs from the moment the first tooth erupts: special toothpaste and very small soft toothbrushes are available for use with babies. It is

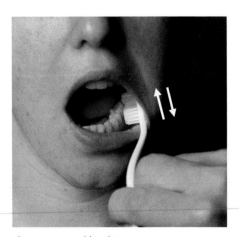

Figure 8.9 Toothbrushing movements

Cleaning a patient's dentures

Cleaning dentures may be a small part or the predominant feature of oral care. The following actions should be incorporated into care where appropriate, based on your assessment.

EQUIPMENT
- Denture container
- Denture brush or toothbrush
- Denture cleaner
- Box of disposable tissues
- A cup of water

Step	Rationale
1 Gather the equipment.	Being organized will allow the patient to feel comfortable that the nurse is confident and competent at the procedure.
2 Clearly label the denture container with patient's name and hospital number.	Lost dentures in hospital can be very inconvenient and distressing for patients, so care must be taken to ensure that these are clearly identifiable when taken from the patient.
3 Explain procedure to patient and gain their consent: negotiate an appropriate time for this procedure, incorporating patient choices.	The patient may initiate this process: otherwise, ensure that the timing of this procedure is appropriate for the patient to minimize any embarrassment.
4 Wear gloves.	To protect yourself from infection/contamination.
5 Provide privacy.	Removing dentures can be extremely embarrassing for individuals, therefore, privacy is vital.
6 Ask patient to remove dentures and place them in a denture container. If the patient cannot do this, use a gauze swab to help grip and manoeuvre the upper plate and then the lower plate from the mouth, placing these into the denture container.	Patients should be involved in their own care as much as possible. It is never wise to put your fingers in the mouth of a patient who may be confused or uncooperative. This carries a potential risk of you being bitten and should only be performed if confident that the patient will cooperate.
7 Offer water to the patient to rinse the mouth and expel into a disposable bowl.	To remove any food debris and accumulated plaque from the gums on removal of the dentures.
8 Visually inspect the gums for any health problems.	The gums may be damaged, ulcerated, and infected through uneven pressure from poorly fitting dentures. This might be particularly so in the case of elderly, confused, and demented patients who do not regularly remove their dentures.

continued

9	Take dentures in their container to a sink and, using the toothbrush and cleanser, scrub clean under warm water (Fig. 8.10).	Hot water could damage certain types of denture. Follow the instructions on the cleanser packaging.
10	If necessary soak badly stained or soiled dentures: sometimes patients routinely do this at night.	To facilitate thorough cleansing.
11	Rinse dentures thoroughly.	Denture cleanser is a strong caustic substance that could irritate the oral mucosa.
12	Rinse denture container.	To remove any soiling from dentures.
13	Return dentures to patient immediately and assist patient to reposition them.	Wet dentures are easier to reposition.

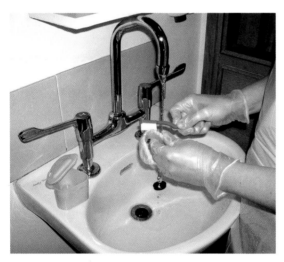

Figure 8.10 Brushing dentures at sink

recommended that they are introduced while the child is very young so that oral care becomes accepted as the norm.

In some people the tongue size can be enlarged, as in Down's syndrome, and in acromegaly. These present different challenges for oral care.

Older adults may have problems with their health that complicate oral care, for example rheumatoid arthritis can severely restrict the fine movement of the hands and fingers and make using a toothbrush difficult. Age-related changes to the mouth and surrounding tissues can increase the risk of developing mouth problems in ill health, for example, there is reduced production and secretion of saliva, and oral mucosa tends to become drier with age.

Confused patients, uncooperative patients perhaps with altered consciousness, and uncooperative children present particular challenges to implementing adequate oral care. Oral care requires full cooperation from the recipient. Where this is not forthcoming, full documentation needs to be made.

8.8 Assisting a patient with dressing

Definition

Clothing of some form is required by every patient, from blankets swaddled around a newborn baby, through theatre gowns, to patients' own clothing. The main functions of clothing are comfort, warmth, privacy, and dignity, and should all be respected. Some patients may wear specific clothing because of cultural or religious beliefs and nurses should assist patients to be clothed as they wish within the limitations of the care environment and the patient's condition.

When to assist a patient with dressing

Patients may not always be able to dress themselves independently. They may be too young, or they may be limited by an acute illness or long-term condition or disability. Wearing appropriate clothing is a frequent issue for people with learning disabilities. At these times, it is necessary for the nurse to assist the patient in dressing, whilst promoting their independence where possible and appropriate.

Procedure

Throughout this procedure, attention must be paid to the holistic needs of the patient and the requirement to respect the individual's level of independence, and to avoid disempowerment.

Preparation

Explain the procedure to the patient and ask if they have any preferences, for example:

- Own clothing—is it appropriate and available? In some circumstances it may be appropriate for a hospital gown to be worn, for example if the patient is to have a diagnostic procedure or surgical operation. The patient may also choose a hospital gown in preference to their own clothes due to excessive soiling, for example, from incontinence or wound **exudate**. The patient's own clothes due to considered, if available and appropriate, as they could help to promote a sense of normality and well-being for the patient. The patient's own clothing will also allow the nurse to assess any difficulties with the procedure of dressing that the patient may encounter when unassisted
- Is assistance required? The patient may have previously been independent in their own environment at home, but due to their condition or treatment now requires assistance

- Patients may prefer a member of their family or carer to assist with their dressing. Children may prefer a parent or guardian—this may be the person who usually assists them or they may wish assistance from someone familiar to them for reassurance. This should be offered if possible and appropriate

The appropriateness of clothing should also be considered when the patient will be going to different environments, for example, going outside. Thin clothing may be appropriate to wear inside, but not appropriate for cold and wet weather.

The nurse should also help guide those patients, for example with mental health issues, whose choice of not wearing clothing is socially and, in some cases, legally unacceptable.

Aftercare

The nurse should ensure that the patient is left comfortable and warm.

The nurse should continually assess the appropriateness of the patient's clothing, for example, if the temperature of the patient's environment increases or decreases, clothing may have to be removed or added. This is also true of the patient's temperature, as it may change because of infection or disease processes. These changes, which are not caused by environmental factors, should be reported to a more senior member of staff, as they may indicate a deterioration in the patient's condition.

Other factors to consider

Working with an occupational therapist

Occupational therapists (OTs) are a professional group and are sometimes classified within the group of allied health professionals (AHPs). Their primary role is to help people improve their ability to perform daily living tasks, such as dressing, cooking, and bathing. Occupational therapists may also work with, and specialize in, particular client groups, for example elderly care, **orthopaedics**, and mental health. You should be aware that occupational therapists are available to

Assisting a patient with dressing

Step	Rationale
1 Explain the procedure to the patient.	To facilitate informed consent.
2 Gain the patient's consent, incorporating patient choice and preferences.	To gain cooperation and respect autonomy.
3 Ensure privacy: curtains or door closed with displayed engaged sign.	To prevent embarrassment and maintain patient dignity.
4 Ensure access to the patient does not pose any physical risk to the nurse or patient.	To protect nurse and patient from injury.
5 After consultation with the patient, collect all clothing required and have ready next to the patient.	To ensure smooth procedure.
6 With patient sitting down, place feet into leg openings of underwear and pull up legs. Trousers, skirts, and hosiery to be worn can then be applied in the same way before standing patient up.	To minimize movement for the patient.
7 Assist patient to stand (using equipment if appropriate and necessary). Adjust pants or knickers and trousers upwards, ensuring correct position.	To maintain dignity and comfort for the patient.
8 For adult female patients place arms into openings of straps of bra and fasten (may be back or front fastening), with patient assisting if able to do so.	To maintain dignity and comfort for the patient.
9 If a vest is required, place head through neck opening of garment, then each hand through corresponding arm openings and adjust into place.	
10 Apply additional clothing in the same way, with patient assisting wherever possible and appropriate. Once garments have been applied, fastenings should be secured and then ensure they are positioned appropriately, to avoid causing trauma or pressure damage.	To ensure comfort and warmth for patient.

assist with the care of their patients and appropriate referrals to them should be made, through your mentor or medical staff.

Patients who have had a stroke or cerebrovascular accident (CVA)

The affected side should be dressed first (that is, first inserted into arm or legs of clothing). This makes the process easier for the nurse and more comfortable for the patient. The nurse should avoid using phrases such as 'bad side' or 'bad arm or leg' when assisting this group of patients, as this can perpetuate potential negative views of the patient's condition in both the patient and other staff or carers.

Patients who have lost a limb

These patients may need very little assistance, depending on their level of mobility and dexterity. The nurse should also consider how long the patient has been an amputee: those who have recently undergone amputation surgery may not yet be able to dress themselves as well as someone who has been an amputee for years.

Patients with limited movement or dexterity

Patients who have impaired fine-**motor** skills, for example, as a result of arthritis in their hands and fingers, may have difficulties with clothing and fastenings, such a small buttons and clasps. Devices such as buttoning aids can help this (see **Fig. 8.11**). Clothing with alternative fastenings

such as elastic waistbands, large buttons, Velcro, and zips may be easier for this group of patients to manipulate.

Patients with a visual impairment

The nurse should describe the clothing available, so that the patient can choose which clothing to wear. Clothing items that complement each other on colour or style can be marked for someone who is visually impaired, by using labels on the clothing that can be felt by the patient. Commercially available tags marked in **Braille** are available for this purpose, or the patient may simply have different shapes cut from clothing labels to match items.

Specialized equipment

The occupational therapist can provide advice and information regarding specialized equipment to aid patients to dress themselves (see **Figs 8.12–8.14**). It should be highlighted, however, that the aim of these aids are to assist a patient who is unable to complete a task independently, not to take any independence from the patient. For example, if a patient is recovering from hip surgery and requires assistance reaching to put on hosiery

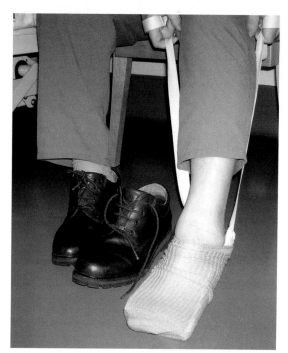

Figure 8.12 Sock aid

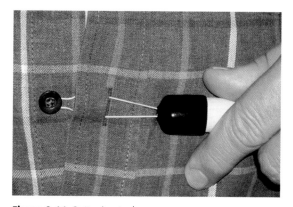

Figure 8.11 Buttoning tool

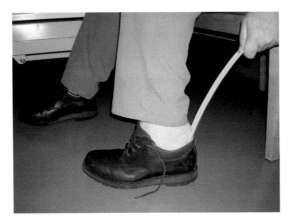

Figure 8.13 Long shoe horn

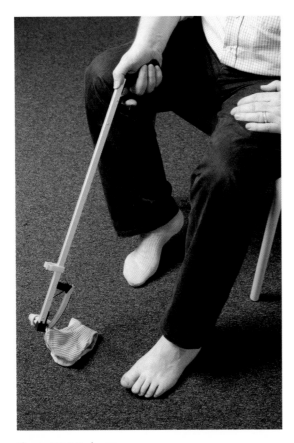

Figure 8.14 Grab arm

and shoes, then a piece of equipment may be appropriate during this interim period. However, on recovery, the patient will hopefully be able to reach again and at this time the equipment would not be appropriate.

8.9 **Wound assessment**

Definition

A wound is described as any breach of the skin that results in the patient losing the protective barrier function of the skin. Wound care is an overarching term and covers a huge range of activities relating to the treatment and management of patients with wounds.

Background

To understand the issues in wound assessment fully you should examine the earlier information on skin care.

Wounds may be acute or chronic in nature and this will determine what care is required by the nurse. The key principles of wound care are to promote healing, prevent infection, and treat any symptoms such as pain, malodour, and exudate levels (Leaper and Harding 1998). Wounds heal by primary or secondary intention. Primary intention describes when the wound edges are brought together by sutures, staples, glue, or clips. This usually follows surgery.

Secondary intention healing refers mostly to chronic wounds, which are 'open' and heal by the formation of granulation tissue in the base of the wound, followed by epithelialization and contraction, during which time infection is a major risk (Leaper and Harding 1998).

Key wound types

Acute

Surgical Either elective or emergency in nature, surgery involves the creation of a wound, in a controlled environment, to access internal structures.

Traumatic Wounds that are sustained as a result of trauma, such as lacerations, road traffic accidents, and falls.

Burns Burns range from minor scalds that only affect the upper layers of the skin, referred to as superficial damage, to more severe burns when the deeper tissues are affected, known as deep tissue damage.

Chronic

Pressure ulcer May be superficial or deep and are often the result of sustained unrelieved pressure, friction, shearing, and moisture on the skin.

Leg ulcer Often occur on the lower limbs and are the result of venous disease, arterial disease, mixed aetiology, or the result of other chronic conditions, such as diabetes and arthritis.

Diabetic foot ulcer May occur as a result of neurological damage in the foot or ischaemia in the limb or a combination of these symptoms. Diabetes affects the **peripheral** perfusion and the neurological function in the feet, resulting in undetected damage. Foot care in diabetic patients is essential to avoid long-term complications of the disease process (Mani *et al.* 1999).

When to assess and treat wounds

Wound assessment is necessary for all wound types and the level of intervention will depend on the wound type. In acute wounds, healing by primary intention, the wound should remain covered for at least 48 hours postoperatively using an **occlusive** dressing. After this time, the protective barrier function of the skin should be re-established.

A patient with a wound that may be **slough**y and at risk of infection or heavily exuding or with an open wound will require a more intensive treatment regime.

Aftercare

Patients with acute and chronic wounds will heal at different rates, and quite often the patient with chronic wounds will require long-term follow-up from the community nursing team. Ongoing assessment of the needs of patients with wounds is imperative and this should include reducing the risk of pressure damage and trauma, which could affect the wound. A diet rich in nutrients should be encouraged to facilitate the long-term healing process; this may last up to 18 months following wound closure.

Other factors to consider

Factors that affect the wound-healing process

For all patients with wounds, nutrition is an important consideration; poor nutrition is relatively common in elderly patients. Patients with wounds will require extra protein, calories, vitamins and minerals, to enhance the wound-healing process. Many patients will also have concurrent illness such as cardiac disease, liver disease, diabetes, and **anaemia**, all of which can lead to slow wound healing.

It is essential that wound care is carried out in the context of the whole patient, and the patient should be treated by the appropriate members of the multidisciplinary team to maximize healing potential (Timmons, 2005).

The role of the specialist nurse in caring for patients with wounds

The tissue viability nurse specialist (TVN) is responsible for advising and educating all staff in pressure relief, wound care, wound infection, and leg ulcers. The TVN should be made aware of patients with problematic wounds that require specialist intervention. The TVN is also responsible for supplying equipment for pressure relief and reduction. Patients who are at risk of pressure ulcers should be referred for specialist equipment.

8.10 **Aseptic technique**

Definition

Aseptic technique is the term given to the process by which a nurse or healthcare professional aims to minimize the risk of introducing infection or contamination to a patient receiving care. This usually involves an invasive procedure, such as catheterization or **cannulation**, and is also applied in the care of wounds. When there is a breach of the normal body defences, there is a risk of

Assessment and treatment of wounds

Table 8.1 is purely a guide and wound dressings should follow local protocol. For leg ulcers, the key therapy is **compression bandaging**, which helps to promote venous return. For pressure ulcers, it is also important to provide regular pressure relief, specialist support surfaces, and seating cushions.

Treatment aims and dressings for different wound types

Wound type	Treatment aims	Primary dressing	Secondary dressing
Acute surgical	Protect and avoid infection	Occlusive film with absorbent pad	Not necessary
Traumatic	Cleanse and avoid infection	Iodine tulle (Inadine Johnson and Johnson) Mepitel	Occlusive dressing with absorbent pad Foam dressing if leaking
Chronic wounds: Dry/necrotic/sloughy tissue	To moisten slough and prevent infection	Maggot therapy Hydrogels	Foam dressing
		Hydrocolloids Honey dressings	
Wet sloughy wounds	To remove slough absorb exudate and prevent infection	Maggot therapy Hydrofibre dressings Alginate dressings (with or without silver)	Foam dressing
Granulating wounds	To protect the tissue from physical damage, maintain moisture levels and prevent infection	Atraumatic wound contact layer dressing (Mepitel, Atrauman)	Foam dressing or film dressing
Epithelializing wounds	To protect the tissue from physical damage, maintain moisture levels and prevent infection	Atraumatic wound contact layer (Mepitel, Atrauman)	Film dressing or foam dressing

infection caused by the transfer of microorganisms. Chronic wounds are never free of bacteria, and although the principles of asepsis still apply, the aim will be to avoid further contamination of the wound and not to promote sterility.

The 'aseptic—no touch technique' (ANTT) is the commonly used term, and describes all procedures during which cross-contamination can occur. The technique described here is based on the use of ANTT (Rowley and Sinclair 2004). There are a number of resources available to support the use of ANTT in a variety of clinical settings. In community settings, nurses may have to adapt the environment to carry out the procedure; however, the basic principles can be followed.

Aseptic technique for wound care

It is essential to gather all equipment before the procedure to avoid interrupting the procedure and risking contamination:

EQUIPMENT

- Clean trolley or bedside table (cleaned with 70% alcohol)
- Apron
- Dressing pack (with or without forceps)
- Cleansing solution (normal saline)
- New dressing or other equipment needed for procedure
- 20 ml syringe and green needle for rinsing wound
- Sterile gloves
- Disposal bag
- Alcohol gel

	Step	Rationale
1	Explain procedure to the patient.	To reduce anxiety, improve comfort, and inform patient.
2	Position the patient as required.	To promote comfort and improve access.
3	Put apron on and wash hands using handwash then alcohol gel.	To prevent cross-contamination.
4	Prepare table or trolley to create 'sterile field'.	To provide clean working area.
5	Open dressing pack and place on surface.	To prevent contamination.
6	Open the pack touching the corners only.	To avoid contaminating the pack.
7	Open other packs and allow to drop onto the 'sterile' field.	To prevent contamination.
8	Pour cleansing solution into the gallipot without touching the gallipot.	To have the solution in a sterile container.
9	Using the forceps arrange the items on the sterile field (see Fig. 8.15).	To help prepare for the procedure
10	Use the same forceps to remove the old dressings and then discard.	To prevent contaminating the field and the environment.
11	Put on sterile gloves handling only the wrist sections and not touching the fingers.	To avoid contaminating the gloves.

continued

12	Cleanse the wound (area) using saline in syringe and needle.	To wash left-over dressing material from the wound.
13	Apply a new dressing using gloved hands.	To avoid touching the wound.
14	Remove gloves and place in disposal bag.	To avoid contaminating environment.
15	Clear the area: sharps in sharps bin and waste in relevant waste bin.	To avoid sharps injury and dispose of soiled material safely.
16	Wash hands using handwash then alcohol gel.	To prevent cross-contamination.
17	Discuss outcome with the patient and reposition patient.	To inform the patient of progress and make patient comfortable.

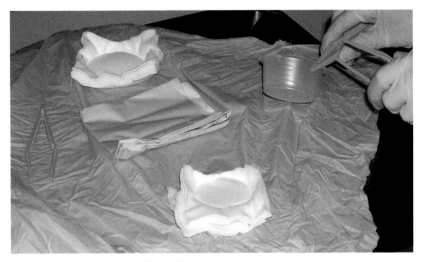

Figure 8.15 Arranging sterile field with forceps

When to use the aseptic—no touch technique

When undertaking any procedure that could lead to infection or contamination, the principles of asepsis should apply. Examples are:

- Wound care
- Catheterization
- Cannulation
- Administration of intravenous therapy
- Central lines
- Administration of **chemotherapy**
- Use of a **Hickman line** or **portacath**
- Peripheral inserted central catheters

Aftercare

Following any aseptic procedure, it is important that local protocol is followed relating to hand hygiene, and cleansing of trolleys and instruments. Any used equipment should be disposed of safely and with regard for local waste disposal protocol.

Other factors to consider

Once the procedure has been carried out, the patient should be made comfortable and fully assessed to avoid relevant complications that may be associated with the procedure.

The value of aseptic technique has been questioned in recent years and yet this has corresponded with a rise in healthcare-acquired infection (HAI). It is, therefore, essential that you take a more cautious approach when caring for patients and use aseptic techniques and good hand washing as much as possible, to reduce the risk of cross-infection.

8.11 **Removal of sutures, staples, or clips**

Definition

Sutures, staples, and clips are put in place to allow the wound to close naturally by opposing the edges of the wound. Depending on the wound site and the surgeon's preference, wounds may be closed using either sutures, staples, or clips during surgery or other procedures.

Background

Sutures are normally composed of silk; however, some man-made fibres are used. Sutures can be **cutaneous** (above the skin and visible) or subcutaneous (beneath the skin surface). Deep wounds may have internal sutures, which will dissolve, as well as skin sutures. Superficial wounds will have cutaneous sutures that require removal. Sutures will have two entry points into the skin and a knot, which will be proximal to one of these. Sutures can be used for wound closure in a number of types of surgery and may be used in a variety of body sites. Sutures may be more time-consuming than using clips for wound closure and the decision should take into account the type of operation, the size of the wound, the body site, and the individual patient's needs.

Clips are used as a wound-closure technique when the wound site may be unsuitable for staples or sutures. **Thyroid** surgery wounds are commonly closed using clips, partly because of the position of the wound on the neck and partly because of the risk of haemorrhage affecting the trachea. Clips can be removed quickly to relieve pressure from **haematoma** to underlying structures.

When to remove sutures, staples, or clips

Timing of suture, staple, or clip removal will vary depending on the operation type, the body site, and whether there are signs of infection. As a general rule, suture removal will be carried out on the seventh post-operative day. This can be earlier for simpler procedures, such as mole removal or closure of surface wounds caused by injury.

Removing sutures

EQUIPMENT
- Trolley (if in secondary care)
- Dressing pack with forceps
- Normal saline
- Suture remover (see Fig. 8.16)
- Gloves (sterile)
- Disposal bag
- Occlusive dressing with absorbent pad (not always necessary)

continued

Removing sutures

 Step   **Rationale**

	Step	Rationale
1	Explain procedure to the patient.	To inform, put patient at ease and gain patient's consent
2	Wash hands.	To prevent cross-infection.
3	Position patient appropriately.	To gain access to the wound.
4	Observe the wound.	To check for signs of infection or risk of **dehiscence**.
5	Open the dressing pack and equipment onto sterile field.	To promote asepsis and provide a sterile working area.
6	Put on the sterile gloves.	To prevent cross-infection.
7	Pour the saline into the gallipot.	To keep as sterile as possible and allow saline to be used to clean the wound.
8	Clean the sutures at the point where they enter the skin.	To reduce risk of bacterial entry into the wound.
9	Using the forceps, lift knot of the suture using the cut end of the suture.	To raise the knot from the wound.
10	Check that the patient is not in pain.	To prevent or reduce pain and allow patient to have analgesia if required.
11	Cut the suture under the knot using the stitch cutter.	To free the suture.
12	Pull on the suture using the forceps.	To remove the suture from the wound.
13	Remove alternate sutures.	To allow further wound assessment.
14	Check the wound for signs of dehiscence.	To ensure that the wound remains intact.
15	Once content that the wound is intact, continue to remove the remaining sutures.	To avoid dehiscence (separation of the edges) of the wound, should healing be incomplete.
16	Check the wound for signs of leakage.	To avoid leakage and discomfort for the patient.
17	If the wound is leaking, apply absorbent occlusive dressing.	To absorb leakage and prevent cross-infection.
18	If the wound remains painful, consult a senior member of staff.	To alert staff to potential wound complications.

19	Advise patient on the signs of wound infection.	To allow the patient to check for signs of infection.
20	Wash hands.	To prevent cross-infection.
21	Record in the patient's notes that the procedure has been carried out, the number of sutures removed, the patient's well-being, and wound assessment post removal.	To ensure that the procedure is recorded accurately.
22	Clear and clean the trolley used, disposing of sharps appropriately.	To prevent cross-infection and allow safe disposal of all materials.

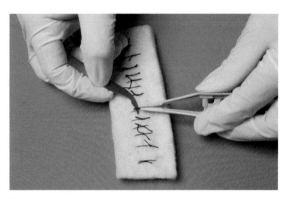

Figure 8.16 Suture remover

Removing staples

EQUIPMENT
- Trolley (if in secondary care)
- Dressing pack with forceps
- Normal saline
- Staple remover (see Fig. 8.17)
- Gloves (sterile)
- Disposal bag
- Occlusive dressing with absorbent pad (not always necessary)

Step   Rationale

| 1 | Explain procedure to the patient. | To inform, put patient at ease and gain consent. |
| 2 | Wash hands. | To prevent cross-infection. |

continued

3	Position patient appropriately.	To gain access to the wound.
4	Observe the wound.	To check for signs of infection or risk of dehiscence.
5	Open the dressing pack and equipment onto sterile field.	To minimize contamination.
6	Put on the sterile gloves.	To prevent cross-infection.
7	Pour the saline into the gallipot.	
8	Clean the wound around the outside where the staples enter the skin.	To reduce risk of bacterial entry into the wound.
9	Using the staple remover, slide the hook under the staple and fully depress the handle, bending the staple and remove the staple from the wound.	To raise the staple prongs and allow safe removal.
10	Check that the patient is not in pain.	To prevent or reduce pain and allow patient to have analgesia if required.
11	Remove alternate clips.	To allow further wound assessment.
12	Check the wound for signs of dehiscence.	To ensure that the wound remains intact.
13	Once content that the wound is intact, continue to remove the remaining clips.	To ensure that all clips have been removed.
14	Check the wound for signs of leakage.	To avoid leakage and discomfort for the patient.
15	If the wound is leaking, apply absorbent occlusive dressing.	To absorb leakage and prevent cross-infection.
16	If the wound remains painful, consult a senior member of staff.	To alert staff to potential wound complications.
17	Advise patient on the signs of wound infection.	To allow the patient to check for signs of infection.
18	Wash hands.	To prevent cross-infection.

19	Record in the patients' notes that the procedure has been carried out, the number of staples removed, the patient's well-being, and wound assessment post removal.	To ensure that the procedure is recorded accurately.
20	Clear and clean the trolley used, disposing of sharps appropriately.	To prevent cross-infection and allow safe disposal of all materials.

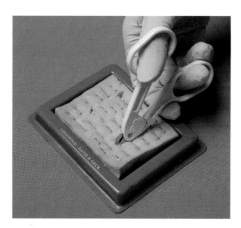

Figure 8.17 Staple remover

Removal of clips

EQUIPMENT
- Trolley (if in secondary care)
- Dressing pack with forceps
- Normal saline
- Clip remover
- Gloves (sterile)
- Disposal bag
- Occlusive dressing with absorbent pad (not always necessary)

Step   Rationale

1	Explain procedure to the patient.	To inform, put patient at ease and gain consent.
2	Wash hands.	To prevent cross-infection.

continued

3	Position patient appropriately.	To gain access to the wound.
4	Observe the wound.	To check for signs of infection or risk of dehiscence.
5	Open the dressing pack and equipment onto sterile field.	To provide a sterile area on which to place equipment.
6	Put on the sterile gloves.	To prevent cross-infection.
7	Pour the saline into the gallipot.	To provide a sterile pot from which to extract the saline for wound cleansing.
8	Clean the clips with saline at the point where they enter the skin.	To reduce risk of bacterial entry into the wound.
9	Using the clip removal insert into the grooves on the clip.	To facilitate safe removal.
10	Check that the patient is not in pain.	To prevent or reduce pain and allow patient to have analgesia if required.
11	Depress the centre of the clip removers.	To assist in removing the clip.
12	Once free from the skin remove the clip.	To remove the clip from the wound.
13	Remove alternate clips.	To allow further wound assessment.
14	Check the wound for signs of dehiscence.	To ensure the wound remains intact.
15	Once content that the wound is intact, continue to remove the remaining clips.	To ensure that all clips have been safely removed.
16	Check the wound for signs of leakage.	To avoid leakage and discomfort for the patient.
17	If the wound is leaking apply absorbent occlusive dressing.	To absorb leakage and prevent cross-infection.
18	If the wound remains painful consult a senior member of staff.	To alert staff to potential wound complications.
19	Advise patient on the signs of wound infection.	To allow the patient to check for signs of infection.
20	Wash hands.	To prevent cross-infection.

| 21 | Record in the patient's notes that the procedure has been carried out, the number of clips removed, the patient's well-being, and wound assessment post removal. | To ensure that the procedure is recorded accurately. |
| 22 | Clear and clean the trolley used, disposing of sharps appropriately. | To prevent cross-infection and allow safe disposal of all materials. |

Aftercare

All wounds should be assessed for signs of infection or dehiscence. The patient should be given information regarding the potential of developing wound infection and the signs and symptoms to look out for. Wound dehiscence or opening of the wound may occur when infection is present or if there is extra pressure on the wound, such as may occur when the patient is coughing or if the patient is overweight.

All patients should have follow-up appointments with a practice nurse, GP, or community nurse after discharge.

Other factors to consider

Patients who have concurrent illness may experience slower healing than younger healthier patients and this should be reflected in the aftercare of the patient. Wounds can affect the patient's ability to self-care and prevent the patient from going back to work. Patients may need advice from social work or other agencies in order to help them return to their home environment.

8.12 **Total patient care**

Definition

This involves the simultaneous performance of several procedures within one nurse–patient interaction. Total patient care is organizational in nature, and requires careful assessment and pre-planning so that it can be performed efficiently, effectively and safely, whilst maintaining a sensitive and caring demeanour.

When to provide total patient care

This method can be used when a patient is unwell, requires bed rest, and has simultaneous needs such as hygiene, shaving, and perhaps wound care, eye care, and oral care. The object of meeting all the patient's needs together is to allow the patient defined periods of intense activity and undisturbed rest. This requires skilful assessment on the part of the nurse, as patients will present with different needs based on their level of dependency and the nature of treatment that they are receiving.

In-hospital settings, post-operative care, and gerontological care are very different and contrast again with domiciliary and childcare settings. No matter how the setting differs and how technical the nature of the care becomes, the objective of total patient care remains: to deliver care in an organized, efficient manner, thus maximizing the patient's undisturbed period to promote rest and recovery. The main requirements for nurses to prepare for total patient care are similar. This brings together in combination many of the skills already mentioned in the chapter, and is, therefore, generally focused, and principle based.

Total patient care

Step	Rationale
1 Assess patient's holistic needs. Refer to multiple sources for your assessment: the patient's care plan, written and verbal handover instructions, and interaction with the patient.	This full assessment will allow anticipated patient activities to be combined in their most logical sequence for your patient.
2 Plan patient care for the immediate period (whether it is morning, afternoon, evening, or night).	Anticipate the patient's needs taking into account the resources that you have at your disposal (help from healthcare assistants, requirements for equipment, such as moving and handling hoists). Poor planning and preparation can lead to interruptions and unnecessary lengthening of care.
3 Discuss with the patient your intentions for delivering care, consider the feedback you receive, incorporate patient choices and gain consent.	It is important that the patient understands the order and intensity of care that you are about to deliver, and actively participates in this. It is also important, for autonomy and dignity, to acknowledge patient preferences.
4 Negotiate assistance from other members of the caring team: integrate planned activity into the overall work of the ward or unit schedule of planned activities.	To provide efficient care for patients with several needs more than one nurse is often required. Timing is crucial and may need to be modified in light of staff availability and other priorities competing for the same resources.
5 Gather equipment and organize immediate environment. For example, hoist, bed-bathing equipment, dressing equipment, shaving equipment, and bedlinen may be required; monitoring equipment, drug administration materials and drugs may be required.	Efficient care requires that all items of equipment required for care delivery are at hand. Take into account health and safety implications for the collection of such equipment in a confined space, and mixing electrical equipment with water (for example, following the bed bath of a patient, you may wish to use an electric shaver, carrying with it a potential hazard).
6 Consider patient safety and ensure that the patient is involved as much as possible.	Patients should be empowered to achieve independence within the limits of their capabilities: this ought to influence pace and sequence of care.
7 Acknowledge that some aspects of total patient care may require special consideration and non-touch or aseptic technique must be used when appropriate. Wash hands and wear gloves as appropriate.	It is possible to contaminate one part of the body with bacteria from another: the eyes, the mouth, the genitourinary tract, and any surgical incision or other wound are particularly susceptible.
8 Respect patient dignity, choice, and consent.	Although many things may be needed to be done efficiently, engaging with the patient effectively through communication is a priority.

Total patient care

9	**Tidy as you go along: remove hazardous material from the immediate environment as soon as possible: for example, soiled dressings, incontinence pads, basins of used bath water.**	Accidents can happen and a de-cluttered care environment is essential for safe provision of nursing care.
10	**Complete procedure by leaving patient comfortable and safe.**	The patient should feel refreshed but may be exhausted and this might be a good time to dim lights and facilitate rest and sleep.

Aftercare

Update the patient's records to reflect your assessment and interventions performed, including changes to care plan.

Improving

This organizational skill requires observation of mentors' and other experts' practice and reflection on your own organizational and prioritizing skills in order to reach perfection.

Other factors to consider

The work of the other members of the care team should be considered, noting any conflicting priorities. Physiotherapists, for example, will manage their workload in light of nursing activities and patient priorities, respecting a patient's need for sleep can be incorporated into a physiotherapist's care plan if adequate warning and consideration are given. Likewise, occupational therapists, radiographers, junior doctors, and any other relevant discipline should be involved in the patient's overall plan of care for any particular period and allowances made for periods of rest and activity.

 ## Scenarios

Consider what you should do in the following situations, then turn to the end of the section to check your answers.

Further scenarios are available at

🌐 **www.oxfordtextbooks.co.uk/orc/docherty/**

 ### Scenario 1

Peter is an 81-year-old man who suffers from dementia and has been admitted to a nursing home. A striking feature of Peter's current state is his unkempt appearance and unclean body odour. You have been asked to assess Peter's immediate needs for physical care. What would your priorities be? How could this be accommodated in a holistic context?

 ### Scenario 2

You are accompanying a health visitor to the home of a large family who have just celebrated the arrival of another baby. While there one of the children, Ethan, a young boy approximately 5 years old, talks to you. You notice that he has a lovely smile, but that it is spoiled somewhat by missing teeth and others that are badly decayed. On leaving, you discuss this with the health visitor who suggests that you develop a strategy for tackling dental health with the parents at the next visit. What would the contents of this 'strategy' be for young Ethan? How would you communicate this to Ethan's parents? How might this affect their approach to the dental care of their newborn child?

 ### Scenario 3

Miriam is a young woman with Down's syndrome. She has been complaining of recurring pain in her eyes, with weeping, and the practice nurse has prescribed some antibiotic eye ointment. Before the practice nurse demonstrates to Miriam how this should be applied, you are asked to 'clean around about the eyes'. What equipment would you need? What explanation would you give? How would you do it? What would you advise Miriam to do before her next application of ointment?

Scenario 4

Billy is a 76-year-old man who has been a resident in a nursing home for the past six months. He is confined to a wheelchair and requires assistance in most aspects of his personal care. He is fully orientated to time and place and has a daughter who visits him four times a week. Billy would like to take a bath. His skin appears very dry, especially on his hands and feet. What factors would you have to consider to take Billy for a bath?

Scenario 5

An 80-year-old man is admitted with a pressure ulcer on his heel, like the one shown in **Fig. 8.18**. He has a history of diabetes, chronic obstructive pulmonary disease (COPD), and peripheral vascular disease. He is undernourished and has had bed rest for six months because of immobility. He receives all care from nursing staff. There is sloughy tissue present on the wound bed and some granulation tissue is also visible.

1 Describe how a pressure ulcer might develop in an elderly patient with this medical history.
2 How may the features of this medical history affect the

development of an ulcer and possibly slow the healing process?
3 Have you used a risk-assessment tool in practice? Which tool have you used?
4 What measures would you take to prevent pressure ulcers from occurring in elderly patients?

Website

🌐 **www.oxfordtextbooks.co.uk/orc/docherty/**

You may find it helpful to work through our short online quiz and interactive scenarios intended to help you to develop and apply the skills in this chapter.

References

Chalmers J and Pearson A (2005). Oral hygiene care for residents with dementia: a literature review. *Journal of Advanced Nursing,* **52**(4), 410–19.

Cooper P, Clark M, and Bale S (2006). *Best Practice Statement: Care of the Older Person's Skin* http://www.wounds-uk.com/downloads/best_practice_older_skincare.pdf.

Ersser S, Maguire S, Nicol N, Penzer R and Peters J (2007). Best Practice in Emollient Therapy: A Statement for Healthcare Professionals. Dermatology UK Ltd, Aberdeen. www.dermatology-uk.com/downloads/Emollient_Therapy_BP.pdf.

Leaper DJ and Harding KG (1998). *Wounds, Biology and Management.* Oxford Medical Publications, Oxford.

Mani R, Falanga V, Shearman CP, and Sandeman D (1999). *Clinical Aspects of Lower Limb Ulceration in Chronic Wound Healing.* WB Saunders, London.

Rowley S and Sinclair S (2004). Infection control: working towards an NHS standard for aseptic nontouch technique. *Nursing Times,* **100**(8), 50–2.

Tanner J, Woodings D, and Moncaster K (2006). Preoperative hair removal to reduce surgical site infection. *Cochrane Database of Systematic Reviews,* **2006**(Issue 3). Art, No: CD004122. D01:10.1002/1465/858. CD004122.pub3.

Timmons J-P (2005). Factors which adversely impact on wound healing. In Gray D, Cooper P, and Timmons J, eds, *Essential Wound Healing: A Guide for Undergraduates,* Wounds UK Books, Aberdeen.

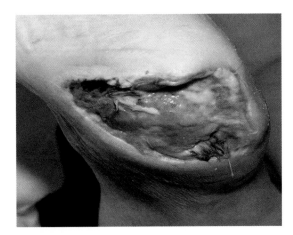

Figure 8.18 Pressure ulcer

Useful further reading and websites

Boon NA, Colledge NR, Walker BR, and Hunter JAA (2006). *Davidson's Principles and Practice of Medicine: With Student Consult Online Access*, 20th edn. Churchill Livingstone, London.

Brawley E (2002). Bathing environments: how to improve the bathing experience. *Alzheimer's Care Quarterly*, **3**(1), 38–41.

This article describes in detail the simple things that can be done to make bathing a pleasure for highly dependent patients: information that can be usefully applied to a number of contexts.

Calianno C (2002). Patient hygiene. Part 2—skin care: keeping the outside healthy. *Nursing*, **29**(12), suppl. 1–11.

Kim S, Mouradian WE, and Slayton RL (2006). What every doctor should know about oral health. *Medical Education*, **40**, 477–8.

Lawton S (2004). Effective use of emollients in infants and young people. *Nursing Standard*, **19**(7), 44–50.

Lodén M, Buraczewska I, and Edlund F (2004). Irritation potential of bath and shower oils before and after use: a double-blind randomised study. *British Journal of Dermatology*, **150**, 1142–7.

Olsen DL, Raub W, Bradley C, *et al.* (2001). The effect of aloe vera gel/mild soap versus mild soap alone in preventing skin reactions in patients undergoing radiation therapy. *Oncology Nursing Forum*, **28**(3), 543–7.

Petersen PE, Bourgeois D, Ogawa H, Estupian-Day S, and Ndiaye C (2005), The global burden of oral diseases and risks to oral health. *Bulletin of the World Health Organization*, **83**(9), 661–9.

Radar J, Barrick AL, Hoeffer B, *et al.* (2006). The bathing of older adults with dementia. *American Journal of Nursing,* **106**(4), 40–8.

Smoker A (1999). Skin care in old age. *Nursing Standard*, **13**(48), 18–24.

Strickland P and Arnold A (2006). Everything you need to know about having happy and healthy eyes. *Health*, (July/August) 124–9.

Walton J, Miler J, and Tordeala L (2001). Elder oral assessment and care. *Medsurg Nursing*, **10**(1), 37–44.

Check **www.oxfordtextbooks.co.uk/orc/docherty/** for changes and new developments. Updated research, guidelines, or equipment will be added every four months.

 Answers to scenarios

 Scenario 1

Your priority would be to assess the extent of physical care that Peter requires and this ought to be done thoroughly and systematically. A verbal history is unlikely to be comprehensive, owing to Peter's dementia. Clearly, there is an immediate need for bathing, so during this process a full visual and tactile assessment can be performed. Peter's preference for bath or shower should be ascertained and his consent gained.

Skin: are there any breaks in skin integrity, sores, ulcers, bruised, or reddened areas? Any signs of itching and scratching or of infestation with body lice? Is the skin dry or inelastic? Are his fingernails and toenails in need of attention? Hair: is it in good condition, or long, untidy, in need of a haircut and shampoo? Are there any signs of an itchy scalp or infestation with head lice? Mouth: does Peter have bad breath? Is his tongue healthily and moist or dry and fissured? Does he have dentures *in-situ* or are these in his belongings?

This full assessment ought to be made while preparing Peter for either an immersion bath or shower, making a mental note of any findings, identifying those areas where priority interventions may be required.

This can be done within a holistic context, for example, by using an activities-of-living model and linking skin condition with mobility, continence, hydration, and mouth condition to dietary intake, dexterity, and so on.

Scenario 2

The strategy would be broadly to monitor and assess Ethan's tooth care practices and to diplomatically educate both him and his parents where necessary.

Key factors to ascertain:

How many sweets and carbonated drinks does Ethan consume?

How are these timed in relation to tooth care and main meals? Does Ethan have an established routine for tooth care and is this monitored by his parents? Does he use the correct size and type of toothbrush, and a fluoridated toothpaste? Does he have a good technique for brushing teeth?

Subtlety and diplomacy are needed when communicating with Ethan's parents: being judgemental would be counter-productive, so emphasize the positive. Establish whether there is an understanding of the link between diet, tooth care, and tooth decay, and of the need to begin good practices in nearly years of childhood. Leaflets from dentists and the health centre may be useful to illustrate and reinforce your message.

This opportunity could be used to discuss the dental care of the newborn child: the use of fluoride toothpaste with the very first tooth, establishing a routine, carefully controlling the quantity and timing of sweet foods and drinks, and the damage caused by sweetened carbonated drinks.

 ## Scenario 3

Equipment: Sterile gallipot, solution (normal saline), swabs, disposal bag, gloves, disposable towel.

This is a simple cleansing procedure to remove dried crusts and sticky material from around the eyelashes and eyelids: the eye itself will not be touched. This will improve comfort and allow the medicated ointment to be more effective. It is painless.

The procedure should begin with the preparation of equipment, arranging everything while maintaining sterility. A moistened swab will be used once only then discarded, sweeping from the inner canthus to the outer, on the lower lid initially. Repeat until crusts are moistened and removed together with any sticky pus.

Miriam would need to check that her eye was clean before applying antibiotic ointment, as any organic material can render the antibiotic ineffective. Having established that she will be required to undertake this procedure, explain that it would be advantageous for her to perform this under supervision, providing encouragement, support, and feedback. It may be that Miriam is slow to learn this skill; therefore, some continued help with this procedure from a carer or a nurse might be required.

 ## Scenario 4

1   Billy may prefer his daughter to assist him in bathing: this could be suggested to him if he wishes—his daughter may have participated in his care prior to admission to the nursing home. If Billy and his daughter wish her to be involved, an appropriate time could be arranged to suit both her and the home.

2   Equipment, such as hoists, and suitably experienced and trained staff need to be available to assist in bathing Billy. It may be appropriate to offer a basin to wash in until the appropriate personnel and equipment are available.

3   If staff and equipment are available then consider the following:

   (a) Assist Billy to the bathroom and into the bath, and ensure his privacy at all times.

   (b) An appropriate emollient to cleanse Billy's dry skin.

   (c) Dry Billy's skin thoroughly to reduce risk of infection, prevent excessive drying and promote comfort.

   (d) Apply emollient to skin and allow it to dry.

   (e) If the environment is large enough, assist Billy to dress—or if he is able to do this independently allow him privacy to do so, and the means to call for assistance when he has finished.

   (f) Refer to nurse in charge, to examine Billy's dry skin, for possible referral to a doctor in case a prescribed topical drug is required.

   (g) Document interventions in the nursing notes and care plan, to ensure communication amongst staff and continuity of care.

 ## Scenario 5

1) Pressure ulcers develop as a result of pressure shear friction and moisture. Excess pressure over bony prominences can create tissue damage as a result of impaired local circulation.

Friction on bed sheets can also contribute to the development of pressure ulcers as can failure to change position and move regularly.

This patient is immobile and has impaired circulation, both of which could assist in pressure ulcer development.

2) Diabetes Patients with long-standing diabetes may develop poor circulation and reduced sensation in their lower limbs.

COPD Patients with pulmonary disease may have a reduced oxygen supply to the minor vessels in the skin and also reduced oxygen saturation.

Peripheral vascular disease The reduced blood supply to the lower limbs can arrest the local tissue perfusion of oxygen and nutrients, this may impact on the development and slow healing of the ulcer.

3) Examples of risk assessment tools are the Waterlow Score and Norton Scoring system.

These tools can lend a degree of objectivity to risk assessment in patients of all ages and in all clinical settings.

4)

- Risk assessment on admission
- Complete skin assessment on a regular basis
- Maximize mobility
- Encourage adequate nutrition and fluid intake
- Change position regularly
- Avoid having patient sit up for long periods.

9 Controlling body temperature

WILLIAM MCDONALD, CLAIRE MCGUINNESS, VALERIE NESS
AND ELIZABETH SIMPSON

Introduction

This chapter introduces the fundamental skills of taking and recording body temperature and helping patients maintain their body temperature within the normal physiological range. Measuring and monitoring body temperature are important nursing skills, as they allow changes in temperature to be detected and management strategies to be put in place, as necessary. Helping the body to maintain a balance between heat production and heat loss (an important factor in **homeostasis**) is another important nursing skill. These skills cannot be viewed in isolation. Adopting a **holistic** approach to care incorporating behavioural and environmental factors enables temperature measurement to be used to guide decisions about treatment.

There are many people who are especially vulnerable to changes in body temperature, such as the elderly and children. Children have difficulty in storing heat because of their small size and larger ratio of body surface to body weight. They also have less insulation as they have a thinner layer of **subcutaneous** fat. Their temperature is usually a little lower in the morning and higher in the evening and can fluctuate with physical exercise. The elderly are vulnerable to extremes of temperature for many reasons, including a slower blood circulation and metabolic rate, changes in their skin and a decrease in heat-producing activities, shivering response, **vasoconstrictor** response, **perception** of temperature, and sweating. Other groups of patients who require careful monitoring are those who have, or are susceptible to, infection, those who have had surgery or are critically ill, and those receiving a blood transfusion.

Learning outcomes

These outcomes relate to numbers 9, 10, 20, and 22 of the NMC's Essential Skill Clusters and specifically to Care Domains 2 and 3 of the NMC's Standards of Proficiency for Pre-registration Nursing (outcomes to be achieved for entry to branch).

On reading this chapter and on interacting with the web pages and undertaking supervised activities, you will be able to:

- Understand the physiology of temperature regulation
- Determine the appropriate equipment to measure temperature
- Measure a patient's temperature,
- Document the patient's temperature accurately
- Recognize deviations from normal body temperature
- Facilitate the maintenance of a patient's temperature within physiological norms

Prior knowledge

To use the clinical skills in this chapter it is important that you have knowledge and understanding of the following, which can be obtained from a range of reference books.

- Anatomy and physiology of the **hypothalamus** (the **thermoregulation** centre in the brain)
- Mechanisms of body temperature regulation (thermoregulation)
- **Cell metabolism** and the effects of temperature change

- The anatomy of where temperature is to be measured
- Factors that can affect heat production and temperature control that arise within the body (intrinsic) and the effects of external (extrinsic) factors, such as exposure, and room temperature (Holland *et al.* 2003)

Background

Normal body temperature

Temperature can be defined as how hot or cold something is. In nursing this refers to the hotness or coldness of the body and is measured with a thermometer. Not all parts of the body have the same temperature. The temperature at the core is around 0.5 °C higher than that at the surface (see **Fig. 9.1**). The definitions given in **Box 9.1** may vary slightly in different reference sources, but can be used as a simple guide.

Temperature regulation

Human beings are very good at maintaining a regular **core temperature** even when the external temperature changes. Body temperature is controlled using homeostasis; heat gain and heat loss are determined and controlled. This balance maintains stability and allows the body's cells to function healthily: any changes to this affect the function of the whole body.

If a patient's heat production increases, the core temperature begins to rise, the hypothalamic **reflex** causes the dilation of arterioles and veins in the skin. This directs warm blood from the core to the skin, increasing heat loss by radiation and conduction. It also reduces blood pressure and increases the heart rate. Sweat glands in the skin are **stimulate**d to increase the production of sweat, which causes increased heat loss from the skin's surface through evaporation. This is enhanced by the hairs on the skin lying flat, allowing the free flow of air across the skin's surface. These are not 'significant' in conserving or losing

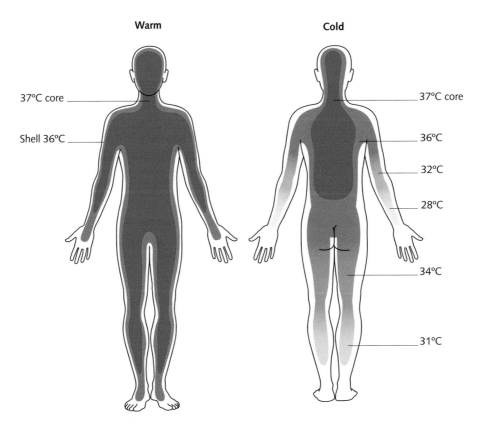

Figure 9.1 Core and peripheral body temperature: (a) in warm surroundings (above 35 °C); (b) in cooler surroundings (20–34 °C)

Box 9.1 Guide to temperature ranges

Temperature, °C	Significance
43 and above	Patient does not usually survive
40–43	Hyperpyrexia
38–40	**Pyrexia**
36–38	Range of normal temperature (**apyrexia**)
27–36	**Hypothermia**
27 and below	Patient does not usually survive

(Hilton 2004)

heat in humans but are important clinical features to recognize and understand.

In some cases, impaired thermoregulatory control can lead to prolonged elevated temperature, or fever. In fever, the hypothalamus temporarily increases its set point. At previously 'normal' temperatures, the patient now feels cold and shivery and seeks warmth. This triggers heat-producing mechanisms, described next, to increase body temperature. This may seem strange; however, when the core temperature reaches the body's new thermoregulatory set point, the patient no longer complains of feeling cold and heat-producing mechanisms stop. This rise in body temperature increases metabolic rate and is the body's way of facing threats to health, for example, through infection.

If a patient's heat production is not sufficient to balance heat loss, body temperature is inclined to drop. In response, the skin's blood vessels constrict, preventing excessive heat loss through radiation and conduction, and blood is redirected to circulate within the vital organs maintaining a steady core temperature. This causes a decrease in oxygen consumption and heart rate and an increase in blood pressure. A further response is for the skeletal muscles to contract and relax involuntarily—a process known as shivering, which causes heat production. Simultaneously the skin stops producing sweat and raises the hairs on the skin to act as an insulating layer to trap the heat—'goose pimples', or 'goose bumps'. When the temperature returns to normal these control mechanisms stop.

Changes in body temperature

When a patient's temperature drops to 35 °C or below, this is known as hypothermia. The patient will begin to shiver to increase heat production. Hypothermia can be caused by exposure to the cold, certain medications, metabolic conditions, and exposure of the body during surgery, and can be exacerbated by other factors, such as **malnutrition** or alcohol intoxication. Neonates and older people living at home are especially vulnerable.

When a patient's temperature rises to 38 °C or above, this is known as pyrexia or hyperpyrexia. This is usually caused by infection but can also be the result of certain medications, allergies, certain diseases, alcohol withdrawal, or malignancy. Measures to increase and decrease body temperature will be discussed later on in this chapter.

9.1 **Assessment of body temperature**

Definition

Body temperature can be assessed in a number of different ways. It may be **invasive**, as in using the rectum but more commonly it is **noninvasive**, as in using the axilla (armpit) or tympanum. Studies to determine the optimal site and measurement device consistently conclude that there is no absolutely correct way. Much depends on the assessment of each individual patient, taking into account their preferences.

Key point: The crucial factor is to use the same route consistently and to report the temperature site used. Changing sites or devices can produce variations in the record that are deceptive or difficult to interpret.

When to assess body temperature

A patient's temperature should be measured on admission to a clinical area, to establish a baseline. This will then allow for comparisons to be made with future measurements. If alterations in temperature occur, the frequency with which these measurements are taken should be increased.

In the community, it is very important that when the community nurse visits older people, their temperature, factors affecting their thermoregulatory system, and their environment are assessed for the risk of hypothermia. As hypothermia is a high risk for elderly people at certain times of the year and in poor housing conditions, the nurse must ensure that a thermometer is selected that is capable of measuring temperatures below 35 °C.

Many different sites and many different devices can be used to measure temperature. These are listed in Tables 9.1 and 9.2.

Key point: The sites in **Table 9.1** are used to measure body temperature because of their accessibility and ease of use (that is, the thermometers can be held in place safely and conveniently) and because they are close to the body's thermoreceptors (these respond rapidly to changes in core temperature).

Procedures: Recording temperature

Preparation

It is essential that the nurse understands the reason for taking the patient's temperature. Following this, all the required equipment should be gathered, prepared, and ready for use. This will ensure that the procedure is carried out with efficiency and minimal disturbance to the patient.

It is vital not to focus purely on the practical skill to be performed. Nurses should use a range of skills prior to, during and post procedure to ensure holistic care. Some of these important skills include:

- Communication:
  - Provide information and gain **consent** for the planned method of recording temperature,
  - Reassure the patient during the procedure,
  - Tell the patient his or her temperature and whether it is in line with expectations,
  - Allow the patient time to ask any questions,
  - Record the patient's temperature and report any unusual finding.
- Observational: look at the patient:
  - Does patient appear warm or sweaty?
  - Does patient appear cold?
  - Is patient pulling covers up?
  - Does patient look comfortable?
  - Is patient telling you that he or she feels hot or cold?
  - Is patient shaking? (Consider **rigor** or shivering.) Remember, children are at risk of febrile convulsion as a result of high temperature. This should always be considered as a possibility when there are signs of shaking or shivering.
  - Observe the patient's posture—is the patient huddled, conserving heat, or open postured, losing heat?
  - Is this an appropriate method of temperature recording to use on this particular patient?
  - Does the temperature recording correspond with the clinical picture of the patient?
- Investigative: are there external factors that may influence the recording? These would include:
  - Time of day
  - Whether the patient has just had a bath or shower
  - Whether the clinical environment is warm or cold
  - Whether the patient has been drinking hot or cold fluid.
- Risk assessment:
  - Assess the patient's physical ability prior to attempting the procedure,
  - Ensure that neither the patient nor the nurse are put at risk during the procedure,
  - Support the patient with pillows if required,
  - Ensure that the patient's dignity is preserved during the procedure,
  - Remove any objects preventing easy access to the patient,
  - Remember to incorporate moving and handling techniques throughout the procedure, to protect both the patient and nurse,
  - Leave the patient comfortable after the procedure.

Table 9.1 Sites for measuring body temperature

Site	For	Against
Aural		
Measures the blood temperature of the **tympanic membrane** (eardrum). Note: readings are slightly higher than oral readings (Farley and McLafferty 2008).	This site has been shown to reflect core temperature very accurately, as it is in close proximity to the thermoregulatory centre in the hypothalamus.	In a constant environment there can be differences in ear temperatures. Difficult in small children as probe does not fit into narrow ear canals.
Oral (sublingual)		
Measures the temperature of tissues that have good perfusion from the lingual and sublingual arteries.	Close to the blood supply of the thermoregulators in the hypothalamus, allowing changes in core temperature to be detected here.	Errors can occur if there is incorrect positioning and allowing insufficient time for an accurate measurement to be taken. It is difficult for patients to maintain the thermometer in position if there is a need for mouth breathing, or if oxygen is being administered. Accuracy can be affected by eating and drinking hot or cold substances, exercise, respiratory rate, and smoking. Patient needs to be fully orientated and cooperative.
Axilla (armpit)		
Measures temperature near the axillary artery. Appropriate devices: Tempa-DOT.	Minimal risk of physical or psychological trauma. Good if oral method is unsuitable, for example, due to injury or general **anaesthetic**.	Precision is difficult. Generally 0.5–1 °C lower than oral temperature as it is not as close to major vessels. Skin surface temperature may vary with changes in environmental temperature. This route can be inaccurate in obese people (an excessive fat layer may prevent thermometer from being close to the underlying circulation). In thin people, the thermometer may not be completely enclosed, but surrounded by air increasing the risk of innacuracy.
Rectal		
Measures temperature of blood within the core of the body well beneath the surface, and is unlikely to be influenced by environmental factors. Insertion to a depth of 5 cm is needed to obtain core temperature.	Research shows this to be more accurate than other sites. It is the best option when a very accurate reading is required.	Not recommended for general use due to cross-infection and a slight risk of lower bowel perforation. Culturally and ethically, this route could be perceived as abusive or unacceptable. The NIHCE guidelines (2007) stipulate that this method should not be used in children unless they are very ill or hypothermic. In these situations the rectal thermometer would be an electronic device.

Table 9.2 Devices for measuring body temperature

Device	For	Against
Tympanic		
(aural route)	This type is fast reading, comfortable and easy to use. It is single use (disposable covers), to minimize infection risk. It is accurate since the tympanic membrane shares its circulation with the hypothalamus.	It is not recommended when precision is essential, for example, for hypothermic patients (Craig *et al.* 2002, Farnell *et al.* 2005). There can be errors from incorrect alignment, unclean lens caps, and variations in conditions (MacKechnie and Simpson 2006). There may be a risk of injury to children under 6 years, or those with ear infection or ear surgery. Two recordings should be performed in the same ear, once the patient has been in a stable temperature environment for 20 minutes.
Tempa-DOT		
The strip should be held sublingually for 1 minute or axillary for 3 minutes. After removing the strip wait 10–15 seconds before reading the colour changes. These strips must be stored in a cool environment and the nurse should refer to the manufacturer guidelines for more detail.	The noted differences in measured temperature between this, glass–mercury and tympanic devices are not clinically significant (Van den Bruel *et al.* 2005). This is also accurate and precise for children younger than 5 years old.	It must be stored carefully at room temperature. It is possible to interpret the reading incorrectly (Creagh-Brown *et al.* 2005)
Electronic		
(oral, axilla, or rectal route)	This is quick and easy to read. **Calibration** is possible. Disposable cover strips are available.	It is more expensive. There is increased risk of cross-infection.
Glass–mercury (oral, rectal, axillary route)		
This device has been withdrawn from many clinical areas and is now rarely used (Commission of the European Communities 2005).	Research still refers to the fact that this is the most accurate standard way of measuring temperature. Disposable covers are available to reduce risk of cross-infection. Low-reading types are available for situations of possible hypothermia.	There is risk of glass breakage and exposure to toxic mercury. It is difficult to read and difficult to maintain the thermometer position. It is slow to respond to temperature changes.

Recording temperature with a tympanic membrane

EQUIPMENT
- Tympanic thermometer,
- Single-use sheath,
- Patient's recording chart,
- Pen.

Key point: Note that tympanic membrane thermometers are not recommended for use in infants younger than four weeks old (NIHCE 2007).

Step | Rationale

Step	Rationale
1 Cleanse hands prior to the procedure.	To prevent cross-infection.
2 Explain the procedure to the patient.	To facilitate informed consent.
3 Gain patient consent.	To gain cooperation.
4 Ensure privacy.	To prevent embarrassment and maintain dignity.
5 Ensure that access to the patient does not pose any physical risk to nurse or patient.	To protect nurse and patient from injury.
6 Switch the thermometer on.	To ensure that thermometer is ready for use.
7 Apply single-patient-use probe cover over the thermometer probe using a non-touch technique.	To prevent contamination and cross-infection.
8 Stabilize the patient's head.	To prevent trauma.
9 Pull ear lobe downwards or pinna up.	To straighten ear canal.
10 Hold the thermometer steady and scan temperature according to manufacturer's instructions (Fig. 9.2).	To ensure that thermometer has reached optimal recording.
11 Accurately record temperature in the chart.	To record as baseline or to compare with previous results.
12 Inform the patient of the results.	To promote patient involvement in care and provide opportunity for patient to ask questions.
13 Leave the patient comfortable.	To prevent complications and prevent harm.
14 Safely dispose of single-use cover according to local infection control policy.	To promote clean environment and prevent cross-infection.

Recording oral temperature

EQUIPMENT
- Thermometer (either mercury, electronic, or Tempa-DOT),
- Cleaning agent for thermometer (if using a mercury thermometer),
- Patient's recording chart,
- Pen.

Step	Rationale
1 Cleanse hands prior to the procedure.	To prevent cross-infection.
2 Explain the procedure to the patient.	To facilitate informed consent.
3 Gain patient consent.	To gain cooperation.
4 Ensure privacy.	To prevent embarrassment and maintain dignity.
5 Ensure that access to the patient does not pose any physical risk to nurse or patient.	To protect nurse and patient from injury.
6 If using a mercury thermometer, shake thermometer to baseline. If using an electronic thermometer or Tempa-DOT: ensure it is ready for use.	To prevent false reading.
8 Place in the posterior sublingual pocket (see Fig. 9.3).	To position in close proximity to the thermoreceptors.
9 Instruct the patient not to talk or bite down but to close their lips.	To prevent trauma and outside air circulating in their mouth.
10 If using a mercury thermometer, leave in place for a minimum of 7 minutes. If using an electronic thermometer, leave in place until thermometer indicates recording complete If using Tempa-DOT, leave in place for the recommended time, for example, a minute.	To ensure that thermometer has reached optimal recording.
11 Remove the thermometer and read the temperature according to the manufacturer's guidelines. If using Tempa-DOT: this will be by observing the dots that have changed colour (be careful not to touch the measuring end), see Fig. 9.4. If using a mercury thermometer, see Box 9.2.	To ensure an accurate reading.

12	Accurately record temperature in patient's chart.	To record as baseline or to compare with previous results.
13	Inform the patient of the results.	To promote patient involvement in care and provide patient opportunity to ask questions
14	Leave the patient comfortable.	To prevent complications and prevent harm.
15	If using a mercury thermometer cleanse with 70% alcohol.	To promote clean environment

Recording axillary temperature

EQUIPMENT

- Thermometer (mercury, electronic, or Tempa-DOT),
- Cleaning agent for thermometer,
- Patient's recording chart,
- Pen.

Step		Rationale
1	Cleanse hands prior to the procedure.	To prevent cross-infection.
2	Explain the procedure to the patient.	To facilitate informed consent.
3	Gain patient consent.	To gain cooperation.
4	Ensure privacy.	To prevent embarrassment and maintain dignity.
5	Ensure that access to the patient does not pose any physical risk to nurse or patient.	To protect nurse and patient from injury.
6	If using a mercury thermometer, shake thermometer to baseline. If using an electronic thermometer or Tempa-DOT: ensure that it is ready for use.	To prevent false reading.
7	Ensure that axilla is dry.	To ensure that reading is accurate.
8	Place in centre of axilla, fold arm down over the thermometer, so that it is surrounded and covered by skin (see Fig. 9.5).	To prevent external factors influencing reading.

continued

9	If using a Tempa-DOT, ensure that the dots are facing the patient's chest. If using a mercury thermometer, leave in place for 7 to 8 minutes. If using an electronic thermometer, leave in place until thermometer indicates recording complete. If using Tempa-DOT, leave in place for the about 3 minutes.	To ensure that thermometer has reached optimal recording.
10	Read the temperature according to the manufacturer's guidelines. If using Tempa-DOT, this will be by observing the dots that have changed colour (be careful not to touch the measuring end). If using a mercury thermometer: see Box 9.2.	To ensure an accurate reading.
11	Accurately record temperature in the chart.	To record as baseline or to compare with previous results.
12	Inform the patient of the results.	To promote patient involvement in care and provide patient opportunity to ask questions.
13	Leave the patient comfortable.	To prevent complications and prevent harm.
14	If using a mercury thermometer, cleanse with 70% alcohol. If using a Tempa-DOT, discard.	To promote clean environment.

Recording rectal temperature

EQUIPMENT

- Electronic rectal thermometer probe,
- Lubricant,
- Gloves,
- Cleaning agent for thermometer,
- Patient's recording chart,
- Pen.

Key point: Note that mercury rectal thermometers have been withdrawn from use in children; an electronic rectal device would always be used and only in situations where hypothermia was suspected or if the child was very unwell. Rectal temperatures should never be taken in infants younger than 6 months unless directly instructed by the doctor. In these situations, you should always seek the advice and support of your mentor and should not proceed unsupervised.

Step

Rationale

	Step	Rationale
1	Cleanse hands prior to the procedure.	To prevent cross-infection.
2	Explain the procedure to the patient.	To facilitate informed consent.
3	Gain patient consent.	To gain cooperation.
4	Ensure privacy.	To prevent embarrassment and maintain dignity.
5	Ensure that access to the patient does not pose any physical risk to nurse or patient.	To protect nurse and patient from injury.
6	Position patient—lying on side—and expose only the buttocks.	To ensure patient comfort and to allow access for thermometer to be inserted.
7	Ensure that the thermometer is ready for use.	To prevent false reading.
8	Ensure rectal area is clean.	To prevent false reading.
9	Lubricate thermometer.	To minimize trauma to rectal mucosa.
10	Continue to communicate with the patient throughout the procedure.	To relax patient.
11	Place the thermometer in the rectum no more than 5 cm.	To prevent trauma.
12	Hold in place with a gloved hand for a minimum of 2 minutes.	To prevent trauma and ensure that thermometer has reached optimal recording.
13	Accurately record temperature in the chart.	To record as baseline or to compare with previous results.
14	Inform the patient of the results.	To promote patient involvement in care and provide opportunity for patient to ask questions.
15	Leave the patient comfortable.	To prevent complications and prevent harm.
16	Dispose of the probe cover.	To promote clean environment.

Recording rectal temperature

Aftercare

After measuring the patient's temperature, it is very important to document it correctly. Each clinical area will have different documentation systems, so you will need to ensure that you are familiar with the chart to be used. Temperature should be plotted over time so that any changes in the patient's temperature are clearly visible (see **Fig. 9.6** for an example). This facilitates evaluation and assists in deciding whether interventions are required or are being effective. You should also document the site that was used, as differences will exist if a variety of sites have been used.

Box 9.2 How to read a mercury thermometer

Mercury thermometers can be difficult to read. Once you have removed the thermometer from the patient, hold it between the index finger and thumb (you should be wearing gloves). Rest it on the back of your hand and raise both hands until the thermometer is at eye level.

Slowly roll the thermometer between your index finger and thumb, keeping your eyes on the numbers etched on the glass; you may have to roll the thermometer backwards and forwards before the mercury line inside the glass becomes clear. When you see this line, read the number and count the graduations to the point where the mercury line stops. This will be the temperature reading you will record on the patient's chart.

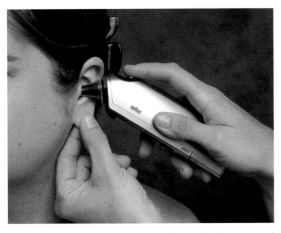

Figure 9.2 Using a tympanic membrane device to record temperature

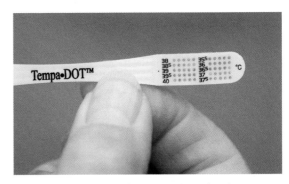

Figure 9.4 How to read a Tempa-DOT: this thermometer shows 36.9 °C

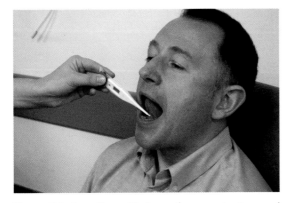

Figure 9.3 Correctly positioning a thermometer to record temperature via the oral route

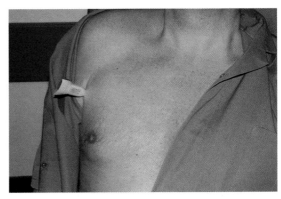

Figure 9.5 Using a thermometer to record temperature via the axilla

Developing your skills

It is essential, as a student nurse, that you practice and become accustomed to recording a patient's temperature. It is also important that the patient is assessed and the appropriate method of recording temperature is used. You should try and practice assessing patient's temperatures on your next placement. Remember to document the temperature correctly and to inform your mentor of any changes or abnormalities.

Other factors to consider

There are certain situations where a patient's temperature should be carefully monitored. Post-operative patients need to have their temperature monitored as they may experience a reaction to the surgery or may be at risk of hypothermia. Patients who are undergoing a blood transfusion can develop severe reactions to the transfusion, which can be detected early by monitoring temperature. A raised temperature can also be an indicator of an infection, therefore, patients with a susceptibility to infection (patients undergoing **chemotherapy** or steroid treatment, or with a low white blood cell count) should have their temperature monitored more frequently. In such high-risk patients, temperature should be documented as it relates to early warning scores (see **Fig. 9.7**).

When a patient is receiving a blood transfusion, it can be normal for the temperature to rise slightly as the body is responding to the introduction of foreign material. If, however, the rise is significant, the medical team should be advised and they may request that the transfusion be

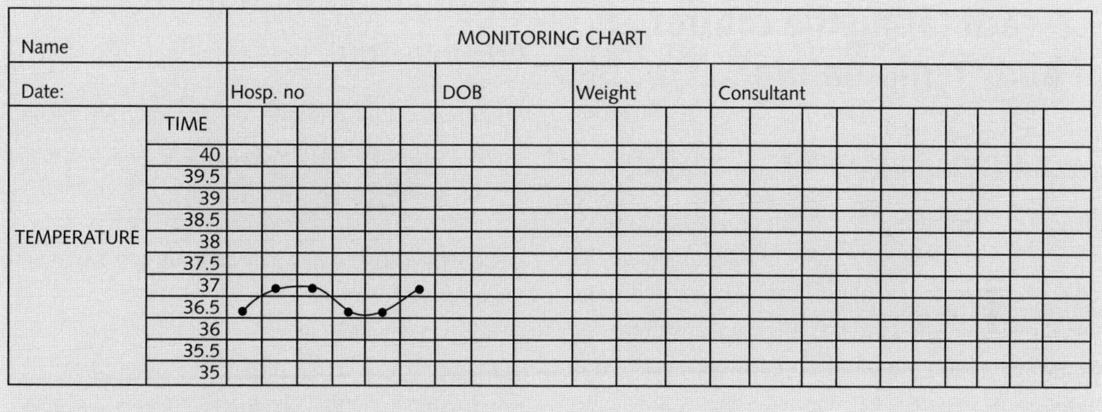

Example of temperature plotted over time
(based on Postoperative Monitoring chart - SIGN guidelines)

Figure 9.6 Graph showing temperature changes over time

SCORE	3	2	1	0	1	2	3
Temp. (°C)		≤35.0	35.1–35.9	36.0–37.4	37.5–38.5	≥38.6	

Figure 9.7 Example of temperature scoring in relation to early warning scoring, based on Modified Early Warning Score (MEWS) scoring

stopped. As a student nurse, it is important that you report to your mentor any temperature that is not within normal limits.

The time of day that a temperature is taken can also influence the reading. This is because of the person's circadian rhythms (the highest body temperature occurs in late afternoon or early evening). Many studies have found that the best time to measure someone's temperature accurately is at about 6 p.m.

There are also other factors that can increase a patient's temperature, such as ovulation (this can increase the body temperature owing to changes in metabolic rate), exercise, and eating.

A temperature reading is only one factor in a patient's assessment. You should always make sure that you use your communication and observational skills to assess the patient fully.

9.2 **Facilitating the control of body temperature**

Definition

There are many strategies that can be used to raise or lower temperature when a patient cannot maintain his or her own body temperature. In some cases one strategy will be enough; however, often a combination of these methods will be used to reach and maintain a normal temperature. The selected strategies will be based on an individualized assessment and will now be discussed.

When to raise or lower a patient's body temperature

There must be an indication that the patient requires some help to maintain body temperature. The most likely indication of this would be a temperature reading that was either above or below normal parameters, or if the patient was showing signs such as sweating, or shivering.

Procedures: Controlling body temperature

Preparation

Before attempting to raise or lower a patient's temperature you must ensure that:

- The patient has been appropriately assessed at the outset,
- The temperature recording obtained is accurate,
- Details of the patient's temperature, pulse, respiration, and any other assessment made, are recorded in the observation chart and nursing notes,
- Advice is sought from a member of qualified staff as to what strategy should be used to raise or lower the temperature.

Strategies to raise the body temperature

Whilst many of the principles of rewarming are the same for adults, children and infants, it is essential to recognize that some aspects differ. The procedures highlighted here are commonly used; however, each patient is an individual and should be assessed fully prior to implementation of any treatment or intervention.

It is also important to realize that raising the temperature too quickly can cause dilation of the **peripheral** blood vessels (vasodilation). (Refer to your anatomy and physiology text for details of this). Vasodilation can lead to a drop in core circulation and, in some cases, acute circulatory failure, or shock (Keane 2001). As such, it is essential to recognize the differences between the two main types of warming;

Passive rewarming

This is the approach of choice if the body temperature is above 32°C but below 36°C and involves taking steps to stop heat loss and rewarm thereafter, as listed in **Table 9.3.** The aim of this is to raise the body temperature gradually and reduce the risks of peripheral vasodilation.

Active rewarming

This approach is used in patients with severe hypothermia, that is, the body temperature is below 32 °C. Here the patient is warmed using one or more of the following: foil blanket, warm airflow blanket, or heater, as described in **Table 9.4**. There is, however, an increased risk of vasodilation, therefore, the methods suggested should be used with caution and the patient must be monitored frequently to ensure that rewarming does not happen too quickly.

Table 9.3 Passive rewarming

Strategies	Adult	Child	Infant
Remove wet or cold clothing and make sure that the patient is dry.	✓	✓	✓
It may be beneficial to cover the patient with a warmed blanket before applying further layers.	✓	✓	✓
Cover the head and neck; heat is commonly lost from these areas.	✓	✓	✓
Put mittens and socks on hands and feet.		✓	✓
Transfer to an **incubator** if the infant is small enough (see **Fig. 9.8**).			✓
Make sure that the patient is in a warm room and that all windows are closed.	✓	✓	✓
If the patient is conscious, and there are no **contraindications**, offer a warm drink.	✓	✓	✓
Continue to monitor temperature frequently to reduce the risk of over-warming.	✓	✓	✓

Table 9.4 Active rewarming

Strategies	Adult	Child	Infant
Remove wet or cold clothing and make sure that the patient is dry.	✓	✓	✓
Make sure that the patient is in a warm room and that all windows are closed.	✓	✓	✓
A heater may be placed in the proximity of the patient. This should not be too close, to prevent injury. An overhead heater is a standard piece of equipment with many incubators. Remember to seek advice from your mentor or a qualified member of staff when setting the temperature on the heater.		✓	✓
A foil blanket may be placed over the patient to reflect heat lost back towards the patient.	✓	✓	
The patient may be covered in bubble wrap to contain heat.			✓
A warm airflow blanket may be used to cover the patient (see Fig. 9.9). This is a disposable blanket through which warm air is pumped. This device usually has a temperature control to facilitate controlled rewarming.	✓	✓	✓
Continue to monitor temperature frequently to ensure that rewarming is both successful and gradual.	✓	✓	✓

Strategies to lower the body temperature

As with strategies to raise body temperature, many of the principles applied to lower temperature are equally relevant to adults, children, and infants; however, there are some differences and individualized assessment remains important when attempting to lower the body temperature (Childs 2006).

There are a number of strategies designed to lower body temperature. It is essential to remember, however, that differing perspectives exist in relation to:

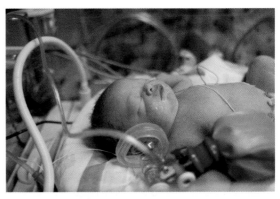

Figure 9.8 Incubator used to maintain body temperature of neonates. Reproduced with permission. © 2001–2006 Sean O' Riordan istock.com

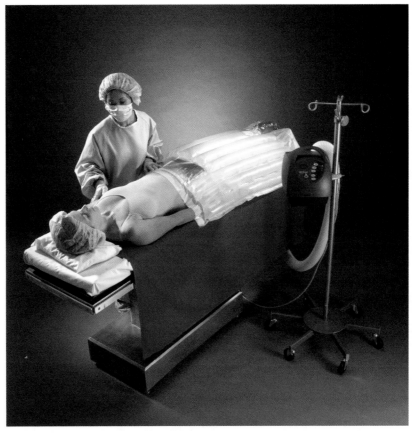

Figure 9.9 Using a rewarming blanket on an adult. Reproduced with permission of Arizona Healthcare.

- The most effective method of cooling
- The optimal route for administering medication to lower temperature. This is most commonly debated when treating children and involves the oral or rectal route
- When intervention is appropriate. There is debate as to the exact body temperature at which attempts should be made to cool the patient
- What the first intervention should be

Table 9.5 lists some suggested methods to treat pyrexia. These methods are not presented in any particular order and depending on the patient's temperature reading, one or more methods may be used. Any decision relating to treatment should be based on a comprehensive assessment (Kayman 2003); this should be undertaken with the support and guidance of your mentor. The important point to note is that nurses must first attempt to establish the cause of the pyrexia before deciding on a strategy to lower it.

Table 9.5 Strategies to lower body temperature

Strategies to lower temperature	Adult	Child	Infant
Rest the patient in a calm relaxing environment, minimizing excitement and unnecessary energy expenditure and heat production. A calm approach to communication and intervention is beneficial.	✓	✓	✓
Remove the bed covers. It may be necessary to do this gradually as the patient may start to shiver. When attempting to lower the body temperature, it is best to avoid shivering as this is the body's mechanism to increase heat generated. Remember to consider the increased risk of febrile convulsion in infants and children.	✓	✓	✓
If the patient is conscious and there are no contraindications, offer a cool drink or some ice to suck.	✓	✓	✓
Lower the room temperature if possible by opening a window but be careful not to place the patient too near as there may be a draught.	✓	✓	✓
A cool fan should be placed in the proximity of the patient to circulate cool air. It may be necessary to cover hands and feet, as these peripheral areas tend to cool before the patient's core temperature drops.	✓	✓	✓
Wash the patient with a sponge and warm water and allow this to evaporate on the skin. Again, it is essential to undertake this procedure with care, as this may cause the patient to cool too quickly.	✓		
NIHCE guidelines (2007) now prohibit the use of tepid sponging in infants and children under the age of 5 years.			
Administer prescribed medication of oral paracetamol, or ibuprofen, which act as **antipyretics**.	✓	✓	✓
NIHCE guidelines (2007) suggest that antipyretic agents should only be given if the child or infant is distressed by the fever. If an antipyretic is given, either paracetamol or ibuprofen should be administered in the first instance. If the infant or child does not respond, then the alternative can be administered as prescribed.			
Administer prescribed medication of rectal paracetamol, which acts as an antipyretic.	✓	✓	✓
Continue to monitor temperature frequently to ensure that cooling is achieved.	✓	✓	✓

Aftercare

It is essential once care has been implemented to reassess the situation; this will include reassessment of the patient's status, and evaluation of the care provided.

Irrespective of the intervention, the practitioner must continually reassess how successful the strategy has been; this will help to ensure that the treatment in progress is appropriate for the patient's needs. In particular, when considering control of body temperature, the risk of warming or cooling too rapidly is of particular concern.

Whilst implementing strategies to warm or cool, the nurse must frequently measure and record the temperature of the patient in conjunction with other observations closely related to temperature regulation, such as pulse, respiration, and blood pressure. This is particularly important in patients who are hypothermic and in danger of excessive peripheral vasodilation, causing acute circulatory collapse. These observations will allow the nurse to monitor the patient's response to treatment, identify complications, and ensure that active measures are stopped when no longer required.

Developing your skills

Experience in managing changes in patient's body temperature will be gained in the clinical area. It is important that you have assessed the patient beforehand to establish the cause of this alteration. Then, through discussion with your mentor and considering your prior knowledge of the management strategies and the rationale for their use, be able to select an appropriate intervention for your patient. Each clinical areas may have different preferred strategies and protocols. Therefore you should ask your mentor about the common practices in their area.

Other factors to consider

Remember, you should try to make the patient as comfortable as possible as, sometimes, the strategies employed to raise or lower temperature can be uncomfortable. You should also communicate regularly with the patient to ensure that they understand what you are trying to achieve. Finally, remember to report any changes to a qualified member of staff.

Summary

This chapter has encompassed measuring and recording a patient's temperature in a number of contexts using the most widely accepted methods. It has also identified strategies and interventions that can help patients maintain their body temperature within normal physiological ranges, given individual differences. It is acknowledged that measuring body temperature and facilitating homeostatic mechanisms in achieving temperature control are important nursing skills and cannot be viewed in isolation. Therefore, a holistic approach to care incorporating behavioural and environmental factors has been adopted, encouraging the best approach for the patient's particular situation, before embarking on the chosen course of action.

Scenarios

Consider what you should do in the following situations, then turn to the end of the section to check your answers.

Further scenarios are available at 🌐 **www. oxfordtextbooks.co.uk/orc/docherty/**

Scenario 1

Daniel is a 6-year-old child admitted to the medical ward of a paediatric hospital with diarrhoea and vomiting. He is unable to eat or drink and is receiving **intravenous** fluids.

The nurse arrives to measure and record Daniel's temperature, pulse, and respiration; at this point he is under the bedcovers, complaining of cold, and crying. His parents are in attendance and are both distressed. The measurements obtained are recorded in **Table 9.6**.

Table 9.6 Daniel's measurements

Temperature	38.5 °C (tympanic)
Pulse	115 beats per minute
Respirations	Unable to measure as Daniel is crying

Once these results have been documented, what would you do next and how can you involve Daniel's parents?

 ## Scenario 2

Mark is a 23-year-old male who is displaying symptoms of hypomania. He has difficulty sleeping, his speech and thought processes appear accelerated, and he continually engages in activities displaying behaviour that often appears to be inappropriate and disinhibited. He does not appear to be able to sit long enough to eat a meal. He denies feeling tired—in fact he says that he is on top of the world—but he appears exhausted.

Consider how Mark's condition may affect his body's responses to try to maintain an appropriate temperature. What might nursing staff do to support him with this?

 ## Scenario 3

You are a student nurse in placement in an orthopaedic surgical ward. You have an 81-year-old patient, Doris, who has just returned from theatre for repair of a fractured neck of the femur. You note that her temperature is 35.2 °C. What action would you take next?

 ## Scenario 4

Andrew is 7 years old. He lives in a downstairs flat with his mother and younger brother. Andrew has autism, is hyperactive, and as a result of this dislikes wearing any sort of clothing—irrespective of the season. He will tolerate a shirt, trousers, and socks in school but no shoes or any form of warmer clothing including pyjamas and bedclothes. The house has no carpets: Andrew destroys carpets, so all the floors are laminated. The windows and doors to the flat must always be locked as Andrew continually tries to escape outside. He never eats warm food or drink. During the summer months, Andrew plays, naked, in the rear garden which is surrounded by a high fence.

What are the main issues in relation to this case and what sort of advice might the community learning disability nurse (CLDN) offer Andrew's mother in relation to the control of his body temperature?

Further scenarios are available at **www. oxfordtextbooks.co.uk/orc/docherty/**

Website

 www.oxfordtextbooks.co.uk/orc/docherty/
You may find it helpful to work through our short online quiz and interactive scenarios intended to help you to develop and apply the skills in this chapter.

References

Childs C (2006). Temperature control. In Alexander MF, Fawcett JTN and Runciman PJ, eds, *Nursing Practice: Hospital and Home*. Churchill Livingstone, Edinburgh.
Commission of the European Communities (2005), 719–736. *Communication from the Commission to the Council and the European Parliament: Community Strategy Concerning Mercury* (COM/2005/20 final). http://ec.europa.eu/environment/chemicals/mercury/pdf/com_2005_0020_en.pdf.

Craig JV, Lancaster GA, Taylor S, Horrox F, Williamson PR, and Smyth RL (2002). Infrared ear thermometry compared with rectal thermometry: a systematic review. *The Lancet,* **360**(9333), 603–7.

Creagh-Brown BC, Armstrong D, and Jackson SHD (2005). The use of the Tempa.DOT thermometer in routine clinical practice. *Age and Ageing*, **34**(3), 297–9.

Farley A and McLafferty E (2008). Nursing management of the patient with hypothermia *Nursing Standard*, **22**(17), 43–6.

Farnell S, Maxwell L, Tan S, Rhodes A, and Philips B (2005). Temperature measurement: comparison of noninvasive methods used in adult critical care. *Journal of Critical Clinical Nursing*, **14**(5), 632–9.

Hilton PA (2004). *Fundamental Nursing Skills*. Whurr Publishers, London.

Holland K, Jenkins J, Solomon J, and Whittam S (2003). *Applying the Roper–Logan–Tierney Model in Practice*. Churchill Livingstone, Edinburgh.

Kayman H (2003). Management of fever: making evidence-based decisions. *Clinical Paediatrics*, **42**(5), 383–92.

Keane C (2001). Physiological responses and management of hypothermia. *Emergency Nurse*, 8(8), 26–31.

MacKechnie C and Simpson R (2006). Traceable calibration for blood pressure and temperature monitoring. *Nursing Standard*, **21**(11), 42–7.

NIHCE (National Institute for Health and Clinical Excellence) (2007). *Feverish Illness in Children*. NIHCE, London. www.nice.org.uk/CG47.

Van den Bruel A, Aertgeerts B, De Boeck C, and Buntox F (2005). Measuring the body temperature: how accurate is the Tempa Dot®? *Technology and Health Care*, **13**(2), 97–106.

Useful further reading and websites

Carroll M (2000). An evaluation of temperature measurement. *Nursing Standard*, **14**(44), 39–43.

Casey G (2000). Fever management in children. *Nursing Standard,* **14**(4), 36–40.

Childs C (2006). Temperature control. In Alexander MF, Fawcett JTN, and Runciman PJ, eds, *Nursing Practice: Hospital and Home*. Churchill Livingstone, Edinburgh. This chapter discusses the regulation of body temperature and disturbances in this regulation in greater detail.

Control of Substances Hazardous to Health (COSHH) (1999). *Management of Health and Safety at Work Regulations*. www.hse.gov.uk/lau/lacs/92-3.htm.

Department of Health (2003). *Getting the Right Start: National Framework Standard for Hospital Services*. DoH, London.

Edwards HE, Courtney MD, Wilson JE, Monaghan SJ, and Walsh AM (2003). Fever management audit: Australian nurses' antipyretic usage. *Pediatric Nursing*, **29**(1), 31–7.

Farley A and McLafferty E (2008). Nursing management of the patient with hypothermia. *Nursing Standard*, **22**(17), 43–6. This simple-to-read article describes the signs and symptoms of hypothermia and its management.

Fawcett J (2001). The accuracy and reliability of the tympanic membrane thermometer, a literature review. *Emergency Nurse*, **8**(9), 13–17.

Holland K (2004). An introduction to the Roper–Logan–Tierney model for nursing based on the activities of daily living. In Holland K, Jenkins J, Solomon J, and Whittam S, eds, *Applying the Roper–Logan–Tierney Model in Practice*, Chapter 1. Churchill Livingstone, London.

Houlder LC (2000). Evidence-based practice. The accuracy and reliability of tympanic thermometry compared to rectal and axillary sites in young children. *Paediatric Nursing*, **26**(3), 311–14.

Khorshi L, Eser I, and Yapucu U (2005). Comparing mercury-in-glass, tympanic, and disposable thermometers in measuring body temperature in healthy young people. *Journal of Clinical Nursing*, **14**, 496–500.

Lees S and Hilton PA (2005). Maintaining body temperature. In Hilton PA, ed., *Fundamental Nursing Skills*. Whurr Publishers Ltd, London.

Marieb EM (2001). *Human Anatomy and Physiology*. Benjamin Cummings, San Francisco.

McQueen S (2001). Clinical benefit of 3M Tempa-DOT thermometer in paediatric settings. *British Journal of Nursing*, **10**(1), 55–8.

Meremikwu M and Oyo-Ita A (2007). Paracetamol for treating fever in children (review). www.thecochranelibrary.com.

Mohammed T (2006). Temperature control. In Trigg E and Mohammed T, eds, *Practices in Children's Nursing: Guidelines for Hospital and Community*. Churchill Livingstone, London.

Molton AH, Blacktop J, and Hall CM (2001). Temperature-taking in children. *Journal of Child Health Care*, **5**(1), 5–10.

Nicoll LN (2002). Heat in motion: evaluating and managing temperature. *Nursing2002*, **32**(5), s1–s12.

Pickersgill J, Fowler H, Bootham J, Thompson K, Wilcock S, and Tanner J (2003). Temperature-taking: children's preferences. *Paediatric Nursing*, **15**(2), 22–5.

Rush M and Wetherhall A (2003). Temperature measurement: practice guidelines. *Paediatric Nursing*, **15**(9), 25–8.

Russell FM, Shann F, Curtis N, and Mulholland K (2003). Policy and practice: evidence on the use of paracetamol in febrile children. *Bulletin of the World Health Organization*, **81**(5), 367–72.

Smith J and Truscott J (2006). Commentary on Khorshi L, Eser I, and Yapucu U (2005). Comparing mercury-in-glass, tympanic and disposable thermometers in measuring body temperature in health young people, *Journal of Clinical Nursing*, **14**, 496–500. *Journal of Clinical Nursing*, **15**, 1340–5.

Spitzer OP (2008). Comparing tympanic temperatures in both ears to oral temperature in the critically ill adult. *Dimensions of Critical Care Nursing*, **27**(1), 24–9.

Walsh A and Edwards H (2006). Management of childhood fever by parents: literature review. *Journal of Advanced Nursing*, **54**(2), 217–27.

Watts R, Robertson J, and Thomas G (2003). Special supplement. Nursing management of fever in children: a systematic review. *International Journal of Nursing Practice*, **9**, 1–8.

Wong DL (2004). *Whaley and Wong's Essentials of Paediatric Nursing*, 7th edn, Mosby, St Louis, MO.

This is a comprehensive paediatric textbook, which includes temperature regulation and also looks at community care and evidence-based practice.

Woodrow P (2003). Assessing temperature in older people. *Nursing Older People*, **15**(1), 29–31.

Check 🌐 **www.oxfordtextbooks.co.uk/orc/docherty/** for changes and new developments. Updated research, guidelines, or equipment will be added every four months.

 # Answers to the scenarios

 ## Scenario 1

- As Daniel is upset and agitated, it is essential to calm him—agitation can increase the generation of heat and will exacerbate his already elevated temperature.
- Daniel's parents can contribute to calming him; therefore, the nurse should try to encourage this approach. This will allow both parents to contribute to the care being provided and may help to reduce parental stress as they will be focused on helping their son.
- Daniel's increased pulse is most probably a direct result of both his distress and his elevated temperature. Accordingly, calming Daniel may help to reduce his heart rate.
- Measurement of respiration is not essential at this point as this may lead to increased distress; this can be undertaken later when Daniel is less upset.
- Daniel's elevated temperature will be making him feel generally unwell; as previously discussed, a high temperature can make the patient feel cold; therefore, it is important to implement the appropriate treatment to reduce Daniel's temperature. Consider the following steps:
  - Remove Daniel's pyjamas.

  - Put socks on Daniel's feet, as extremities tend to become cold when the temperature is elevated.
  - Cover Daniel with a cotton sheet—this may help to reduce his distress and will protect his modesty. Additionally, it may help him to feel less cold.
  - Discuss Daniel's elevated temperature with a qualified member of staff.

 ## Scenario 2

- Mark's accelerated activity levels are likely to cause him to use calories rapidly and to feel hot, perspire, and appear flushed.
- Excitability and poor concentration on mundane matters, such as eating and fluid intake, may result in weight loss, **dehydration**, and exhaustion.
- A lack of consideration regarding appropriate clothing may also contribute to raised temperature.
- Adopting a gentle, calm approach, using a soft tone and even rate of speech is less likely to add to Mark's level of excitability. It is unlikely to be helpful to engage with him in arguments about his behaviour and attire.
- Caring for Mark in a quiet, less stimulating environment should help begin to address distraction, mood changes, and excessive **motor** activity.
- Try to provide ways of eating and drinking that meet Mark's required needs but do not involve sitting in communal areas for long periods of time, for example, offering smaller amounts of food and drink more frequently.
- Mark can be gently encouraged to participate in considering how his temperature may be influenced by his actions and attire, with a rationale offered in a way that does not encourage conflict.

Scenario 3

Use the previously mentioned nursing skills to assess Doris:
- Professional and ethical:
  - Recognize your limitations and report your findings to the nurse in charge,
  - Report to medical staff.
- Care delivery:
  - Observational:
    - How does Doris look?
    - Is she shivering?
    - Is she cold to touch?

- – Communication: ask Doris how she feels.
    - – Diagnostic and **therapeutic**: repeat the recording.
- Care management:
    - – Gradually begin to introduce passive rewarming methods,
    - – Continue to record temperature at 15–30 minute intervals,
    - – Ensure that the rewarming is a slow process.
- Professional development:
    - – Reflect on experience,
    - – Identify knowledge gaps and plan how to fill these,
    - – Discuss with your mentor.

 ## Scenario 4

- The average parent may not understand the basics of human anatomy and physiology and the community learning disability nurse may be able to explain the issues relating to the safe control of Andrew's body temperature.
- Students may consider any related physiology—for example, mechanisms of shivering or nonshivering and thermogenesis
- Andrew's hyperactivity is liable to result in his body temperature rising whilst he is active, and falling when he is at rest. Lack of clothing is liable to be a specific issue in terms of excessive heat loss.
- Internal temperature of the house may be unusually warm during the winter, while there may be ventilation problems during the summer months.
- Behaviour modification programmes may prove to be of benefit to enable Andrew to tolerate additional clothing.
- Whilst there may be social acceptance of a naked *child* staying cool in the garden, this is likely to prove problematic as Andrew matures.

10 Mobilizing

VALERIE NESS AND JOHN MURRAY

Introduction

This chapter introduces the fundamental skills relating to the activity of mobilizing. The ability to mobilize relies on functioning **motor** and nervous systems. Therefore, injury or disease to any part of these systems may affect the person's ability to move. Any loss of mobility, even if for a very short time, can have devastating effects on an individual's independence and health.

Movement is learned and developed from the basic functions present at birth: the degree of movement and the ability to mobilize become unique to the individual. It follows then that the assessment of an individual patient's mobility is a vital first step in delivering patient care. These essential assessment skills will be discussed in this chapter.

As a nurse, you will encounter many patients who have very different and often complex mobilizing needs. Some of these needs will be discussed in this chapter; however an individual assessment is essential as your patients' requirements are often unique. Handling aids can often assist both the patient and the nurse in mobilizing and should always be considered during a patient assessment. Following on from this assessment, and using the skills discussed in the mandatory skills chapter, the remainder of this chapter will focus on the skills required to assist patients to mobilize in a safe and efficient manner, with this essential activity.

Key point: The words handler, carer, and operator are often used in the moving and handling literature. As this is a book aimed at nursing students, the word nurse will be used instead of these, but this could mean any person involved in moving and handling the patient.

This chapter will help you to gain the skills required to assess patients, recognize those who need assistance in mobilizing and provide you with the skills to make this possible.

Learning outcomes

These outcomes relate to numbers 2, 9, and 10 of the NMC's Essential Skill Clusters and specifically to Care Domains 2 and 3 of the NMC's Standards of Proficiency for Pre-registration Nursing (outcomes to be achieved for entry to branch).

On reading this chapter and on interacting with the web pages and undertaking supervised activities, the student will be able to:

- Discuss and implement an individual's mobility assessment
- Understand the influencing factors affecting an individual's ability to mobilize
- Demonstrate knowledge of the risks associated with immobility
- Demonstrate and carry out active and a range of **passive movement** exercises on patients
- Relate the principles of efficient movement to practice
- Describe a range of different types of equipment that are available and when and how they should be used
- Identify individuals with complex mobilizing needs and understand the risks associated with moving these people
- Understand how patient care can be enhanced through appropriate moving and handling

Prior knowledge

It is important that you have the knowledge and understanding of the following, which can be obtained from a range of reference books.

- The general advice in Chapter 2.2 on movement and handling
- Biomechanics: the physical stresses and considerations of human movement
- The clear, detailed guidance on a range of techniques in *The Guide to the Handling of People* (Smith 2005). Patient handling, however, should not be attempted without first undertaking practical training on an approved course. This particularly applies to the use of any moving and handling equipment
- Local moving and handling guidelines
- Chapter 6, which discusses breathing, Chapter 8, which discusses skin care, and Chapter 3, which discusses the unconscious or **dependent** patient
- Basic musculoskeletal anatomy and physiology related to the alignment and normal range of motion of major joints. For example; a patient with an otherwise healthy appearance may have significant joint pain owing to old age or wear and tear (osteoarthritis), or to an **autoimmune** (heightened or exaggerated immune reaction) inflammatory process rheumatoid **arthritis**. (*Arthro* means joint or point of articulation and *itis* denotes inflammation)
- Range of motion terminology (for example, **adduction, abduction, rotation, extension**, and **flexion**)
- Core communication skills to support clear explanations and encourage patient cooperation as appropriate (Section 2.1 and Chapter 4)
- Special considerations and local or national guidelines for **neurology** (stroke, paralysis, **sensory** deficit) or orthopaedic (bone fractures, joint surgery) patients

Background

The entire musculoskeletal system is involved in movement, balance, and mobility. Ideally you will understand the normal range of motion of the major joints and limbs, the normal shape and range of motion of the spine, and the musculature supporting the limbs, the neck, and the spine.

While the skeleton acts to provide strength and rigidity of posture and allow articulation at the joints, the muscles act to move and to stabilize the body. Balance is a further important factor in mobility and this is governed by nervous system components that provide constant information and feedback about the body's position, orientation, and pace and direction of movement.

Conditions affecting a person's mobility include any disorder of the musculoskeletal system—for example, fractured bones, torn muscles, **ligaments**, or **tendons**, or joint problems. In addition, mobility will be affected in neurological conditions, such as stroke, multiple sclerosis, and altered levels of consciousness, as balance and sensation of sensory feedback may be impaired. Any period of prolonged immobility will also result in reduced capability—the patient will need support, assistance, and perhaps equipment to return to their previous level of indepedence.

10.1 **Assessment of the patient's ability to mobilize**

Definition

A full assessment of a patient's ability to mobilize is an essential part of a **holistic** assessment and should be an ongoing process. Hospital patients should be assessed on, or prior to admission and the assessment should be updated at regular intervals, determined by the condition of the patient or change in environment. Observational skills and the ability to obtain a detailed history are the keys to a good assessment. Motor function has a major impact on quality of life and life expectancy.

When patients are assessed in terms of their mobilizing needs, or indeed any care, the same criteria should be used. These include the factors influencing the ability to carry out an activity of living and can be divided into physical, psychological, sociocultural, environmental, and politico-economic factors. In general, this will cover the patient's ability to mobilize, the patient's physical and psychological situation, details of any handling aids, or techniques that should be used and the number of staff required to assist the patient.

Alongside assessing a person's ability to mobilize, a moving and handling assessment is often carried out to optimize a patient's ability to mobilize and to keep staff safe. The assessment should incorporate the patient's bed mobility, ability to move in and out of bed, ability to transfer to and from chairs, **commodes**, and trolleys, any hygiene issues (for example, toileting, showering, bathing), and ability to walk. This should be documented using the local clinical area's standard form (see **Fig. 10.1**) and should be safe for the most inexperienced nurse.

This assessment must involve the patient and relatives or carers, where appropriate. It may also be important to involve other health professionals, such as physiotherapists (see Section 2.2).

Patient's Name: Hospital Number:

Ward:

Weight: Height: Age:

INDIVIDUAL MOVING AND HANDLING ASSESSMENT
ABILITY CODES
A. Able to weight bear and balance independently
B. Able to weight bear and balance with supervision
C. Able to weight bear and balance with equipment and assistance of one operator
D. Able to weight bear but unstable - requires assistance of two operators
E. Unable to weight bear - requires hoist and two operators

ASSESSMENT ONE						
PATIENT ACTIVITY	ABILITY LEVEL					RECOMMENDED MANOEUVRES
Date:	A	B	C	D	E	
General Mobility						
Bed > Chair Chair > Bed						
Toileting						
Standing/sitting						
Bathing						
Manoeuvring in bed						
Signature of Assessors:						

ASSESSMENT TWO						
PATIENT ACTIVITY	ABILITY LEVEL					RECOMMENDED MANOEUVRES
Date:	A	B	C	D	E	
General Mobility						
Bed > Chair Chair > Bed						
Toileting						
Standing/sitting						
Bathing						
Manoeuvring in bed						
Signature of Assessors:						

Figure 10.1 Example of a moving and handling assessment form

Table 10.1 The influencing factors in patient mobility

Influencing factors	
Physical	Injury, for example, fractures, swellings
	Dependence—require aids or assistance
	Past medical history, for example, cerebrovascular accident (CVA), arthritis, amputation, Parkinson's disease
	Pain, perhaps increasing on movement
	Range of movement
	Weight
	Posture and **gait**
	Balance (both sitting and standing)
	Physical disabilities—sight, hearing, speech
	History of falls—vertigo, epilepsy, spasms, dizziness, faintness
	Tissue viability
	Motor nervous function
	Osteoporosis
Psychological	Conscious level
	Capacity to comprehend and cooperate
	Depression or anxiety
	Knowledge of ability, importance of mobility
	Fears, for example, fear of falling
	Motivation
	Mood—aggression, agitation
Sociocultural	Ability to carry out activities
	Lifestyle—drive, walk, public transport
	Social activities, exercise
	Social support
	Employment
	Cultural or religious considerations
Environmental	Place they live—type of home, space, safe, obstructions, furniture
	Stairs
	Day and night variations—does patient's ability change during the day?
	In hospital—change of environment
	Attachments—IV lines, catheters, oxygen therapy
Politico-economic	Finance—means to pay for aids
	Leisure facilities, local transport

When to assess the patient's ability to mobilize

An assessment of a patient's ability to mobilize should be carried out as part of the general individual patient assessment. A specific moving and handling assessment should also be carried out in those patients who are considered to be at risk. It is vital to consider the implications to the patient of prolonged immobility—see Section 10.2.

Procedure

Preparation

Ensure that you have all the required documentation and a moving and handling assessment tool if one is being used.

The information should be thorough, for example, if equipment is to be used, such as a hoist, then both the type of hoist and size of sling should be documented.

Table 10.1 lists the influencing factors in patient mobility. All of these should be considered when assessing your patient.

Aftercare

It is very important that the document is completed and included in the clinical notes.

If the patient is at risk, then appropriate action should be taken. This assessment document should be referred to before any care takes place. If new staff are involved in the patient's care, they should be shown this documentation before nursing this patient.

Since the factors influencing a patient's ability to move can change at any time, reassessment is vital and this should also be documented and shared with all concerned.

Developing your skills

It is essential that you become practised in the skill of assessing a patient's ability to mobilize both in hospital and in the community. You should try and practice this skill on your next placement. You may require assistance from your mentor or another qualified member of staff to address their needs fully.

Try assessing a patient on your own: then repeat the assessment with your mentor and compare results, considering what has been omitted or enhanced. Discuss the rationale behind each aspect of the assessment.

Other factors to consider

There are other specific assessment documents, which should be used in specific situations, for example, fall-risk assessment and pressure-sore risk assessment. These are both covered in Chapter 3.

There are also specific moving and handling assessment tools, which are used in the community. These look specifically at the patient's home environment and ability to mobilize within and out of the home. Risk assessment documents should also accompany the patient on transfer, discharge, and to other areas, such as X-ray or investigation areas, where they will be moved.

Patients who need special consideration during the assessment process are heavy (bariatric) patients. The World Health Organization (2000) has described obesity as one of today's most significant health problems. It now affects two-thirds of the global adult male population and more than half of the global adult female population.

The health organization's moving and handling advisors should be consulted at the initial point of contact with the healthcare environment to ensure that the correct advice and equipment is made available. Often the maximum load that a hoist will safely accommodate is 190 kg. There are specialized pieces of equipment to manage heavier patients. It is, therefore, the manager's responsibility to ensure that appropriate equipment is available as these types of patient are becoming more and more common (Health and Safety Executive 2007). Consider that a patient whose weight exceeds the safe limit of the hoist may also need a specially reinforced bed, chair, or wheelchair.

10.2 **Recognizing and preventing the major complications of immobility**

Definition

Understanding the causes of the major complications of immobility will help the nurse to assess the patient's risk status thoroughly. Prevention of complications forms a large part of planning the nursing care for every patient.

When to intervene to manage major complications of immobility

Key point: Good assessment will always include consideration of the risk of developing complications as a result of the patient's condition. You must recognize and be alert for the potential that any complication will arise. A sound knowledge of what those potential complications might be is vital to planning good care.

During and following assessment, the nurse can plan appropriate care measures to prevent these complications occurring and observe and manage the signs and symptoms of these complications should they arise.

These complications primarily arise from being immobile; therefore, patients at risk will be those who, for example, are confined to a bed or chair as a result of illness, a neurological condition, such as stroke or paralysis, or a musculoskeletal disorder, such as a fractured hip or leg. Look for patients at risk in any care environment. Common complications of immobility are listed in **Table 10.2**.

Developing your skills

When a patient is identified as being at risk of complications related to immobility, the plan of care must reflect a structured approach to reducing the risk and managing those complications. This must be clearly documented and regularly reviewed so that a consistent approach to patient care is adopted. Develop your skills in patient assessment and problem identification by considering which patients will be most at risk of these complications.

Other factors to consider

Other potential complications of immobility not included in Table 10.2 are:

- Psychological isolation and depression
- Disorientation
- Fear and resentment of dependence
- Loss of employment
- **Urinary stasis** (incomplete bladder emptying and static positions can mean a greater likelihood of bacteria colonizing the urinary tract)
- Loss of muscle strength
- Orthostatic (or postural), hypotension (blood pressure drops with upright postures)
- Loss of appetite and dehydration

When performing patient assessment of immobility also be aware of the tools that exist for measuring how much at risk a patient is—these are discussed in Chapters 2, 3, and 5.

By its nature, we consider immobility to be a condition of people who can't get around well, however, numerous patients in the community manage independent lifestyles with quite severe levels of disability—for example wheelchair users may be able to live independently in an adapted environment but should be regularly assessed for the above complications of immobility as they are seated all day. Patients with **dementia** or depression may seem active when visited by carers but can be very immobile when with their spouse or someone they are accustomed to—moderate exercise is important for health regardless of age or condition.

Patients with mental health problems or clients with autism can and may tolerate long periods of immobility and discomfort. All clients should be given physical assessments at regular intervals even when they appear to have no physical disorders.

Table 10.2 Common complications of immobility

Complication	Main causes	Management
Constipation A slowing of frequency in bowel movements, generally associated with a hardening of stools and sometimes discomfort and a need to strain when defecating.	Gravity and general activity play a significant part in the normal transit of bowel contents. The large bowel extracts fluid from its contents, so the slower the transit time of the faeces, the drier the content. Apart from reduced mobility, the most common causes of constipation are **dehydration**, lack of fibre, and opioid **analgesics.** Severe or unmanaged constipation may result in impaction where the faeces are so dry and consolidated that the bowel may need to be evacuated manually (Baillie and Arrowsmith 2006).	It is important to document bowel motions properly in those at risk of constipation and act earlier rather than later to relieve constipation. Exercise and a diet rich in fibre will reduce constipation. Where these are not practicable, there are a number of simple medicines both **oral** and rectal that will **stimulate** the bowel and or soften the contents. Manual or digital evacuation of faeces should be undertaken with care as a last resort and then only by experienced staff (Kyle 2006).
Deep venous thrombosis Formation of a blood clot in the deep veins of the legs, usually in the calves. Presence of the clot impairs the circulation leading to local swelling, redness, and surface dilation of nearby blood vessels. If the clot detaches it can travel to the lungs causing an often fatal blockage. This is known as a **pulmonary embolism** or PE. Symptoms of PE are chest pain that is worse on **inspiration,** usually of sudden onset, often accompanied by coughing—sometimes of blood (haemoptysis)—and breathlessness or, in more severe cases, sudden collapse and sometimes death.	Venous stasis (sluggish blood flow in veins) as a result of immobility and decreased **vasomotor** tone (vein flaccidity). Compression of blood vessels in some areas, usually caused by pressure on back of legs in lying position. Increased **coagulability** (tendency for clot formation) caused by underlying illness, dehydration, some drugs, and high **oestrogen** levels.	Mainly prevention, through use of: Anti-embolic stockings: these elastic stockings uniformly compress the tissues around flaccid veins and increase velocity of blood flow through them. Passive limb movements will encourage increased blood flow and have musculoskeletal benefits, administration of an **anticoagulant** (anticlotting drug) will also reduce risk of clot formation. If a deep venous clot has formed, attempts are made to prevent it from growing bigger and allowing the body to dissolve it by using infused or injected drugs progressing then to a tablet form. (Crowther and McCourt 2005)
Pressure ulcers These are areas of localized damage to skin and underlying tissues primarily caused by pressure. They occur mainly in areas where there are bony prominences, such as the heels, side of ankle, sacrum, hips, shoulder blades and back of head (EPUAP 2007).	When an immobile patient remains in a static position, the pressure placed on tissues beneath the patient impedes the circulation to these tissues and they effectively begin to die though lack of vital nutrients and build up of waste products. Additional factors that contribute to damage are **friction** and **shearing forces**—where tissues wish to slide but are stopped from doing so—for example,	Prevention is, as always, the best solution. Regular positional change will help significantly and it is vital that patients are carefully assessed and those at risk identified early. It is vital that at-risk patients' skin surfaces are continually reviewed. The use of specialized pressure-reducing and pressure-relieving mattresses and cushions is recommended for those at high risk or who have already developed pressure ulcers (Royal College of Nursing and National Institute for Clinical Excellence 2005)

the deep muscles and bones of a seated patient will want to slide downwards owing to gravity but the superficial skin may be fixed and immovable—thus, there is a force similar to tearing or shearing present.

Other major factors are poor nutrition, generally impaired circulation from underlying illness, and the presence at the skin surface of moisture, for example, urine.

Hypostatic pneumonia The pooling and collection of secretions in the lungs secondary to immobility and reduced coughing.	An immobile patient with reduced lung expansion and little or no ability to cough will accumulate secretions in the lungs. Areas of lung become nonfunctional. Plugs of mucus can also significantly block branches of the respiratory tree, particularly in the dehydrated patient. The presence of the collected fluid can also act as a focus for bacteria and lead to significant respiratory infection.	Regular positional change helps reduce pooling of secretions and more upright positions generally facilitate greater lung expansion than **supine** (on the back) positions (Geraghty 2005). Oropharyngeal or tracheal suction through a thin catheter inserted via mouth or nose may serve to remove some secretions in the higher part of the respiratory tree, but more importantly can stimulate the cough **reflex** and usefully mobilize some of the deeper secretions (Lynn 2008).
Muscle wasting	After prolonged immobilization, for example, in a cast, the muscles decrease in size and will be very weak and it will be painful to start using them again.	Mobilize the limb to the greatest extent possible and permitted by the medical team. The plaster should always be applied so as to avoid immobilizing neighbouring joints unnecessarily.
Contracture Immobile muscles may progressively shorten and become contracted.	Muscle tissue is very adaptable; consider the different physiques of those undertaking different sports. Incorrect positioning, especially when some form of tension is created within a muscle group, can result in adaptation of those and reciprocal muscle groups. This adaptation is usually seen as a **contraction,** or shortening and twisting of a limb (Martini 2006)	Range of motion exercises (described in Section 10.6) will reduce the development of contractures caused by immobility. Occasionally oral medicines are given and sometimes botulinum toxin (Botox) is injected into contracted muscles to relieve pain or loss of range of motion caused by contractures.

10.3 **Recognizing and selecting common handling aids**

Definition

By developing their knowledge of the handling aids available, nurses should be able to recognize patients who may benefit from access to certain types and understand how and when to use these aids.

Table 10.3 describes the most commonly used handling aids available and their advantages and uses and precautions to be taken when using them. Individual patient assessment is paramount in selecting the most appropriate aid.

When to suggest a handling aid for a patient

A number of patients with a long-term or short-term disability will, with access to appropriate devices and equipment, be able to function more independently. These may, among others, include the frail elderly, those with neurological deficits, such as stroke or cerebral palsy, and those with fractures or sprains.

Knowledge of what equipment is available will greatly help you in advising the patient and liaising with departments such as occupational therapy and physiotherapy on your patient's behalf. Often a minor piece of equipment can greatly increase a patient's level of independence and likelihood of rehabilitation.

Key point: Some immobile patients can be repositioned with greater safety and comfort, for patient and nurses, when appropriate equipment is used.

Aftercare

If a patient has been allocated a new item or a change of equipment, clear instructions should be given on how to use it most effectively and safely. Attend to the precautions and issues described above. It is also important to then assess the patient's understanding

and ability to use that item safely. For example, when starting a patient with a walking frame or Zimmer, it is important that the patient learns to keep the weight forwards and only move the frame forwards when satisfied with their foot positioning. For wheeled walking frames—their patient must be able to prevent them rolling away either through manipulation of brakes, or, for some, by pushing down. Patients employing a transfer board will have to demonstrate satisfactorily that they have the sitting balance and coordination to use it safely.

Competent patients should then be regularly reassessed for continuing competence or the need to progress to a more or less supportive device as their conditions improve or deteriorate.

Developing your skills

Where possible empathize with your patients by using these pieces of equipment on yourself. During equipment training sessions, see how you feel when moved by a hoist. Is it comfortable? Do you feel secure? What makes you more or less comfortable or secure?

Consider using smaller pieces of equipment with an additional disability, for example use a crutch while keeping one foot off the floor, or try to use a walking frame with one arm held to your chest.

Consider how this experience will enhance the advice and guidance you might give to a patient trying a handling aid for the first time. Some of these aids are referred to in the next section.

Other factors to consider

Patients can associate some mechanical lifting aids, such as hoists, with a degree of discomfort. Minimize this by using good sling application technique and chiefly by reducing the time during which the patient is solely supported by the sling to a few seconds.

In a domestic setting, some equipment may be difficult to use—for example aids that roll easily across smooth ward floors can be very hard to use on carpets. Some hoists can be too bulky for use in small rooms. Fortunately, there are hoists specifically designed for the community—these are usually smaller and more manoeuvrable than the heavy-duty hoists found in hospitals. Some of these hoists are very portable and can easily separate into three or four parts for easy transport by a visiting carer. Some hoists will be permanently based at the patient's home through equipment management or leasing schemes.

Residential care homes are usually equipped with similar devices to hospitals; however, devices are usually selected with carpets in mind, albeit low pile ones.

Patients in the community with long-term handling needs and suitable environments can have ceiling-track hoists fitted (providing the ceilings are suitable). These tracks can electrically transfer patients between rooms, for example, from bed to toilet and then to sitting area. An advantage of the ceiling track is that furnishings, carpets, or obstacles are easily avoided, although to move between rooms, door frames and lintels will need adaptation.

There are also specialized pieces of equipment to manage heavier patients. Choosing a sling for these patients is not merely dependent on their weight and size; it is also necessary to know their body shape and weight distribution, that is, where do they carry most weight, for example the thighs or gluteal region (Rush 2006).

Understandably, some patients are nervous when suspended by a lifting device—you can reduce their anxiety by being as competent and skilled as possible with the equipment. Practice on colleagues before practising on patients!

Table 10.3 The most commonly used handling aids

Handling aids and their uses	Precautions or issues to bear in mind
Walking stick Widens base. Transfers some weight from leg to arm.	Limited stability. General balance and arm or wrist strength must be good. Can stigmatize the user. The correct size is required.
Elbow crutch This gives greater stability of grip. Wrist strength is not as important as with a stick, therefore, the patient can bear more weight through the arm.	Stability is still limited. Definitely gives the patient an appearance of disability.
Walking frame (Zimmer) As above but larger base, so greater stability.	The correct size is important. The patient should have a comfortable slight bend in elbows when standing upright. Offers no protection should the patient lean backwards.
Forearm walker (Pulpit Zimmer) As above but allows more weight to be transferred from the legs to the device (see **Fig. 10.2**).	There is better stability, and arm and wrist strength is less critical. With minor modification it can be used with one arm.
Wheeled frame As above but it can support those less able to lift and lower the frame. Some are designed to cope with slightly rougher outdoor terrain, such as pavements (see **Fig. 10.3**).	Terrain cannot be very rough. It can roll away from the patient's control. Some versions have brakes.
Grab rails, handles, and bed rails These allow patients to move, balance, and stabilize themselves in various settings.	Must be within easy reach, at the correct angle and secure enough to bear the patient's weight.
Lifting and transfer pole (monkey pole) This allows the patient to adjust position in bed and to redistribute pressure on their tissues (see **Fig. 10.4**).	The patient must have sufficient upper body strength and balance. Need to exercise caution during movements, so that skin under the patient is not dragged under friction and against resistance—especially the heels and buttocks.

Transfer board

This comes in a variety of shapes and materials. It is used as a bridge on which to slide from bed to chair or commode and back. It can be used with a sliding sheet to reduce friction. It can also be used to break a standing transfer from bed to chair into stages or as a 'safety net' during standing transfers.

Transfer surfaces need to be of equivalent heights (see **Fig. 10.5**). Apply caution with any sliding device to prevent sliding on to floor—especially if used with sliding sheet. The patient needs upper body balance and postural control.

Turning disc

Some are designed to be stood on and some to be sat on. With a seated patient, this will facilitate the swinging of legs into a bed or a car (see **Fig. 10.6**). This eliminates the friction and shearing that could occur between the skin and the support surface. Turning discs for standing patients particularly assist the patient who struggles to shuffle their main weight-bearing leg around the weaker one.

Generally there is a soft or padded version for sitting on and a rigid one for standing on.

A soft version may be left in place beneath the patient during, for example, a meal or car journey but care must be taken that it does not represent a hazard to the skin owing to ridges or prominent seams compressing the tissues.

When used to help the turn of a standing patient, the patient must be able to bear weight, at least through one leg and movements should be slow to reduce the patient's reflex postural stiffening associated with changes in balance and weight distribution.

Bed blocks

These are used by patients to facilitate their own movement up or down the bed.

The broad base of the blocks reduces the depth to which the hands would sink down into the mattress. In addition the handles lengthen the patient's arms and allow greater clearance above the mattress (see **Fig. 10.7**).

The patient will need reasonable arm and wrist strength to hold the blocks and raise up off the mattress. It is vital that heels are not dragged over the sheets, so knees must be bent up at the start of the move upwards, or a sliding sheet should be put beneath them. Good technique makes this manoeuvre much easier. Sitting upright with knees bent, the blocks will be held by the patient securely on the mattress behind themselves. The patient should then relax down and initiate the movement backwards by leading with their head—this erects the spine and makes movement of the torso and structures around the shoulder girdle much easier than if they attempt the manoeuvre with chin on chest.

Lateral transfer board (patient slide)

A typical patient slide for transfer from trolley to bed and vice versa will be about 1.8 m long (see **Fig. 10.8**). It acts as a low-friction bridge from one support surface to another across which a patient can be slid (refer to Section 10.4 for further details).

As with all sliding devices, care must be taken that the patient does not slide out of control. It is additionally very important that the two surfaces are anchored or braked to prevent their separation during the manoeuvre. The board may be used in conjunction with sliding sheets if appropriate. Movements should be coordinated and controlled with sufficient personnel to ensure patient and nurse safety.

Sliding sheets

These are low-friction fabric sheets of varied size, shape, and design that can help to slide patients, usually up and down beds. Their use in patient handling is strongly recommended so that manual manoeuvres are made more manageable for nurses and to reduce any drag or friction on patients when they are being repositioned.

The low-friction nature of the sheets means that the patient is at risk of slipping unless supervised. Moving these sheets from bed to bed in residential or hospital environments may lead to cross-infection, so patients should have their own sheets allocated for their stay and organizations must have good laundering arrangements.

Shower trolley

This is used to shower patients who are too immobile for a conventional shower or cannot sit safely in a bath—this may include the spinally injured or unconscious patient. See **Fig. 10.9**. The patient can be transferred laterally onto the waterproof trolley, sides raised, and then cleaned thoroughly with a shower head. A special bathing area with space, shower head and a drainage point to connect the trolley to is recommended.

A wet patient will very quickly lose body temperature. The process needs to be carried out efficiently in a sufficiently warm environment. Care must also be taken to protect the vulnerable patient's airway and neck.

Mobile hoist

There are numerous models available; one example is shown in **Fig. 10.10**. Lifting range is generally from as low as the floor to a point sufficiently high to manoeuvre a patient onto a bed. A sling is placed around a patient and then connected to the hoist for lifting. There are a range of slings for different purposes, for example, flat lifting, bathing, sitting, and for amputee patients. Owing to the risk of used slings transferring infection from patient to patient, most patients will be allocated their own sling, whether they are in hospital or a residential home setting.

There are also disposable slings available for single patient use. These are used throughout a patient's stay and discarded at their discharge or when any signs of wear are detected.

Ensure that the patient does not exceed the maximum weight limit. Use the correct size and type of sling. Always scrutinize slings for any signs of damage before use.

Many patients are nervous when asked to trust any mechanical device—good communication skills on the part of nurses and competence and assurance in the use of the devices will allay some concerns. Always ensure proper training on the hoist and its accessories has been given before using them.

Standing and raising hoist

This usually brings a patient to a standing position by a process of blocking the knees and then levering the patient up from a chair or bed (see **Fig. 10.11**).

These can be extremely useful when dressing or toileting patients as the patient is supported without impeding access to the lower body.

There must be no reason why a patient should not bear their own weight through the legs and feet.

Often a wide band is placed around the patient's torso to help raise the patient. This must be positioned to support the rib cage and not to drag the patient from beneath the arms.

Walking hoist

An overhead attachment is linked to a chest harness. This allows a patient to develop walking ability, yet be secure in the event of a fall (see **Fig. 10.12**).

This also significantly protects the nurse involved in the rehabilitation of patients.

Correct harness size and application are vital for patient comfort, safety and confidence.

Ceiling hoist

Tracks can be secured to suitable ceilings, allowing patient movement in certain directions, as shown in **Fig. 10.13**.

All considerations that apply to mobile hoists and slings also apply to ceiling hoists. However, while mobile hoists need fairly large clear areas of floor space to move around, ceiling hoists are well out of the way. The full mechanization of transfer means that some disabled patients can often become more independent in a well-designed environment.

Patient handling sling

A broad band that can fit around a patient allowing nurses to hold onto the sling rather than grip part of the patient.

The sling also lengthens the nurse's arms so they can begin a manoeuvre in a more comfortable or upright position.

The sling is *not* a lifting device and clearly does not reduce the load borne by the nurse. Rather it improves patient security and comfort, while often facilitating better nurse positioning. A handling net may be used in place of a sling in some areas.

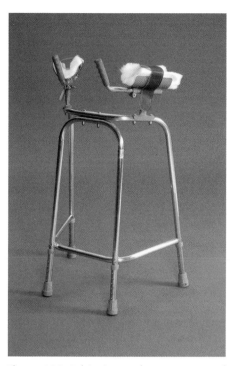

Figure 10.2 Pulpit Zimmer frame. Courtesy of Homecraft Rolyan Ltd.

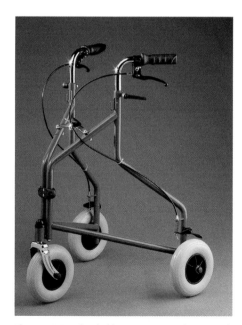

Figure 10.3 Wheeled frame. Courtesy of Homecraft Rolyan Ltd.

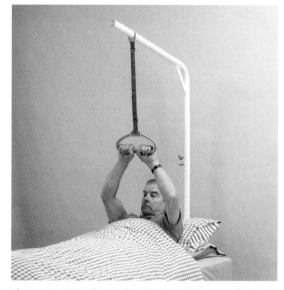

Figure 10.4 Monkey pole. Courtesy of Homecraft Rolyan Ltd.

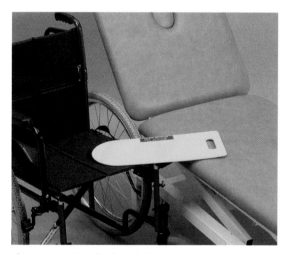

Figure 10.5 Transfer board. Courtesy of Homecraft Rolyan Ltd.

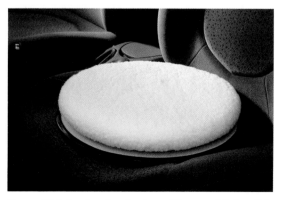

Figure 10.6 Turning disc. Courtesy of Homecraft Rolyan Ltd.

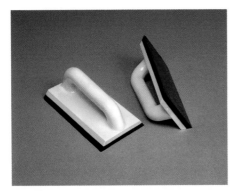

Figure 10.7 Bed blocks. Courtesy of Homecraft Ryan

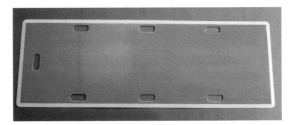

Figure 10.8 Patient slide. Courtesy of Homecraft Ryan

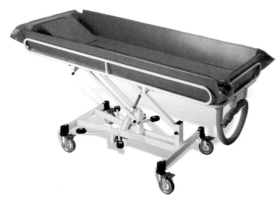

Figure 10.9 Shower trolley. Courtesy of Homecraft Ryan

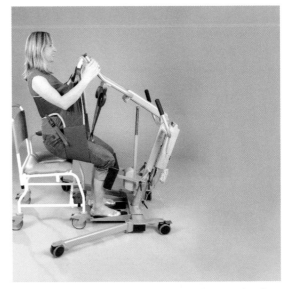

Figure 10.11 Standing hoist. Courtesy of Homecraft Rolyan Ltd.

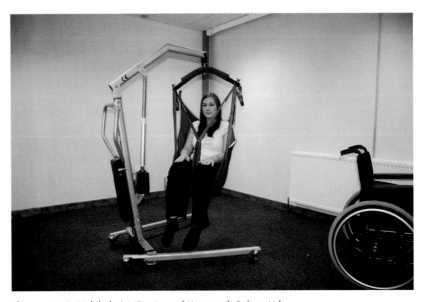

Figure 10.10 Mobile hoist. Courtesy of Homecraft Rolyan Ltd.

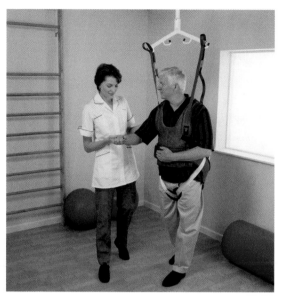

Figure 10.12 Walking hoist. Courtesy of ARJO

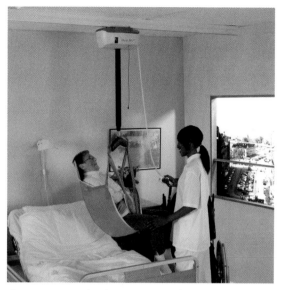

Figure 10.13 Ceiling hoist. Courtesy of ARJO

Not all patients can safely use one of the smaller aids; however, for those who can, there may be significant psychological benefits in relation to increased feelings of independence. Some patients may alternatively be very resistant to the use of aids because of the stigma that they may carry. For example, a crutch may be associated with being disabled. Significant communication and persuasion skills may need to be used to encourage a patient even to attempt some devices.

Some items can be coloured, accessorized or decorated to make them less clinical and possibly more acceptable to children or teenagers. Never use equipment specifically designed for adults on children or vice versa—proper sizing and measurements must be made depending on the item.

10.4 **Practical handling of bedbound patients**

Definition

If, because of impaired consciousness or physical ability, a patient cannot effectively move unaided, assistance will need to be provided. Sometimes this assistance will be given mechanically through the application of appropriate handling equipment, but sometimes, when assessed as

safe to patient and nurse, some manual assistance can be given—this is only appropriate with cooperative patients where the patient or environment do not put the nurse at risk of injury.

This section considers four of the most common manoeuvres that might be undertaken with a bedbound patient:

1 Moving a patient from lying to sitting in bed,
2 Repositioning a patient when in bed,
3 Moving a patient horizontally in bed,
4 Lateral transfers—trolley to bed: bed to trolley.

When to move a bedbound patient

Any patient who is in bed should be encouraged to be as independent as possible, some of the aids described in Section 10.3, such as bed blocks and monkey poles, may help patients to move themselves and these should be promoted where appropriate. Some patients are so dependent that it will not be safe to handle them manually and hoists or other devices must be used according to a handling assessment.

Attention must be paid to good positioning in bed when caring for dependent patients or patients whose ability to adjust their own position is impaired. These may include unconscious patients, those with a neurological impairment such as stroke or spinal injury, or simply anyone who is too infirm or frail to reposition themselves successfully.

Good positioning can reduce many of the complications associated with immobility. Proper comfort promotes rest. Any reduction in stress and fatigue will enhance the body's capacity for self-healing. Family and friends will be considerably reassured when care has clearly been taken to make their loved one comfortable.

Alternative interventions

Electronic beds

For more dependent patients, in or out of hospital, special beds that will alter their profile electronically should be considered in a balance between the safety of the nurse and the movement capacity of the patient. It may be that a healthy, well-trained community healthcare nurse can manage the patient at home with ease but a frail spouse will be unable to provide the same support during the hours between visits. Equipment that allows the patient to be well cared for at home offers multiple advantages over hospitalization. Numerous patients in the domestic or home setting are cared for on sophisticated electronic beds that facilitate positional change at the press of a button, though a domestic hoist may be more versatile for some situations.

Hoists

A hoist is an effective and often underused tool for changing a bedfast patient's position in the bed. With careful application of the sling, the patient can be comfortably repositioned. Raising them in a supported position over the bed will facilitate the changing or straightening of sheets and optimal positioning of pillows prior to settling the patient in their new position. This can actually take less time than manual techniques that may involve effort, risk and ultimately be less effective.

Procedures

Preparation

Before any handling manoeuvre, you should mentally rehearse it before undertaking it, even when using handling equipment such as hoists.

Consider ELITE:

- Equipment
- Load
- Individual
- Task
- Environment

(For details see Section 2.2.)

Questions to ask include:

- Is there any risk of pain or injury to the patient?
- How will you position yourself—what are the start and finish points of the manoeuvre?
- Can the surrounding environment be improved?
- How will you protect and support the patient?

Whatever the technique, it should allow close observation of the patient for any signs of discomfort during movement.

Special considerations

Special care must be taken with certain categories of patient. For example; the patient with impaired consciousness will need assistance to protect the neck and head. A rapid slide from trolley to bed can jar the patient's hip as it arrives—this can destabilize the internal fixation performed on a repair of a hip fracture.

Patients with neurological conditions, such as cerebral palsy can often begin to contract into the shapes they are habitually placed in—particularly if placed in a contracted (curled up) position overnight. Regular positional change is, therefore, important, particularly to maintain and sustain more upright postures. Try to set these patients in a comfortable position but with limbs and spine as straight as possible for sleeping—for example on their backs but with a **30° tilt** to alternate pressure from side to side.

Key point: Some patients are connected to numerous tubes and **drains** and the manoeuvre may need additional members of staff to ensure these accessories are also safely transferred.

Procedure: moving from lying to sitting up in bed

This is certainly one of the most common manoeuvres to be performed in assistance of the bedbound patient. It is a movement from the supine (lying on the back) to **semi-recumbent** (sitting against a support of pillows or a back-rest). A sling may be used to assist in this manoeuvre, as shown in **Fig. 10.14**.

One of the most common reasons to move a patient into a sitting position would be to facilitate eating and drinking.

Key point: Shearing forces occur when the body's weight and deeper tissues move under gravity but the superficial skin remains stationary. This can disrupt the microcirculation to the superficial tissues (Pellatt 2005).

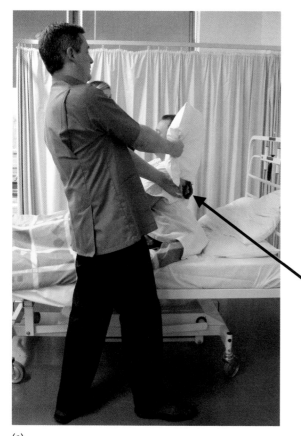

(a)

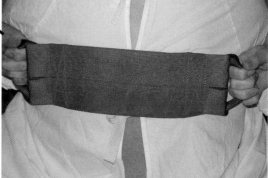

(b)

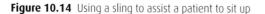

Figure 10.14 Using a sling to assist a patient to sit up

Moving a patient from lying to sitting up in bed

Step	Rationale
1 Complete a full assessment and additionally consider: **Is there any aspect of the patient's condition that will influence the safety or feasibility of the manoeuvre? For example, injuries, pain or capacity to comprehend and cooperate. What can the patient do unassisted with instruction and supervision or with small aids?**	To determine risks. Providing something secure for the patient to pull on such as a bed ladder or lifting pole (see handling aids) may contribute significantly to the patient's ability to either help or to move independently. Some people, while not able to sit up directly from the prone position, can move into a seated position from lying on their side—often they can also wriggle up the bed more effectively when on their side.
2 Where possible, work with a colleague.	A single nurse will always be at risk when assisting a patient to move. This risk can only be controlled when it is certain that the patient will do nothing unpredictable and the nurse limits effort to offering slight support and assistance in a position of comfort and stability.
3 Any approach to the patient in bed (or in a cot) must permit you to adjust your base so that you can comfortably shift your weight in the intended direction without losing balance and stability. Twisting should always be avoided. In practice this usually means avoiding being parallel to the side of the bed and instead taking a more oblique or diagonal approach to the patient (Foss and Farine 2007).	The bed itself represents a hazard to the operator. It will distance you from your load and can force you into stooped postures with locked knees.
4 On no account should a dependent patient be dragged upright by the arms or shoulders (see banned manoeuvres, Section 2.2).	This commonly results in pain and injury for the patient and the nurse (Fragala *et al.* 2005).
5 By gently raising alternate shoulders, position a patient-handling sling or net beneath the patient's shoulders.	The sling or net can give two nurses the added reach to adopt a comfortable upright starting position and a point to hold on to that supports rather than endangers the patient's shoulders.
6 Slightly bend the patient's legs.	Sitting up will always be easier for the patients if their legs are slightly bent, that is, not locked in a position of resistance.

7	Nurses hold the sling facing the opposing top corner of the bed: transferring their weight from the front foot and stepping back will raise the patient.	Good starting positions mean the manoeuvre should be accomplished without twisting and by using your own weight as a counterbalance to the patient's.
8	Either ask the patient to tuck the chin onto the chest, or hold a pillow lightly behind the patient's head in each operator's free hand.	Care must be taken to ensure that the patient's head and neck are well supported during movement.
9	Have pillows or wedges ready to support the patient in a sitting position.	Having sufficient pillows or alternative supports such as foam wedges to place behind the patient will reduce the need to sit him or her nearer to the back of the bed for support.
10	Verify that the patient is comfortable, ensuring bedclothes are smoothed beneath and secure above and limbs are comfortably positioned.	Minor areas of discomfort will prevent the patient from fully relaxing and possibly disrupt sleep. Cloth folds under the patient will result in discomfort and may compromise circulation. The patient should be sufficiently covered to maintain a comfortable body temperature. Limb positioning is important in reducing a number of complications, such as drop foot, contractures and joint pain. Appropriate spread and distribution of the patient's weight will reduce shearing forces acting on the tissues.

Aftercare

Review the patient's ability to maintain sitting balance and consider the need for bed safety rails. Plan for regular positional change and communicate the next planned movement to the rest of the care team and the patient.

Procedure: Repositioning the patient when in bed

This involves the optimum positioning of immobile or dependent patients when in bed to promote comfort and reduce the incidence of complications associated with immobility and bed rest. It mainly involves a simple repositioning of limbs.

Preparation

A sliding sheet may be needed for movement up, down, or to the side. Pillows may help to support the patient in the new position.

Key point: The low-friction nature of the sliding sheets means that the patient could be at risk of slipping to the floor, so care must be taken to prevent this. An additional concern is that using the sliding sheets between patients can result in cross-contamination and spread of infection. A patient should have sheets allocated for their use only and there should be robust laundering provisions for reusable materials.

Repositioning the patient when in bed

Step	Rationale
1 Assess the patient's ability to protect his or her own airway (ability to breathe easily). For example; how alert is the patient? Can the patient move voluntarily to prevent choking? Is there a risk of vomiting?	Position will be determined by the need to prevent aspiration (inhalation of fluid) and occlusion (blocking) of the airway by, for example, the tongue. An unconscious patient with an at-risk airway would normally be positioned in the recovery position (Resuscitation Council of the UK 2005).
2 Assess patient's skin for areas of tissue damage, redness, or impaired circulation.	Final positioning should remove or relieve pressure on any damaged or vulnerable areas.
3 Formally assess the patient's pressure ulcer risk factors, using an evidence-based risk assessment tool (see Chapter 3).	The patient may require a specialized mattress if at high risk of developing pressure ulcers. Proper use of assessment tools can give a more consistent and objective measurement of risk than using an unstructured approach.
4 Consider additional factors, such as the presence of IV infusions, wound drains, traction devices, and plaster casts.	Position should not interfere with the free flow of infusions or drains. Traction devices and plaster casts will themselves limit movement and can create additional points of pressure on the tissues.
5 When possible, discuss and explain what you plan to do and why, with the patient, and where appropriate, the relatives.	Involving patients in, and explaining, care can reduce anxiety and increase cooperation.
6 Choose position. Often a semi-recumbent (reclining but not flat) position is best for breathing.	Being fully supine (flat on one's back) can compromise the lungs' capacity to fully inflate (Geraghty 2005). Numerous recommendations have been made suggesting that, for the recumbent patient, the best angle for the backrest to improve respiration is 45° (Griffiths and Gallimore 2005).
7 A lateral recumbent (lying on the side) position, however, may be required for the patient who cannot protect their own airway.	In this position, the patient's airway is less likely to be occluded by the tongue and secretions can drain freely from the mouth.

8 Limbs and head should be carefully and comfortably aligned, within the restrictions posed by the patient's condition. Align head and neck with the spine. Position limbs gently flexed and with support for joints.

Good alignment and support should prevent tension in muscles and strain at joints. Both can lead to joint injuries, pain, contractures, and foot and wrist drop (Carpenito-Moyet 2004).

9 Assess areas of pressure and position the patient so that pressure is not placed directly on bony areas, such as the outside of the knee or ankle, the sacrum or shoulder blades, the hips or shoulder tips, and even the ears and base of skull. A 30° tilt is often the optimum one for prevention of pressure sores (see Chapter 3).

Pressure is more likely to cause interruption to normal circulation and tissue damage in areas directly compressed beneath hard surfaces such as bony prominences.

10 Ensure linen creases are smoothed from beneath patient.

Lying on creases may result in interruption to circulation and normal fluid drainage of tissues in that area.

11 Smooth out the skin beneath the patient as far as is practicable.

Small pulls and tugs on the surface of the skin generate sensations that can stimulate tension in the muscles nearby and so lead to tension, discomfort, and a reduced capacity for deeper relaxation and rest.

12 Check that any equipment, tubing, or drains have not been disturbed during movements and that they are also well positioned.

Tubes, catheters, and drains can easily become dislodged during patient movement. Additionally, they may become kinked or twisted and so stop functioning.

13 Finally assess the patient's level of comfort by asking those who are able to respond. Some may not be able to respond clearly, for example, the unconscious patient, patients with a speaking difficulty or a language barrier and very young children. For some patients, assessment of discomfort will be made by noting the presence of any facial tension or grimacing and any sounds, which may be incomprehensible yet still reflect discontent with the new position. Respirations may increase and some patients in pain may become flushed, while some may become pale. They may also become sweaty or clammy.

Conscientious and thoughtful use of good observational skills will alert the nurse at as early a stage as possible when further attention is required.
Don't leave until you have ascertained, to the best of your ability, that the patient is safe and comfortable.

Replace bed safety rails if necessary.

Aftercare

Seek advice regarding any potentially adverse observations you have made and document any significant details, such as the presence of skin discolouration or signs of pain. Decide on the planned time for next repositioning and ensure that this is effectively communicated to the rest of the team and the patient.

Procedure: Moving a patient horizontally in bed

In most examples, this means either up and down or onto and off the bed. Usually, the patient is flat and is repositioned by the use of sliding sheets (low-friction sheets placed beneath the patient). This skill is usually required when nursing a dependent patient. The patient may be slid up the bed to allow use of a built in backrest at the top of the bed, or slid down to lie flat. Some patients will be slid across the bed for more central positioning or to allow positioning on their side. Some patients will simply have a sliding sheet placed beneath the heels to prevent drag and friction injuring the heel tissues during movement, as shown in **Fig. 10.15**.

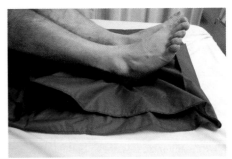

Figure 10.15 Sliding sheet beneath heels

Moving a patient horizontally in bed

Key point: The low friction nature of the sliding sheets means that the patient could be at risk of slipping to the floor, so care must be taken to prevent this. An additional concern is that using the sliding sheets between patients can result in cross-contamination and spread of infection. A patient should have sheets allocated for their use only and there should be robust laundering provisions for reusable materials.

Step	Rationale
1 Prepare and gather equipment: all lateral movements should generally be assisted with low-friction sliding sheets (Hignett 2003).	It is vital that the patient's skin and soft tissues are not dragged to and fro creating friction, as this will damage the skin's surface (Pellatt 2005). Attention must be paid to this risk during any manoeuvre. These sheets are designed to slide easily over themselves and each other so that friction is applied to the sheets and not the patient's skin.
2 To roll a person efficiently, you should ask the person to look in the direction of the roll, move the arm that will be below out from the body in a forwards direction and take the upper arm across the body in the planned direction of movement.	As long as there are no **contraindications** to rolling the patient, the sliding sheets can easily be positioned beneath the patient during a slight roll to either side. Most patients can be easily rolled on to their side by carefully aligning the limbs and controlling the pelvis.
3 When you then move the leg from what will become the upper side across in the direction of intended movement the hips and centre of gravity will easily follow and the patient will be on their side.	While standing upright, a person's centre of gravity is usually within their pelvis. However, when lying flat, although in a different plane, the centre of gravity will still be in the pelvis (Foss and Farine 2007).

4 With sheets in position the nurses should then be able to slide the patient up or down without significant effort.

With sliding sheets in position, flat movement of the patient will usually be smooth and without strain. Heavy patients will always be more difficult and more nurses or equipment should be considered for moving them.

5 Attention must be paid to how the patient will be handled. Some sliding sheets have handles, some are held directly and in some cases the patient is manoeuvred by gently pushing the hip or shoulder.

Direct fingertip gripping and tight grasping of sheets by nurses unnecessarily increases tension through their arms shoulders and neck and should be avoided (Brown and McLennan 2007),.

6 Once the patient is repositioned, the sheets can be easily removed, either in the reverse direction of their insertion or by peeling them under themselves and away from the patient.

Peeling the sheet away from the patient directs any friction away from the skin and onto the low friction surface of the sheet.

Aftercare

It is important to confirm that the patient is safe and secure in this new position. Determine a time for the next positional change and communicate this to the remainder of the care team and the patient.

Procedure: lateral transfers

Patients are mostly transferred laterally when moving from trolley to bed or vice versa. Going from the ward, onto an X-ray table and then back to bed will involve four separate transfers of this nature.

Moving a patient on or off the bed can also be done with sliding devices. However, to prevent the patient slipping between, for example trolley and bed, the gap must somehow be bridged. This is generally done with a slim plastic board (see **Fig. 10.16**) across which the patient slides. There are several other devices that can be used and examples are given in Section 10.3.

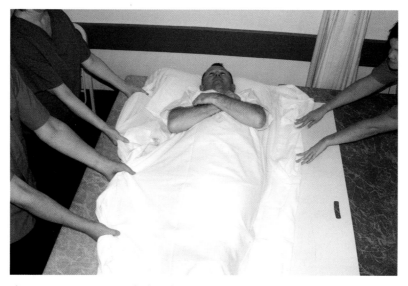

Figure 10.16 Using a transfer board to move a patient

Lateral transfers

EQUIPMENT

- Transfer board or patient slide,
- Sound (strong and intact) bed sheet, preferably with a sliding sheet beneath as the strength of sheets cannot be guaranteed,
- Possibly a folded blanket for padding.

Step	Rationale
1 Where possible explain the transfer to the patient.	A sideways slide can startle those who are not prepared.
2 Position bed and trolley as close together as possible. Use height adjustment to match the two surfaces. Apply bed and trolley brakes securely.	In all cases, care must be taken to ensure that the trolley and bed will not slip apart during the manoeuvre. A slight slope down in the direction of travel may facilitate the transfer but anything more than a few centimetres will affect the anchoring of the edge of the slide—it could rock up and down.
3 Usually the patient will be pulled across on his or her own sheet with the sliding sheets and transfer board beneath.	Advantages of this are that the patient arrives on a sheet and the sheet will usually be broad enough to give nurses a comfortable hold. Straps, handles, or the sheet should allow the operators to adopt comfortable upright positions and not strain over the bed or trolley. Caution must be exercised in ensuring that the sheet is in good enough condition to allow this, although, because the patient's weight is evenly distributed, this is usually not a problem.
4 Nurses should try to take a palm-uppermost hold.	This keeps the elbows in and reduces shoulder and neck tension.
5 The transfer should be made in two or more stages with good communication between nurses and patient.	Care must be taken not to move the patient too briskly as this can be frightening and could also result in the patient brought close to or over the far edge of the bed or trolley.
6 Ensure patient comfort throughout. Bony prominences such as vertebrae should be padded with a folded blanket beforehand.	Sliding across a rigid board, particularly for a thin patient, can be uncomfortable and scrape bony projections.
7 Slightly roll the patient to remove the slide—this should be easy.	Usually the patient will have slid completely across the bridging slide, making it simple to remove.
8 Position the patient for comfort and safety.	The transfer has only helped the patient from trolley to bed or vice versa. Now the patient will need to be properly positioned.
9 Adjust the height of the bed.	Leaving a patient in a bed at a raised level makes a fall out of bed more dangerous, and may additionally not suit relatives who wish to hold a conversation with the patient from a chair.

Aftercare

Use of the patient's own sheet to pull on means that the bed will need to be remade. Use this opportunity to assess skin condition for signs of redness, abrasion, or breakdown.

Developing your skills

As with all equipment, first practice on colleagues until you feel competent and confident.

Experience being transferred in this manner yourself, so that you are aware of what the patient will experience. Take account of this personal experience when explaining the procedure to the patient.

Other factors to consider

Being immobile in bed for lengthy periods can result in isolation from others. Prolonged isolation can lead to the patient becoming withdrawn and depressed. Patients should be regularly engaged in conversation when able and as far as possible included in any surrounding activity and discussion.

Being confined to bed can be particularly frustrating for children and may have an impact on their behaviour, **emotional** state, and concordance with treatment. It will be important to consider how to occupy and divert the child. Parents, teachers, and play specialists may all contribute.

10.5 **Positioning the patient in a chair**

Definition

It is important to assess and select the best type of seating for the dependent patient. The patient should be safe and comfortable once seated.

When to position the patient in a chair

Attention must be paid to good positioning in chairs when caring for dependent patients or patients whose ability to adjust their own position is impaired. This may include those with a neurological impairment, such as stroke, those with musculoskeletal injury, or simply those who are too infirm or frail to successfully reposition themselves.

Whenever possible, patients should move to a seated position for mealtimes, as swallowing safety and digestion are considerably enhanced.

Key point: To position a nonweight-bearing patient in a chair use a hoist. The manual handling of nonweight-bearing patients represents an unacceptably high risk of injury to nurses (Hignett 2003).

Procedure: Positioning the patient in a chair

Preparation

Choosing the correct chair

Assess the patient's capacity to remain seated safely. The patient should, with moderate support, be able to maintain a comfortable position when seated. If there is a risk of pressure sore development, it may be made worse when the entire weight of the torso rests on the ischial tuberosities (bony prominences at the bottom of the pelvis) (Hampton 2003). Recumbent (lying) patients will spread their weight over a greater area than seated patients.

Select a chair of the correct height for the patient. If a chair is too low, the patient may struggle to stand. This may impair the patient's potential for independence or put nurses at risk. When a chair is too high, the patient's legs will 'dangle'. The soft tissues at the back of the knee and lower thigh then support the weight of dependent lower limbs and feet. This can compromise circulation and drainage and compress nerves—leading to disturbances of sensation and discomfort.

Bearing weight through the ball of the foot rather than the whole sole for sustained periods stimulates nerves responsible for maintaining balance and posture and can result in muscle tension that in the long term may cause shortening or contraction in the calf and hamstring muscles (Martini 2006). The height of the chair, therefore, should allow the patient to place both feet flat on the ground without unduly compressing the tissues at the back of the knee (Pheasant 2001). Chair raisers are available that allow some modification to meet individual needs.

Positioning the patient in a chair

EQUIPMENT

- Possibly chair raisers,
- Possibly a patient hoist with sling.

Step	Rationale
1 A weight-bearing patient should face forwards and be positioned close to the seat with the back of one or both calves or knees lightly touching the front of the seat.	Being close to the seat means the patient is more likely to find a secure position on sitting. Feeling the chair from behind will reassure the patient and increase their confidence when moving backwards.
2 The patient should be guided to place the hands on the armrests of the chair.	This will steady the patient and allow the arms to take some weight and so help in controlling the rate of descent. Also, it will reassure the patient.
3 One or two nurses can, if required, position themselves at the side of the chair, slightly behind the patient, facing forwards, though angled obliquely towards the patient (see Fig. 10.17).	As the patient bends his or her knees the trunk will move towards the back of the chair. If the nurses are slightly behind they can provide a very light touch to facilitate a gentle guidance into sitting. Standing at an oblique angle to the patient reduces the likelihood that the nurses will be forced into a twisted posture as they gently relax down with the patient.
4 The nurse's involvement should be very minimal and aim to guide gently rather than control the patient's descent.	Gravity will take the patient into the chair. Patients with muscle weakness may control their sitting up to a certain point and then abruptly descend. The nurse should not be liable to be dragged or unbalanced by this very likely occurrence.
5 Once seated, the patient may need support to lean or rock from side to side to enable the movement of the buttocks back in the chair.	If the patient leans to one side, the weight is partially lifted off the other, and so this side, once released in this way can more easily be moved backwards. It may be that the patient can do this with guidance or they may need some assistance. If the assistance required becomes significant it may be that the use of equipment is indicated (Alexander 2005).
6 Ensure that the patient is positioned well in to the backrest with feet flat on the ground and evaluate for the factors above.	Confirm that the criteria that apply to good seating are met for the patient.

Select a chair with the correct depth of seat for the patient. If the seat is too deep, the patient's back may not reach the support of the backrest, leading to strain and tension in the lower back. Too deep a seat may also lead to compression of the tissues at the back of the knee as described above. Tension on hamstring tendons behind the knee leads to contraction of the hamstring muscles—prolonged and sustained tension leads to shortening of these muscles (Martini 2006). Additionally, an over-deep seat may compromise the patient's ability to move from sitting to standing. A seat that is too shallow will simply not allow the patient to be secure and comfortable when seated.

Assess the height, shape, and size of the armrests for comfort and function. The patient's forearms should be comfortably supported without points of excessive pressure. The level of armrest should not result in raised or dropped shoulders, which will ultimately result in muscle tension. Good, well-positioned armrests can significantly assist some patients in rising from sitting as they can use them to bear some weight through their arms and then push themselves upright (Thomas 2005).

Aftercare

Once seated, evaluate the patient's ability to expand and relax the lungs comfortably and effectively. This may be noted while the patient speaks or by close observation of respiration (see Chapter 5). Also once seated, assess the patient's ability to maintain sitting balance safely and in a comfortable upright position. Additional support may be required: having insufficient support for the back will result in tension and back discomfort for the patient (O'Sullivan *et al.* 2006).

Key point: Good posture allows good lung expansion. Generally an upright position, in contrast to a reclined position, allows better lung filling and consequently, during speech, more syllables per breath (Redstone 2004).

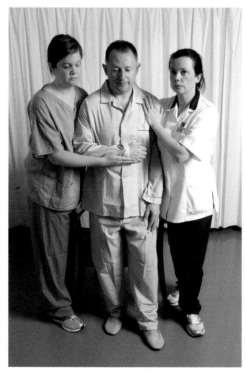

(a)

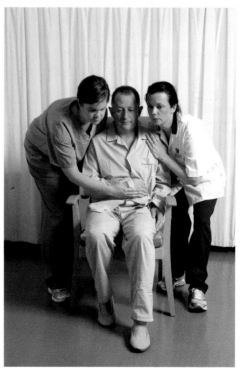

(b)

Figure 10.17 Assisting a patient to sit

Developing your skills

Regularly evaluate the comfort of the seated patient. In the frail patient, the change from being in bed to sitting up can, at first, be quite fatiguing. Time spent sitting should, therefore, be monitored and controlled as appropriate. Document the time spent sitting and any associated observations as relevant.

Other factors to consider:

Special pressure-relieving cushions are available and should be used in those at risk of developing pressure sores.

Some wheelchair patients will spend the bulk of their waking hours in their wheelchairs; these must, therefore, be correctly sized for them. Children will grow and need wheelchair upgrades. Adults may put on weight or need increasing support. There are specially designed wheelchairs for disabled sports. Wheelchairs also need regular maintenance and safety checks, so the patient should have planned time intervals for these services—often a sticker is placed on the chair indicating the time for next check. Again, the patient's ability to operate the chair safely should be regularly assessed, as should the competence of any relatives or carers who will also be operating the chair.

As with lying down, patients with neurological conditions such as cerebral palsy can often begin to contract into the shapes in which they are habitually placed. Regular positional change is important, particularly to maintain and sustain more upright postures.

Simply moving from being bedbound to sitting can be very beneficial to the patient psychologically. It represents another step towards normality.

10.6 **Performing a range of motion exercises**

Definition

Exercise can be active or passive. Patients who can independently move their limbs should be encouraged to do so (active) as they will benefit from the exercise. Those patients unable to move their limbs themselves will benefit when a nurse takes their joints and muscles comfortably through their normal range of motions for them (passive exercises). See **Fig. 10.18** for examples. This can be very beneficial in reducing stiffness and muscle wasting.

When a muscle is held immobile, the tissues remodel to their new resting length. This is termed adaptive shortening and will limit the range of motion (Everett 2001) that can be achieved. Exercise also enhances the circulation. In the legs, this decreases the risk of developing deep venous thrombosis (a blood clot in a vein in the leg).

When to assist a patient with exercise

The patients most likely to need assistance with active or passive exercise will be those that have a barrier to normal voluntary movement. The main barriers that might reduce the patient's ability to move the affected limb without assistance will be:

- Muscular—damage to a muscle, muscle group or tendons
- Skeletal—damage to bones, joints or ligaments
- Neurological—impaired or absent nerve messages to the affected area

Alternative interventions

There are a number of active exercises that patients can perform themselves when the above barriers do not restrict them from doing so. A physiotherapist should be consulted for specialist advice.

Working gently and smoothly and stopping at the point of any pain, discomfort, or fatigue, patients can take their own limbs through their normal range of motion to regain or retain that range. They can perform gentle muscle-stretching exercises but should always consider opposing muscle groups, for example when a stretch has involved the flexion of a limb (bending it towards the midline), it is good to balance that with a stretch that involves extension of the limb (straightening it away from the midline).

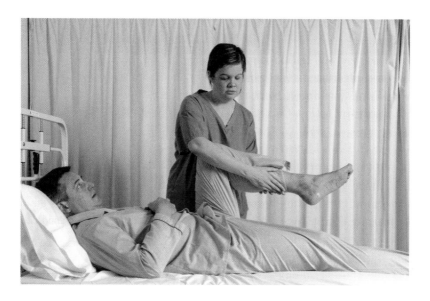

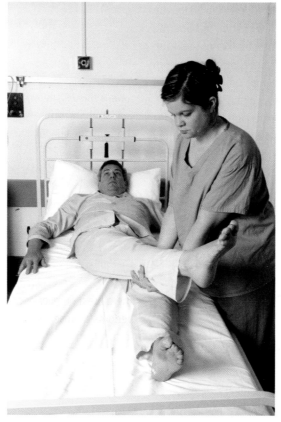

Figure 10.18 Passive movements: (a) flexing the leg at the knee; (b) adduction of lower limb (caution: this movement should *not* be performed on any patient with recent hip surgery)

Passive exercising

Usually no equipment is needed, but a specialized continuous passive motion device may be required in special circumstances.

Step	Rationale
1 Assess the patient's need for pain management measures.	Pain will reduce a patient's capacity to participate effectively in any form of exercise.
2 Ensure that the environment and the patient are sufficiently warm.	When cold, circulation is impaired and muscles and ligaments are less able to relax and stretch comfortably and, thus, more prone to injury and discomfort (Dowds 2007).
3 Ensure that there are no contraindications to performing exercises and establish any underlying cause for reduced mobility.	Performing exercises immediately after an injury may lead to increased inflammation. Tears in muscles or ligaments should be given a few days to heal. If the area is one where a recent fracture has been repaired, again a short period of healing must be allowed so that the repair is not destabilized. Patients with recent hip fixation should avoid adducting (bringing a limb to the midline) the femur beyond the midline for up to two months after surgery—this stresses the repair unnecessarily.
4 Where possible discuss, explain and agree the plan of care with the patient and the care team.	An involved patient given clear explanations and the rationale for interventions is more likely to cooperate with a programme that may involve effort and discomfort. Passive exercise is very valuable in the unconscious patient, so inform relatives if appropriate and confirm the validity of the plan of care with the other professionals caring for the patient.
5 Draw screens around the bed and adjust the patient's clothing to retain modesty.	Satisfy requirements for privacy and the maintenance of the patient's dignity.
6 Hold the limb gently without direct gripping and give support on either side of the joint. Perform movements slowly and smoothly.	Stimulation from gripping, jerky movements, and poor support can all lead to muscle tension and spasm.
7 Be very clear about not exceeding the normal range of motion for that area and closely observe the patient for signs of discomfort. Never force a joint beyond a point of resistance without due consideration of the potential for damage and pain.	Some joints, for example the elbow, can easily be damaged by overstretching.

8	The speed and duration of the movement should be considered against the level of effort, resistance, and discomfort encountered.	Smooth but brisk movements can enhance circulation but can over-stress areas not fully loosened off.
9	Place limbs in a comfortable supported position.	Maintain good alignment and reduce stress on joints.
10	Evaluate fatigue level of patient.	You will need to decide if the level of exercise should stay the same or be increased or reduced next time.
11	Consult with the patient about any need for further analgesia.	A patient who feels able to influence and gain control over pain is more likely to cooperate and participate again.
12	Consider whether a patient with, for example, one unaffected arm could perform some exercises unaided.	Participation in their own care can give patients a sense of empowerment. Ensure, however, that the patient moderates the activity and does not become overzealous.

Within the limits of their conditions; seated patients can extend and flex their lower limbs and arms while seated. Bedbound patients can stretch muscles, move limbs, and rotate ankles and wrists.

This type of purposeful activity may alleviate some of the boredom and frustration felt when restricted and may increase patients' engagement with their rehabilitation by involving them. Some patients, however, may need to be discouraged from attempting too much, too soon.

A machine can provide continuous passive movement, usually of a joint. The continuous passive motion device can be attached to an arm or leg and will mechanically move back and forth to a set range or angle and at a set number of movements per minute. Patient tolerance of the device must be closely monitored. For increasing muscular contractures, it may be necessary to prescribe the use of splints and a range of drugs, sometimes progressing up to local injections of botulinum toxin (Botox), which can be used to reduce excessive muscle tension (Pellat 2005).

Aftercare

Assess the need for additional analgesia or the need to increase the dose for subsequent sessions. Discuss this with the prescriber if necessary. Document the scope and duration of the activity and any relevant information, such as the presence or absence of pain, the range of motion

achieved, and any limiting factors. Limiting factors other than pain can include swelling, disturbances of circulation, or excessive muscle spasm.

Developing your skills

Ask a friend or colleague to perform passive movements of your limbs and assess your own level of discomfort and ability to cooperate during the procedure.

Other factors to consider

It is very important to value the specialist advice provided by the local physiotherapist in deciding what will be best for each patient.

For a child, and for many adults, it may help to make the active, or assisted active, exercises fun in some way, for example by using a ball in throwing or kicking games, or by having targets to achieve like stretching to ring a bell or buzzer. Slow rehabilitation can drain motivation, so having lots of small achievable targets or goals is much better than having abstract, distant ones.

Sometimes, young children or patients with a learning disability may not have the communication skills to let you know clearly that they are experiencing pain or discomfort. Good communication skills on your part will be necessary as well as close observation for signs of discomfort and intelligent interpretation of nonverbal cues (see Chapter 4).

10.7 **Managing more complex mobilizing needs**

Definition

Every patient is different and some may have quite individual mobilizing needs. Many types of patient can pose specific challenges to the delivery of effective care. This can be because of one or many influencing factors, as discussed previously. For example, those with hip fractures, spinal injuries, or amputations, or those who have had strokes, are unconscious or have disabilities. Another group of patients who have specific needs are those who are at risk of falls or who have fallen.

There are many different ways of moving these patients and many different pieces of equipment that can be used. It is not possible to discuss all of these here; however, if a thorough assessment has been carried out and the safe principles in the moving and handling section have been adhered to then most complex situations can be managed.

This section considers four of the most common complex mobilizing needs:

1 The falling patient,
2 The fallen patient,
3 The unconscious patient,
4 The uncooperative patient.

Preventing falls and assisting during a fall

Step		Rationale
1	Assess the patient and look at the patient's notes.	To ensure nurse and patient safety.
2	Have the patient sit.	To assist with the assessment.
3	Ask the patient to raise the lower part of the legs from the knee downwards until straightened.	A patient who is able to do this should be able to bear weight.
	If the patient can straighten the legs, stand the patient up.	This will allow you to assess if the patient can bear weight.
4	If the patient starts to fall, allow the patient to do so in a controlled way: • Release your hold of the patient, • Move behind the patient, • Open your hands and step backwards, • Allow the patient to slide to the floor, slowing their descent, where possible, with your arms/body.	It is safer for both the patient and the nurse to let the patient fall than to try and catch the patient.
5	The priority is to maintain the safety of the patient's head by cushioning it with your hands and ensuring that it does not hit any inanimate objects or the floor.	To protect the patient from a head injury.

Key point: The nurse or carer should be aware and prepared for the fact that every patient is different. Patients with complex needs require thorough moving and handling assessments to be carried out regularly and up-to-date records kept in their notes.

Procedure: The falling patient

It is important to assess an individual's capacity to bear weight before attempting any move, to prevent the patient from falling once standing. A patient is considered to be able to bear weight if they have the muscle power and joint range to stand and take weight through one or both feet, without the intervention of another person to provide support for the duration of the task being performed.

The patient's ability to bear weight is not always clear. You should also assess whether one side is weaker and whether any aid or assistance is required, and for how long the patient is capable of bearing weight.

Procedure: The fallen patient

Some patients may fall or collapse in hospital, the care home or their own home environment. Appropriate solutions should be in place; these may include hoists or inflatable systems.

Aftercare

If the patient has fallen, a falls risk assessment should be made and recorded in the patient's notes (see Chapter 3).

It may also be useful to request a physiotherapy review of the patient or to have the patient's medication reviewed. The initial priority is to ensure that the patient is as comfortable as possible. If there is no obvious injury, then do not rush the patient into standing, and follow the guidance given in this chapter. If there are signs of injury, assess the patient's level of coherence and understanding, reassure the patient, and wait until help arrives.

The patient should be reassessed and monitored to ensure that he or she is comfortable and to detect any changes in condition. The patient should be reassured and given an opportunity to discuss the events with the nurse. An incident or accident form should then be completed by the nurse and any witnesses, and the patient's moving and handling assessment form and nursing notes should be updated.

Procedure: The unconscious patient

Unconscious patients are at risk of many complications unless they are moved and repositioned regularly. There are also many risks associated with poor moving and handling practice. The unconscious patient should be considered as flaccid. Appropriate equipment can reduce the amount of nursing effort required. When moving the unconscious patient, the nurse must use hoists or horizontal transfer methods. Care must be given especially to the head and airway. Below is a summarized guide to positioning the unconscious (**unintubated**) patient (see **Fig. 10.19**).

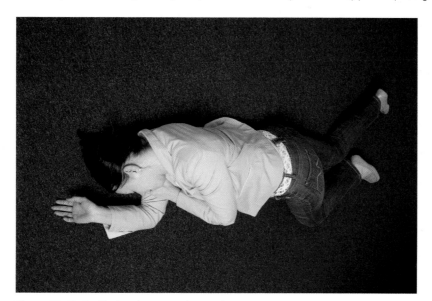

Figure 10.19 Positioning the unconscious patient

Assisting a patient who has fallen

This is the safe moving and handling procedure for moving the patient off the floor, if it is appropriate to do so.

Step		Rationale
1	Assess the situation and approach if safe.	To ensure nurse safety.
2	Assess the patient—are there signs of life, conscious level, obvious injuries?	To ensure priority care is given.
3	Make the patient comfortable—place a pillow under the head if appropriate.	To maintain patient comfort and dignity. Only use a pillow if no neck injury is suspected.
4	Get medical or nursing help.	To carry out patient assessment and to establish if it is safe to move the patient.
5	Treat any obvious injuries.	To reduce pain and prevent further injury.
6	Reassure the patient.	To ensure cooperation and reduce anxiety.
7	If the patient is able to get up from the floor, assist the patient to roll onto hands and knees. Place a chair beside the patient to lean on before standing up.	To encourage independence and increase confidence. To assess for postural hypotension.
8	If the patient is unable to get up, use a hoist. Alternatively, if patient is aware and has some balance, an inflatable system may be used to get to chair height (Smith 2005).	To prevent injury to the patient or nurse.

Positioning an unconscious patient

Step	Rationale
1 Assess patient fully.	To ensure nurse and patient safety.
2 Position patient in the lateral or semi-prone position.	To prevent airway blockage caused by tongue falling back. This will not be necessary if the trachea is intubated.
3 Place head in a neutral position with the aid of a pillow if required (the head of the bed may also be elevated slightly).	To ensure patient comfort, keep airway open, and allow venous drainage.
4 Keep the trunk straight (spinal alignment). Pillows may be needed.	To promote patient comfort and maintain alignment.
5 Bring the uppermost arm forwards in front of the patient, bend the elbow slightly, keep wrist extended.	To promote comfort.
6 Bring the lower arm alongside the face with the palm upwards.	To promote comfort.
7 Flex the uppermost leg: bring it forwards and support on pillows. Keep lower leg straight, in line with the spine and not touching the upper leg.	To promote comfort, prevent pressures sores, and prevent internal rotation of the hip.

Aftercare

The unconscious patient should be repositioned as required. This will depend on the individual patient and the pressure-relieving devices that are available. This will help prevent the complications of immobility that have been discussed in this chapter. It may be appropriate to think of other interventions that can help prevent the complications of immobility, for example, passive exercises (as discussed earlier) and anti-embolic stockings.

Procedure: The uncooperative patient

Patients can be uncooperative for a variety of reasons. The emphasis, as with all patients, needs to be on communication with the patient and risk assessment. Some of the common groups of people who fall into this category are those with learning disabilities, acute mental health needs, dementia, disorientation, disturbed behaviour through drugs or alcohol, or a personality disorder. They may have had previous bad experiences when being mobilized or are anxious, frightened, confused, or in pain.

If the patient chooses to lie on the floor, it is often safer to leave him or her there, provided that this is safe.

Every situation requires individual assessment and planning; however, some of the following solutions may help in certain situations.

Developing your skills

To help in moving and handling in these situations, communication skills are very important. Read over the

Moving an uncooperative patient

Step	Rationale
1 Assess patient fully.	To ensure nurse and patient safety.
2 Be encouraging, confident, and reassuring to your patient.	Reduces patient anxiety, which should improve cooperation.
3 Take a calm approach.	Reduces patient anxiety, which should improve cooperation.
4 Orientate the patient to the environment.	Reduces patient anxiety, which should improve cooperation.
5 Tell the patient what is expected of them.	Increases patient cooperation and so reduces the workload for the nurse.
6 Clearly and repeatedly state the instructions.	To increase patient understanding and, therefore, cooperation.
7 Assess the environmental factors and change them where possible, for example, floor patterns.	To ensure nurse and patient safety. To enhance a calming environment.
8 Give the patient as much control as possible over his or her own movements.	Increases patient cooperation and so reduces workload for the nurse. Enhances patient independence.
9 Guide the patient with the palm of your hand, that is, no gripping or sudden movements.	To maintain calm approach and cause no harm to the patient.
10 Keep close to the patient.	Maintains a feeling of security.
11 Take your time, especially when introducing patient to a new move or piece of equipment, for example, a hoist.	Time spent initially to make this a good experience will save time in the future.
12 Use appropriate moves based on your assessment.	To maintain nurse and patient safety.

information from nursing and psychology classes and practise your communication skills in the clinical area with patients and members of the multidisciplinary team.

When you are assessing a patient, with or without your mentor, always think about the patient as an individual with individual needs. Ask to see the local policy for moving these types of patient and discuss with your mentor any other needs that may need to be considered in patients with complex mobilizing needs.

Other patients to consider

Patients with spinal injuries

These patients should not be lifted manually or in a conventional hoist, as this would cause the patient to bend which could cause further injury. It is extremely important to maintain anatomical alignment of the vertebral column. Patients with a cervical spine injury are normally nursed in a supine position in bed. They are cared for in a Stryker bed with cervical traction that can allow the patient to be rotated (Griffiths and Gallimore 2005). These patients should only be moved under the direction of an experienced nurse.

Patients with hip fractures or who have had hip surgery

These patients cannot be rolled from side to side in the normal way, as the hip should not twist. They should, therefore, be moved with their affected leg held straight and without twisting their hip. Frames and special hoists can be used to help move these patients (Griffiths 2006). Early mobilization after surgery is vital to prevent the complications associated with immobility from arising and to encourage the rehabilitation of the patient.

Patients who have had strokes (cerebrovascular accidents)

A patient who has had a stroke is often not fully aware of sensations from one side of the body. A thorough assessment of these patients is again imperative to manage mobilizing needs appropriately. The nurse should help the patient control the affected side and be aware of this at all times when moving the patient to allow safe mobilization. Mobilization is very important for these patients as they are sometimes prone to **spasticity** (an increase in muscle tension or tone), which may lead to contractures. These contractures have a long-term damaging effect on mobility and the other activities of daily living and should be avoided. The physiotherapist will be actively involved in special therapy for these patients (Gibbon 2002).

Once, and if, these patients are able to bear weight, their environment should be assessed and be free of obstacles and they should be wearing appropriate footwear. Depending on their visual ability, they may need visual aids, such as eye patches to eliminate double vision. They will be referred to the physiotherapist and occupational therapists to assist in meeting their needs and in providing appropriate aids.

The patient who has had an amputation

The patient may have had a limb amputated as a result of trauma, vascular disease, or infected sores. Again, the assessment of these patients is vital to establish, amongst other things, the strength of the remaining limb, whether the patient has an artificial limb and how well it is used. Walking with an artificial leg requires much more energy than walking normally.

If the patient has just had the limb amputated then specific post-operative mobilizing techniques can be adopted. If the amputation is near the knee, sliding sheets can be used. Obviously, if the patient is unable to assist or is heavy, a hoist with a special sling should be used instead.

A pneumatic post-amputation mobility aid can be used to aid in early mobilization but nurses must be aware that the patient is a risk of falls owing to a change in the patient's centre of gravity and phantom sensation in the amputated limb. These patients will often require help to remain motivated and so nurses should be positive but realistic in their process of rehabilitation (Gibson 2001).

 ## Scenarios

Consider what you should do in the following situations, then turn to the end of the section to check your answers.

Further scenarios are available at **www.oxford-textbooks.co.uk/orc/docherty/**

 Scenario 1

Mrs Jones has been admitted to your ward with a broken hip. She is frail and 78 years old. Following repair of this fracture, she had a small stroke. Plans for early, active mobilization have been significantly disrupted, as she is unable to bear weight and now has difficulty in communicating.

Mrs Jones lives with her husband Joe. He, too, is frail and elderly and a little forgetful. He is very worried about his wife. They have two daughters in their forties, though one lives in New Zealand.

- In relation to her immobility, what will be the greatest risks faced by Mrs Jones?
- How could these risks be managed?
- Is any support available for her husband?

Scenario 2

William Rose is 68 years old and has dementia. William is unsteady when walking and frequently uncooperative.

Because of his problems mobilizing safely, the care home staff where he lives are concerned that he may fall and suffer a serious injury. William, however, is determined to investigate anything and everything of interest to him. He has had several small 'tumbles'.

How might William be managed with respect to:

- His risk of falling and sustaining an injury?
- His uncooperative behaviour?
- His need for exercise?

 Scenario 3

James Young is 7 and has **Down's syndrome** and mild learning disability. James has been hospitalized following a severe chest infection. James is now mobilizing freely in the ward area and loves attention. He is sometimes tearful but very affectionate and constantly asks to be picked up, hugged, and carried by the nurses. James weighs 30 kg, and while the nurses enjoy playing with him, two or three are finding that they are developing lower back discomfort

related to lifting and carrying him around.

- Should health and safety at work prevent nurses from comforting a young child?
- Are there ways to comfort James without bearing his weight?

Scenario 4

Tracy Whitman is 7 She has a broken leg in a cast and needs to use crutches to walk. It is very important to Tracy that she be able to return to school with her classmates despite her injury. In addition, Tracy is a very active child and she and her parents are concerned that she may suffer long-term impairment from this injury.

- Can Tracy return to school?
- What can be done to restore her to her previous flexibility and fitness?
- What other factors should be considered?

Website

www.oxfordtextbooks.co.uk/orc/docherty/

You may find it helpful to work through our short online quiz and interactive scenarios intended to help you to develop and apply the skills in this chapter.

References

Alexander P (2005). Sitting to sitting transfers. In Smith J, ed., *The Guide to the Handling of People*, 5th edn, pp. 159–87. National Back Pain Association and Royal College of Nursing, Teddington, UK.

Baillie L and Arrowsmith V (2006). Meeting elimination needs. In Baillie L, ed., *Developing Practical Nursing Skills*, 2nd edn, pp. 277–349. Hodder Arnold, London.

Brown A and McLennan A (2007). Moving and handling. In Jamieson EM, Whyte LA, and McCall JM, eds, *Clinical Nursing Practice*, 5th edn, pp. 213–18. Churchill Livingstone, Edinburgh.

Carpenito-Moyet LJ (2004). *Nursing Care Plans and Documentation: Nursing Diagnoses and Collaborative Problems*, 4th edn. Lipincott, Williams and Wilkins, Philadelphia.

Crowther M and McCourt K (2005). Venous thromboembolism: a guide to prevention and treatment. *The Nurse Practitioner*, **30**(8), 26–43.

Dowds M (2007). Exercises: active and passive. In Jamieson EM, Whyte LA, and McCall JM, eds, *Clinical Nursing Practice*, 5th edn, pp. 135–8. Churchill Livingstone, Edinburgh.

EPUAP (European Pressure Ulcer Advisory Panel) (2007). *Pressure Ulcer Guidelines*. www.pressureulcerguidelines.org/prevention/page12817.html.

Everett T (2001). Joint mobility. In Trew M and Everett T, eds, *Human Movement: An Introductory Text*, 4th edn, pp. 85–104. Churchill Livingstone, London.

Foss M and Farine T (2007). *Science in Nursing and Health Care*, 2nd edn. Pearson Education, London.

Fragala G, Fragala M, and Pontani-Bailey L (2005). Proper positioning of clients: a risk for caregivers. *AAOHN Journal*, **53**(10), 438–42.

Geraghty M (2005). Nursing the unconscious patient. *Nursing Standard*, **20**(1), 54–64.

Gibbon B (2002). Rehabilitation following stroke. *Nursing Standard*, **16**(29), 47–52.

Gibson J (2001). Lower limb amputation. *Nursing Standard*, **15**(28), 47–52.

Griffiths H (2006). Manual handling risk management: critical care beds and support systems. *Nursing Standard*, **20**(32), 45–53.

Griffiths H and Gallimore D (2005). Positioning critically ill patients in hospital. *Nursing Standard*, **19**(42), 56–64.

Hampton S (2003). The complexities of heel ulcers. *Nursing Standard*, **17**(13), 68–79.

Health and Safety Executive (2007). *Risk Assessment and Process Planning for Bariatric Patient Handling*. Loughborough University for the Health and Safety Executive. www.hse.gov.uk/research/rrhtm/rr573.htm.

Hignett S (2003). Systematic review of patient handling activities starting in lying, sitting, and standing position. *Journal of Advanced Nursing*, **41**(6), 545–52,

Kyle G (2006). Assessment and treatment of older patients with constipation. *Nursing Standard*, **21**(8), 41–6.

Lynn P (2008). *Taylor's Clinical Nursing Skills: A Nursing Process Approach*, 2nd edn. Lippincott, Williams and Wilkins, Philadelphia.

Martini F (2006). *Fundamentals of Anatomy and Physiology*, 7th edn, international edition. Pearson Education Inc. and Benjamin Cummings, San Francisco.

O'Sullivan PB, Dankaerts W, Burnett AF, *et al.* (2006). Effect of different upright sitting postures on spinal–pelvic curvature and trunk muscle activation in a pain-free population. *Spine*, **31**(19), 707–12.

Pellatt G (2005). Caring for people with impaired mobility. In Baillie L. ed., *Developing Practical Nursing Skills*, pp. 155–86. Hodder Education, London.

Pheasant S (2001). *Bodyspace: Anthropometry, Ergonomics and the Design of Work*, 2nd edn. Taylor and Francis, London.

Redstone F (2004). The effects of seating position on the respiratory patterns of preschoolers with cerebral palsy. *International Journal of Rehabilitation Research*, **27**(4), 283–88.

Resuscitation Council of the UK (2005). *Basic Life Support Guidelines*. www.resus.org.uk/pages/bls.pdf.

Royal College of Nursing and National Institute for Clinical Excellence (2005). *The Management of Pressure Ulcers in Primary and Secondary Care: A Clinical Practice Guideline*. www.nice.org.uk/nicemedia/pdf/CG029fullguideline.pdf.

Rush A (2006). *Overview of Bariatric Management*. Disability Living Foundation. www.dlf.org.uk/pdf/professional/Overview%20of%20Bariatric%20Management.pdf.

Smith J, ed. (2005). *The Guide to the Handling of People*, 5th edn. National Back Pain Association and Royal College of Nursing, Teddington, UK.

Thomas S (2005). Sitting to standing. In Smith J, ed., *The Guide to the Handling of People*, 5th edn, pp. 123–39. National Back Pain Association and Royal College of Nursing, Teddington, UK.

World Health Organization (2000). *Obesity: Preventing and Managing the Global Epidemic*. WHO, Geneva.

Useful further reading and websites

Allan D (2002). Caring for the patient with a disorder of the nervous system. In Walsh M, ed., *Watson's Clinical*

Nursing and Related Sciences, 6th edn, pp. 665–745. Balliere Tindall, London.

Athorn S and Hilton PA (2004). Mobilizing. In Hilton PA, ed., *Fundamental Nursing Skills,* pp. 20–42. Whurr Publishers Ltd, London.

Donnell C (2007). Mobility and immobility. In Brooker C and Waugh A, eds, *The Foundations of Nursing Practice: Fundamentals of Holistic Care,* pp. 501–29. Mosby Elsevier, Edinburgh.

This is a general nursing textbook for all nursing students undertaking the common foundation programme.

Hignett S, Crumpton E, Ruszula S, Alexander P, Fray M, and Fletcher B (2003) Evidence-based patient handling: systematic review. *Nursing Standard,* **17**(33), 33–6.

Hignett S and McAtamney L (2005). Rapid entire body assessment: REBA Appendix 1. In Smith J, ed., *The Guide to the Handling of People,* 5th edn, pp. 291–6. National Back Pain Association and Royal College of Nursing, Teddington, UK.

Moody P, Gonzales I, and Cureton VY (2004). The effect of body position and mattress type on interface pressure in quadriplegic patients: a pilot study. *Dermatology Nursing,* **16**(6), 507–12.

Moore Z (2005). Pressure ulcer grading. *Nursing Standard,* **19**(52), 56–64.

Office of the Public Guardian (2008). *Additional Publications and Newsletters.* www.publicguardian. gov.uk/mca/additional-publicationsa-newsletters.htm.

Royal College of Nursing (2001). *Manual Handling Assessments in Hospitals and the Community: An RCN Guide.* Royal College of Nursing, London.

This guide gives general practical advice on the topic of manual handling risk assessments, both in hospital and in the community, to prevent back injuries to staff involved in patient handling.

Royal College of Nursing (2002). *Code of Practice for Patient Handling.* Royal College of Nursing, London.

This code offers a framework for implementing the Manual Handling Regulations and the recommendations for lifting from the Health Services Advisory Committee.

Ruszala S (2005). Controversial techniques. In Smith J, ed., *The Guide to the Handling of People,* 5th edn, pp. 273–84. National Back Pain Association and Royal College of Nursing Teddington, UK.

Scottish Executive (2008). *Adults with Incapacity.* www. scotland.gov.uk/Topics/Justice/Civil/awi.

Smith J, ed. (2005). *The Guide to the Handling of People,* 5th edn. National Back Pain Association and Royal College of Nursing Teddington, UK.

This is an excellent book for all nurses and covers how to move patients safely as well as legislation, risk assessment, and **ergonomics**. It is written in line with the Royal College of Nursing's code of practice for 'a safe patient-handling policy'.

Van Duersen RWM and Everett T (2001). Biomechanics of human movement. In Trew M and Everett T, eds, *Human Movement: An Introductory Text,* 4th edn, pp. 37–68. Churchill Livingstone, London.

Welch E (2005). The assessment and management of venous thromboembolism. *Nursing Standard,* **20**(28), 58–64.

Check 🌐 **www.oxfordtextbooks.co.uk/orc/docherty/** for changes and new developments. Updated research, guidelines, or equipment will be added every four months.

Answers to scenarios

Scenario 1

- In relation to her immobility, what will be the greatest risks faced by Mrs Jones?
  - Deep venous thrombosis is a significant risk after major surgery,
  - Mrs Jones will be at a high risk for development of pressure ulcers,
  - It is likely that Mrs Jones will tend towards dehydration and malnourishment if a strategy to supplement her voluntary intake is not adopted. She may also have swallowing difficulties secondary to the stroke,
  - A chest infection is possible, especially if Mrs Jones has swallowing problems,
  - Mrs Jones is likely to suffer some degree of constipation,
  - Mrs Jones will lose muscle strength,
  - Mrs Jones may become disoriented.
- How could these risks be managed?
  All these risks will be reduced through pursuing a programme to increase mobility and exercise.
  - For deep vein thrombosis, also use elastic stockings and anticoagulants,

- For pressure ulcers, formally assess Mrs Jones's risk and regularly reposition her. Consider a special pressure relieving mattress.
- For nutrition and hydration, carefully monitor Mrs Jones's input and output and supplement as necessary. In the short term, **intravenous** fluids may be required.
- To prevent chest infections; encourage movement, deep breathing, and coughing. Analgesia may be required if pain is further restricting Mrs Jones's desire to move and cough. Her swallowing capability should be assessed; in case she is at risk of aspirating (inhaling) her food.
- Some passive movements will retain some muscle strength, but are no substitute for weight-bearing exercise.
- Orientation can be improved with good clear communication and ensuring she is regularly engaged in conversation.

- Is any support available for Mrs Jones's husband?
  - Mr Jones's capacity to cope by himself at home should be considered.
  - It may be necessary to explore options for Mr Jones's continuing support with various agencies providing social services.
  - Their daughter should be involved closely in this assessment. She should consider her capacity to support her father in his own home and alternatives to this.
  - There is a high risk that Mrs Jones will die in hospital of one or several complications.
  - If Mrs Jones survives, she may need long-term residential care. Mr Jones and her daughter need to consider the implications of this to them.
  - The daughter in New Zealand should have the gravity of her mother's condition clearly explained, in case she wishes to visit her sooner rather than later.

😑 Scenario 2

- How might William be managed with respect to his risk of falling and sustaining injury?
  - A structured falls risk assessment should be carried out to formally identify William as a patient at risk of falling.
  - This status should be clearly communicated to all the care staff and William's relatives.
  - The environment in which William mobilizes should be made as safe as possible. Ensure no trip hazards, such as cables and uneven flooring. Remove or pad sharp-edged furniture and fittings.
  - Consider whether William will tolerate wearing hip protection pads.
  - The likelihood of William experiencing a fall injury should be discussed with his family, explaining that not restraining or sedating him is a positive choice in his interest. An almost inevitable risk of injury should not be seen as negligence but rather as a probable consequence of not trespassing against his human right to basic freedoms.

- How might William be managed with respect to his uncooperative behaviour?
  - Caring for a patient with dementia can be frustrating. Staff must retain a calm and patient approach.
  - Having a rota system for staff to supervise more awkward residents will spread the workload more fairly and avoid overstressing any single nurse.
  - Enlisting the support and cooperation of loved ones recognized by William will be most effective in gaining his trust.
  - A firm but nonconfrontational approach, using diversion rather than authority, is more likely to win his cooperation.
  - Sedation should be considered as a last resort in the elderly, as it tends to exacerbate confusion.

- How might William be managed with respect to his need for exercise?
  - It is not permissible to restrain a patient simply because there is a fear of falling. Exercise is necessary to reduce the complications of immobility.
  - Setting aside times when William can specifically receive one-to-one care and be encouraged to mobilize with supervision will give him set episodes of exercise: this may reduce his need for wandering outside of these sessions.
  - Stimulation and distraction through other activities may reduce his need to seek stimulation in wandering about.

Scenario 3

- Should health and safety at work prevent nurses from comforting a young child?
  - No. However, an injured nurse will not be caring for anyone.
  - Loads come in all shapes and sizes: human beings can represent the most awkward of these. However, whether your job involves people or boxes, there should be systems and ways of working that minimize the risk of injury.
  - Just as in industry, it may be possible for the care team to agree a system for coping with the handling demands presented by James.
  - This could be described as a frequently occurring hazard in this type of environment.
- Are there ways to comfort James without bearing his weight?
  - Rather than picking James up for a hug, the nurse should drop to one knee and hug him. Care of the knees will have to be considered though!
  - A mobile child should be encouraged to walk rather than be carried.
  - Taking James by the hand and diverting him with conversation and activity should easily substitute for carrying.
  - With a consistent approach by all the staff, James should come to accept in a short time that he is not going to be lifted and carried—simply saying to him that your back is sore should suffice as explanation.
  - With sensitive management he should become aware that he is receiving the same amount of attention and affection as before. In fact, he may end up with more if the nurses are no longer worried about hurting themselves.

 Scenario 4

- Can Tracy return to school in time with her cast?
  - With most simple breaks, as soon as Tracy is plastered she can go home. After a short period to allow pain and inflammation to abate, she should be encouraged to mobilize to prevent further complications of immobility.

- Some assessment and selection of optimum crutch style and size—usually elbow crutches—and some coaching in their proper use, will be of benefit.
- Propelling herself over long distances will be fatiguing and can result in falls or strain on wrists, elbows, and shoulders. Therefore, a strategy of using the bus or getting a lift to and from school may be necessary in the short term.
- Most schools are designed, or have been modified, to facilitate students, and teachers, with disabilities.
- Clearly, Tracy's ability to participate in physical education will be limited, but she should be able to manage most classes.
- What can be done to restore Tracy to her previous flexibility and fitness?
  - Maintaining activity is important.
  - The muscles of the plastered leg will lose strength and the joint will stiffen. At this age, though, Tracy should easily recover to regain full function.
  - Moderate activity will keep Tracy reasonably fit—overdoing things while in a cast can result in strains and sometimes back pain. Tracy should be sensible.
  - Once the cast is removed, Tracy should progressively increase movements that enhance her range of motion, always paying attention to discomfort.
  - For keen sports fans, specialist physiotherapy may be worth pursuing and there a number of physiotherapist working in the health service with this interest.
  - Any interruption to the integrity of Tracy's now quickly growing skeleton may mean that the injured leg, while healing well, may not grow as efficiently as her uninjured leg. Tracy will need ongoing monitoring to ensure that this is not the case—if it is, she may require additional surgery and perhaps bone grafting to lengthen that limb.
- What other factors should be considered?
  - Strong psychological and emotional factors are likely to motivate Tracy to not miss school. Many social partnerships and alliances will be forged in the early days and Tracy will not want to miss this.
  - Tracy will not want to stand out as significantly different from her peers, so will have to consider strategies to minimize her disability.

- The use of humour may help her to de-emphasize her broken leg and support the fact that this is only a temporary setback. She could collect signatures on the cast.
- One advantage may be that when meeting many new faces, Tracy will be memorable.
- Individual self-expression is important; this is frequently done through dress. Tracy may need to focus on her upper half while she wears old torn jeans around the leg casts—skirts would be good but might not fit into the prevailing fashion.
- As an active child, Tracy will find being unable to participate in physical activity very frustrating.
- While striving for independence Tracy is going to have to concede that she is slightly dependent— acceptance of this will reduce her frustration.

Working and playing

PETER JOHNSTONE

Introduction

Working and playing are central to human development. Working is associated with paid employment, but not all jobs, occupations, or businesses are well paid, and some are even voluntary. It must also be remembered that work can also mean craft, diversion, hobby, interest, pursuit, or recreation; so work may have a **therapeutic** role, as does play.

At the most simplistic level, there are parallels in what work and play can offer the developing person:

- Physiologically, work provides the adult physical and mental stimulation, as well as potential to acquire skills. The same is provided to the child through play, with gross **motor** skills being acquired prior to fine motor control
- Developmentally, both work and play encourage **cognitive** progression
- Psychologically, both work and play encourage association and interaction
- Spiritually, both encourage/promote a sense of belonging, and play may promote morality
- Socioculturally, both promote cooperation, integration and communication

All of the above can be affected by short- and long-term illness, physical and cognitive impairments, and mental illness, no matter what the age of the individual.

This chapter introduces the basics, to assist you in assessing the developmental stages of play and to facilitate the organization or facilitation of suitable play and recreational activities, no matter what the age of the patient.

Many topic areas in foundation nursing programmes, such as first aid, moving and handling, infection control, and therapeutic management of aggression and violence, are generic in nature, to be relevant to all client groups. The underlying principles relating to the skills in this chapter similarly apply to whichever branch of nursing the student embarks on, although most of the examples will apply to child and learning disability branches.

Learning outcomes

These outcomes relate to numbers 9 and 11 of the NMC's Essential Skill Clusters and specifically to Care Domains 2 and 3 of the NMC's Standards of Proficiency for Pre-registration Nursing (outcomes to be achieved for entry to branch).

On reading this chapter and on interacting with the web pages and undertaking supervised activities, the student will be able to:

- Understand the different stages of play and the ages at which children normally achieve them
- Know which healthcare professional to consult if you suspect a child is not at the developmental age expected
- Be able to select toys and activities suitable for infants, toddlers, and children of any age
- Question adolescents and adults to assess their preferences for activities and facilitate access to their preferred pastimes
- Suggest and monitor group play or social activities appropriate for children, adolescents, and adults
- Be able to select activities that will help a patient develop particular abilities

- **Sensory** skills, that is, stimulation of the senses-vision, listening, talking, touching, and smelling,
- Fine or gross motor skills,
- Cognitive skills,
- Social skills.

Prior knowledge

It is important that you have the knowledge and understanding of the following, which can be obtained from a range of reference books (see, for example, Brooker and Waugh 2007; Grandis *et al.* 2003; Hinchcliff *et al.* 2003; Heath 2001; Hubband and Trigg 2000).

Developmental physiology

- Self-awareness: eyes—see; hand—reaches; mouth then hand—feels
- Sensory-motor development: tactile, auditory, visual, and kinaesthetic stimulation
- Gross and fine motor skills acquisition: head control precedes the ability to sit, stand and walk. There is a developmental sequence, hence, grasping a crayon precedes holding a pencil with a pincer movement
- Creative skills: creativity can be developed and nurtured in early life and skills transferred to an alternative context or setting as the child grows, that is, skills developed as a child may lead to greater potential to be imaginative, ingenious, inventive, adaptable, or talented, depending on the opportunities that were made, or that were available when young

Developmental psychology

- **Attachment**: how parents, family, and infants bond (Ginsburg *et al.* 2007)
- Self-awareness concepts: the process of self-identity
- Intellectual development: numbers, colours, spatial relationships, and even abstract concepts
- Creative skills development: experimentation, exploration, fantasy, and make believe

Developmental sociology

- Self-awareness concepts: testing abilities and learning the effect that behaviour has on others

- Development of social and moral values: fairness, honesty, self-control, and learning to consider others
  - Intellectual development: developing new **perceptions** and relationships by assimilating past experiences,
  - Creative skills development: listening to others, re-exploring own ideas, developing something new.

Background

The importance of play

Play is one of the most important activities in a child's development. Through it, the child gradually experiences the skills, attitudes, and modes of behaviour appropriate to adult life. It must be noted that the development of your play skills will be ongoing throughout placements in any appropriate setting, whether a children's ward, nursery, school, family-based placement, or even web-based/simulated settings.

Play is important in a child's life, so that the child may:

- Learn self-awareness
- Learn to deal with the stresses of daily living
- Develop sensory or motor activity
- Develop intellectual skills
- Develop **socialization** skills and moral values
- Develop creative skills

Without the stimulation and activity of play, any or all of the above can be affected. Play is important because children may not be capable of verbally expressing their anxiety or confusion: play can aid an adult's understanding of what the child is thinking and feeling. Its use as an assessment and intervention tool can only happen if there is good communication through trust built over time, requiring effort and sensitivity on the part of the adult (Darbyshire 1994).

The educative role of play in hospital prepares the child for a hospital stay and any unpleasant experiences that treatment may involve. Through play, explanations can be provided in a way that the child can understand. The therapeutic function of play is primarily aimed at alleviating the child's stress, but it can also help reduce the parent's anxiety (Ginsburg *et al*. 2007). Finally, play as a means of physical exercise improves health and can be great fun.

Play can be incorporated into many procedures and nursing interventions, for both diversional and educational purposes. As a diversion in potentially stressful situations, play can aid relaxation and cooperation. It also helps to promote security, releases tension and may allow for expression of feelings. Play enhances interaction and may aid in the development of a positive attitude towards others while providing a means for accomplishing therapeutic goals. It also provides the child the opportunity to express choices and be in control (Ginsburg *et al*. 2007).

In a similar vein, the physical, mental, social, sexual, **emotional**, and spiritual life of adults can be affected by employment or unemployment. This is linked to the notion that through being gainfully employed, an individual is making a contribution to the wider community. Societies promote and encourage conformity to socially accepted norms. Within this context, it is worth considering the negative effects of inadequate social and educational integration of children and young people with special needs within the wider society, attitudes towards individuals with mental health problems, as well as the general attitude towards people who are dependent on state benefits.

Motor, sensory, cognitive, and social skills develop throughout life. Whether a skill develops or not depends on opportunities to practise. This is easily understood when motor skill development is considered: cycling, skateboarding, skiing, knitting, sewing, and calligraphy must all be developed and practised until they are mastered. So too with sensory skills: exposure to altered sensory states tends to increase tolerance, as exemplified in bungee jumping, exposure to addictive substances, and other thrill-seeking behaviour. With cognitive skills, brain-training programmes are becoming increasingly popular. Finally, social skills are acquired and honed through praising and rewarding conformity to socially and morally acceptable behaviour (Townley 2002).

Sensory abilities

Touch, smell, vision, hearing, and vocalization are all present from birth and their nature and importance evolves as we develop (Hinchcliff *et al*. 2003):

- Touch, without permission, becomes a problem as we grow older
- Smell becomes more important, as taste for food and attraction to others develops
- Vision is important to the sighted, as aestheticism matters in today's world
- Hearing matters: among other things, it allows the young to learn and to develop linguistic skills, so being deaf can impede speech acquisition. Loss of hearing that may occur with age can lead to frustration and marginalization

Loss of any of the senses can lead to safety issues:

- Loss of touch, feeling, sensation can reduce awareness of burns or other skin damage
- Loss of smell can reduce awareness of burning, or malodorous decomposing foodstuffs
- Loss of vision may reduce awareness of smoke or fire, or traffic when crossing the road
- Loss of hearing may reduce awareness to fire alarms, door bells, or telephones

In addition to these safety issues, loss of sensory input from any of the above can lead to the individual being unable to articulate thoughts and feelings and reduces the individual's capability to express opinions or choices concerning an aspect of life.

Senses require stimulation to develop or just to be maintained; hence, brain training and memory games can be popular with all ages.

In all sectors of healthcare, there are many therapists who contribute to sensory development or its maintenance, for example, occupational therapists, physiotherapists, audiologists, optometrists, and speech and language therapists.

Motor abilities

In natural development, gross motor skills precede the ability to develop fine motor skills (Heath 2001; Hinchcliff *et al*. 2003). Without the ability to control the neck and head, it is not possible to sit. The ability to sit allows for standing; standing precedes walking, initially with a wide **gait**, then developing into a more refined gait.

Gross motor skills can be maintained with walking, dancing, and aerobics, even in an armchair. Maintaining movement is essential, as inactivity is associated with obesity, muscle wasting, and depression, amongst other potential problems

Fine motor skills can be maintained by writing, painting, knitting, dominoes, and other games.

Group activity and sports encourage cooperation and camaraderie as well as offering diversion. Activity develops self-worth and releases feel good chemicals called endorphins.

Cognitive abilities

Cognitive skills can develop with age, in the absence of learning disability or mental health issues, but opportunities for cognitive engagement must be made available for this to happen (Brooker and Waugh 2007; Heath 2001). The tendency is for increasing age to lead to diminution of cognitive skills but this is not inevitable and is often associated with physical health problems and decreased social interaction. This can be minimized by stimulation such as reminiscence therapy and other forms of brain training or stimulation.

Social abilities

An individual's lifestyle and social functioning may be affected temporarily or permanently by disability, dependency, and economic constraints, such as becoming redundant, or immobile with limited access to transport (Brooker and Waugh 2007; Grandis *et al.* 2003). Many health-related factors can lead to social isolation and stigma, as exemplified in people with mental illness, learning disabilities, and those with disfigurement and disease. Social inclusion and acceptance of variability is the mark of a civilized society.

11.1 **Assessment of developmental stage for play**

Definition

Children of different ages will need very different play activities. To select appropriate toys and activities for

children, nurses need to be able to recognize a child's developmental stage. This can normally be determined by the child's age, but it must also be recognized that skill acquisition cannot occur in a vacuum or nonstimulating environment (Price and McNeilly 2006).

This section covers normal child development within the first year, a critical time when nurture may alter nature: without the correct opportunities a child may not reach full potential (Taylor *et al.* 1999).

Background

Typical stages of development

To understand play and be able to carry out an assessment of the child's development it is important to understand what the different stages of development are. These are shown in **Table 11.1**.

Birth weight doubles by five or six months and trebles by one year. The length of the infant increases by 50% in the first year, and usually doubles by four years of age. Any inappropriate inputs or interventions in the first five years (but especially the first two years) can have a long-term or even permanent effect on the developing person. Please also refer to the work of Freud, Piaget, and Erikson for theories of continuing development (Brooker and Waugh 2007; Heath 2001).

In the earliest phases of social development, the infant does not conceive of objects as being external to him or her; for the infant there is no outside world. It is only through sensory experience that the child comes to recognize the external world as other to him or herself. Though child's play is initially solitary, it is through play that children develop contact with other people. While playing, children practise language, communication, and interpersonal skills and learn to cooperate with each other, share, and compete.

Toddlers have very little interest in other children; they tend to be interested only in their own activities and not in those of others. Everything is 'me'. At this age, children think that the world revolves around them, and only exists for them. Between the ages of two and three years, the child begins to exhibit parallel play, in which he or she plays next to but not with other children. As shown by this type of play, children at this age are self-centred

Table 11.1 The stages of growth and development in the first year of life

Age	Development
Birth to 3 months	**Motor, sensory:** primitive reflexes, sucking, grasp, startle response to sudden sound.
	The infant cries, grimaces, and extends limbs when agitated and distressed.
1–3 months	**Motor, sensory:** holds head up momentarily, makes crawling movements when prone.
	Social, understanding: smiles responsively.
3–4 months	**Motor, sensory:** lifts head from prone position for short periods, turns head towards sounds.
	Social, understanding: smiles.
	Speech: makes sounds when spoken to.
	Manipulative: begins to watch own hands, can grasp a rattle or toy.
4–9 months	**Motor, sensory:** rolls from side to side when lying on back, turns head to talking person.
	Social, understanding: shows pleasure with crowing and cooing.
	Speech: vocalizes, grunting, says 'da', 'ma'.
	Manipulative: begins to pass objects from hand to hand, also able to manipulate objects.
9–10 months	**Motor, sensory:** sits up from lying.
	Social, understanding: recognizes and rejects strangers, shouts for attention and imitates.
	Speech: babbles and vocalizes, says single words like 'Mum Mum' and 'Da Da'.
	Manipulative: Picks up objects between fingers and thumb, (pincer movement).
10 months to 1 year	**Motor, sensory:** crawls well, pulls upright, may walk with support.
	Social, understanding: obeys simple commands and imitates adults, shows variety of emotions.
	Speech: says single words like 'dog', 'bus' and sibling's names.
	Manipulative: holds cup to drink.

and have difficulty sharing with others. They interpret toys, not in terms of general properties, but in terms of their use.

A pre-school child progresses from solitary play through parallel play to cooperative play. During cooperative play, the nature and verbal exchanges of the child become much more adult-like (minus adult understanding). During this time, the children play with each other instead of just next to each other, and they talk and listen to what others in the group have to say, and then answer appropriately.

The acquisition of social norms may start for some children at this age.

Social skills develop early. By the age of three months, an infant can recognize familiar faces, and acquire social skills and eye contact through play. When spoken to by an adult, a child will respond by cooing and smiling. From six to nine months, a baby enjoys mirrors and simple games with people, such as peek-a-boo and clapping hands. The child is capable of looking and reaching at this stage. To the child, objects that cannot be seen, heard, or touched do not exist.

As children's ability to master physical objects improves, they become much more interested in their peer group, that is, they prefer playing with children who have had the same or similar experiences to themselves. Playing with children of the same age, the child learns how to compete, cooperate, and compromise. In cooperative play, the children work towards a common goal, which is determined by them. A lot of organization goes into the achievement of the goal. There is a great sense of awareness either of belonging or not belonging to a group. Social inclusion and exclusion can occur with toddlers and pre-schoolers for the most obscure of reasons. By school age most children can offer some sort of explanation for socially excluding a peer, but as before this can be somewhat obscure.

Cooperation occurs in games. such as football, rounders, 'tig', and hide and seek, and other culturally specific forms of team play. In these games, each child must know the rules of the game, and where team effort, competitiveness, and organization are essential. If you do not conform to group norms and you break the rules, you may find yourself excluded from the group. Cooperation applies equally in the learning disability, mental health, and adult elderly sectors.

When to assess a child's developmental age for play

Nurses should assess the child's developmental age for play at each and every opportunity. In certain situations, a play therapist would do this instead, for example in a developmental assessment unit; but in an outpatients department or pre-admission programme, play will be overseen by nursing staff.

Special considerations

There are many reasons why children might not show normal development, and most would already be known when assessing developmental age for play, for example, if the child has a learning disability, or an illness that affects sensory or motor skills (Hinchcliff *et al.* 2003). The experience of being in hospital and being unwell may also affect the child's normal behaviour patterns and social skills. Please note that medications and treatment can affect cognitive skills too.

Procedure: Assessing stages of play development

The nurse should assess a child's developmental age for play by observation or interaction with the child and parent or carer. **Table 11.2** outlines what skills the baby or child is developing at each stage, and these stages are also depicted in **Fig. 11.1** While this model of play development is primarily influenced by the work of Parten, developed during the 1930s. The works of Piaget, Vygotsky, and Mead are relevant too (Brooker and Waugh 2007; Heath 2001).

Aftercare

If the student suspects that a child is not ready for toys or activities typical of his or her age, a referral should be made to someone more senior for an assessment or observation. Initially, students would refer to their mentor or facilitator for this guidance.

Table 11.2 Stages of play development

Stage of play (typical age at which it is reached)	What to look for
Parent and baby play Usually up to one year of age	Senses being developed: sight, hearing, touch, and smell. Also essential for pre-vocalization and socialization.
	Some autistic spectrum patients may not appear to develop beyond this stage.
Solitary play 1–2 years, or more	The child plays alone with different toys, despite other children being in the room. The child makes no attempt to interact, and is totally absorbed in his or her own activity. This is a stage of great independence and self-reliance.
	Sharing and being sociable is unlikely at this stage. Some individuals with a learning disability may appear to be stuck at this stage.
Parallel play 2–3 years	The child is quite happy to watch others at play, shows great interest and may even copy, but does not necessarily participate.
	The initial stages of being sociable are developing, but at a safe distance.
Spectator play 3–4 years	The children play independently of each other, even though they may have the same toys. This is characteristic of toddlers and is the beginning of being sociable.
	The children learn to be much more sociable. They play as a group and discuss what they want to do, that is, play becomes organized. The children learn to share at this stage. They learn ground rules and there is a marked sense of belonging or not belonging. Leaders may emerge.
Cooperative play 4–5 years	Although an adult is depicted in Fig 11.1, a group of pre-school children may learn to play cooperatively on their own.
	Depending on the children's mental, social, or emotional age, some may falter here.
	Theoretically antisocial tendencies may begin at this stage.
Group play 4–5 years, and beyond	The children are advancing much more socially; they are not just learning the rules, but must learn to stick by them.
	Not even all adults play by the rules, and some may never be group players.

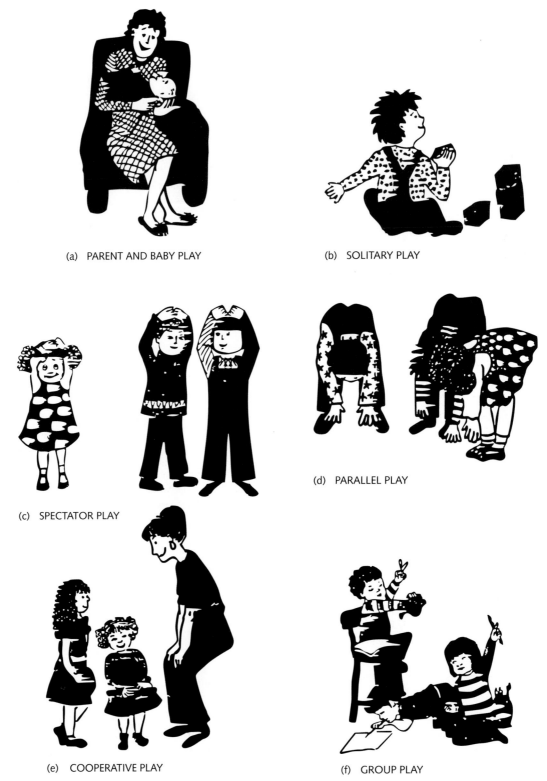

(a) PARENT AND BABY PLAY

(b) SOLITARY PLAY

(c) SPECTATOR PLAY

(d) PARALLEL PLAY

(e) COOPERATIVE PLAY

(f) GROUP PLAY

Figure 11.1 (a) Parent and baby play, (b) solitary play, (c) spectator play, (d) parallel play, (e) cooperative play, (f) group play

Other factors to consider

Working with other members of the healthcare team

No matter the setting, inputs from other members of the interdisciplinary team are essential. You will work with play leaders, physiotherapists, occupational therapists, speech and language therapists, and others, as you progress in your studies and beyond.

- Play leaders or play therapists have specialist training in both the recreational and therapeutic uses of play in a variety of care settings and can be a great resource in any team caring for younger patients
- Physiotherapists supply treatment programmes not only in hospital settings but also in wider community settings
- Occupational therapists can be found in a variety of settings and may have a role in maintaining present functionality or facilitating acceptable adaptations. While many occupational therapists work in the adult sector, and in mental health and learning disabilities, some specialists work with children. Adult and community-based occupational therapists will have to know a wide range of issues concerning their clients, for example, living arrangements, physical limitations, occupation (present and any future), and even finances
- Speech and language therapists can be found in both hospital and community settings, facilitating speech, language, and communication skills as well as ensuring that sucking, swallowing, and breathing are coordinated

Availability of the above therapists depends on each Area Health Authority's economics and priorities.

Working with play leaders

The following points are some of the aspects that the play leader (in a hospital setting) should know about the child to ensure maximum benefit from play (Grandis *et al.* 2003). Equally, therapists in the learning disability, mental health and elderly settings will benefit from similar information:

Name This should include preferred name. Not all children (or adults) use their first name and some shorten their name.

Chronological age This normally indicates the expected or socially accepted norms of a person that age: this may not always be the case, for example, in an individual with learning disabilities.

Mental age This is generally a reasonable indicator of intellectual development and is particularly useful in learning disabilities.

Any physical limitations Knowing this prevents an individual from being asked to do the impossible. It also reduces the potential for embarrassment and the possibility of a patient's misplaced anger.

Any prosthesis The presence of an artificial limb should be known.

Dietary restrictions (if any) While some dietary issues may only lead to gastro-intestinal upsets, for example, lactose intolerance, some can be potentially fatal, for example, peanut intolerance.

The play leader can give feedback to the nursing and medical staff regarding the social interactions of the child and the effectiveness of the prescribed therapy, if any. Similar communication occurs between occupational therapists, physiotherapists, and nurses for all client groups, whether in hospital or community settings.

11.2 **Suggesting suitable play and recreational activities for patients**

Definition

In all care settings, the aim is to maintain and develop the skills and senses of perception that an individual possesses, while preventing their deterioration in those at risk. Therefore, it is important to be able to select the most appropriate play and recreational activities for the individual no matter what the age or development.

Selecting toys and activities suitable for babies up to 6 months old

Toys or activity	Developmental benefit
Birth to 3 months	**Physical**: sight
	Cognitive: sensory, novelty, enhances perception
Rattles: Note that rattles must not be shared between babies to avoid transmitting infection	**Motor, sensory**: holds head up momentarily, makes crawling movements when prone
	Social, understanding: smiles responsively
Music boxes	**Physical:** stimulates hearing; music can soothe and lull infant to sleep and can cover household noises; provides sensory novelty
Rubber and teething rings and rubber animals (no sharing)	**Physical:** provides **oral** stimulation and exploration, assists with grasping and holding; can soothe painful gums during teething
Soft cuddly toys, and stuffed toys (no sharing)	**Physical:** stimulates sense of touch, texture, warmth
	Emotional: stimulates sense of comfort and security, warmth and sensory novelty

When to suggest play or recreational activities

A nurse needs to observe patient's normal activity and recognize any drop in interest in activities as an important indicator of possible problems. When to suggest activities and when not to intervene is a decision that needs to be carefully considered. The decision to intervene may be guided by:

- The availability of toys or activities,
- The patient's choices and preferences, or
- The therapeutic aim of developing a particular skill.

More often than not, organizing and facilitating these activities is likely to be the responsibility of a specific member of the multidisciplinary team, who may be your mentor or facilitator.

Procedure: Selecting activities suitable for adolescents

Adolescents may 'conform by nonconformity', for example, being a member of a group or gang, such as Goths, Emos, Preppy (Label worshipper), Geeks. While in hospital, the adolescent's position in a ward can play a big part in making him or her feel part of the team, thus avoiding isolation. The methods suggested to discourage social isolation in when selecting activities suitable for adults (see later) can also be used with adolescents (Russell-Johnson 2000).

Adolescents should be enabled to make choices when at all possible. Encourage independence and allow them to explore the environment. Introduce adolescent patients to the ward staff, and make regular ward routines known to them as soon after their admission as possible. Ensure that there is a suitable place for storing personal belongings.

Selecting toys and activities suitable for babies of 7 to 12 months

Toys or activity	Developmental benefit
Dolls	**Emotional:** can be used to promote a sense of security and for hugging
Peek-a-boo	**Social:** discovery stimulates social development; teaches that objects endure beyond their initial perception. Some babies giggle with glee in anticipation of parent or sibling appearing from behind an object
Large ball	**Physical:** helps gross motor development and coordination; teaches visual displacement
	Physical, cognitive, and social: teaches unified activity; encourages self-imitation and mobility; teaches repetitious experimentation and anticipation of events
Stuffed animals or soft toys (no sharing)	**Physical, cognitive, and emotional:** Stimulates observation of objects; raises awareness of other (objects); aids in developing a sense of self as an entity separate to other objects in the environment
Mirror	**Physical:** stimulates sense of touch
	Cognitive and social: stimulates curiosity; stimulates social development and imitation
Pots and pans	**Physical:** stimulates gross motor development skills and begins causal relation between movement and sound
Stacking toys	**Physical:** stimulates coordination, spatial perception, and balance
	Cognitive: teaches experimentation, trial and error

Assess the effect that the illness is having on the adolescent, taking into account the following points:

- The nature of the illness
- The timing
- The new experiences imposed by the illness
- Will there be any change in body image?
- Will it affect future expectations?

Key point: The adolescent is already experiencing the effects of hormonal influences on growth acceleration, skin, and structural appendages and body image is important.

A good nursing history is essential, and should include the following information:

- Hobbies
- School
- Family
- Illness
- Previous hospitalization
- Eating habits
- Recreation

Procedure: Selecting activities suitable for all adult patients

As well as the many types of activities that patients may choose to do individually, the following are ways of discouraging social isolation. This applies to adults and adolescents with or without a learning disability, individuals with mental health challenges, and the elderly (with suitable adaptations).

- Organized sports involving team play (including chair activities)
- Dancing, sports (any unsupervised activity)
- Drama groups, going to social events

Selecting toys and activities suitable for toddlers aged 13 to 24 months

Toys or activity	Developmental benefit
Pull toys	**Physical and cognitive:** stimulates gross motor development and awareness of presence of object even when out of the line of sight
Picture book	**Cognitive and social:** Stimulates guided language development; teaches remembered properties for objects, for example, form and colour; provides social experience when assisted
	Physical: teaches page manipulation and fine motor control
Book and rhymes	**Physical:** provides fine distinction in hearing
	Emotional and social: social experience and humour
	Cognitive: stimulates language development
Toys as symbols of adult activity	**Cognitive:** symbols represent actions (for example, vacuum cleaner equals cleaning the carpet)
Scribbling on paper	**Physical and cognitive:** stimulates creativity and fine motor development
Small push and pull toys	**Physical:** stimulates gross motor development and walking
	Cognitive: provides active experimentation with toys, objects, and self-expression
	Physical and social: develops gross motor skills and self-expression
Large crawl-in boxes	**Physical:** teaches gross motor skills
	Cognitive: creates own environment
Large blocks	**Physical:** stimulates two-handed movement, lifting, placing, and stacking
	Cognitive: stimulates self-expression
Stuffed animals blanket, or blanket substitutes (no sharing)	**Cognitive, emotional, and social:** comforts and provides security through familiarity in smell, touch and texture
Filling and empting toys	**Physical, cognitive, and emotional:** provides self-satisfaction with repetition
Puzzles with squares and pegs	**Cognitive:** provides awareness of simple shapes; increases spatial awareness

Selecting toys and activities suitable for pre-school children aged 3 to 5 years

Toys or activity	Developmental benefit
Clay	**Physical:** enhances fine motor skills
	Cognitive: teaches representations of reality
Plastic scissors and paste	**Physical and cognitive:** stimulates creativity and fine motor skills
Dolls	**Emotional:** provides opportunities for fantasy and role play, parental mimicking
Chalk and chalkboards	**Cognitive:** stimulates creativity, concept of eraseability, writing
Building a city of blocks	**Cognitive:** stimulates creativity and reality representation
	Cognitive and social: fosters higher levels of thinking and social interaction
Sandcastles	**Cognitive:** stimulates creativity
Transport toys (trucks and wagons)	**Cognitive and social:** teaches basic rules governing 'driving', walking on streets, and crossing roads: provides social interaction
Simple jigsaw puzzles	**Cognitive:** stimulates problem solving; causes preoccupation with parts—not the whole
Colouring books and sets	**Physical and cognitive:** stimulates creativity; teaches colour; how to colour between the lines, and fine motor coordination
Tricycle and transport toys	**Physical:** teaches motor skills and coordination. Also helps increase fine motor skills
Crayons (nontoxic)	**Cognitive:** stimulates memory of objects, shapes, colour, and creativity
Puzzles	**Cognitive:** teaches problem solving and abstraction
Simpler electronic games	**Cognitive and physical:** stimulates problem solving and teaches a variety of physical skills or memory skills dependant on the game; a wide range of games are available

Selecting activities suitable for children aged 5 to 10 years

Game or activity	Developmental benefit
Word games	**Cognitive and social**: stimulates social communication and language skills
Group games	**Cognitive and social:** stimulates competitiveness, self-control, and social conformity, develops relationships to rules, teaches cooperation, and pre-social behaviour
Hide and seek	**Physical:** teaches motor skills through movement
	Cognitive and social: teaches problem solving, group interaction, and cooperation through group rules. Object permanence. Teaches play, work, and fantasy as coequal activities
Team games	**Social:** teaches rules, fair play, and team effort, teaches how to be fair and adhere to established standards
	Cognitive: rules become more variable and complex and play becomes more intellectual
Board games	**Social:** teaches fair play and competitiveness
	Cognitive: intellectual and experimental
Table games	**Cognitive:** teaches ability to apply rules, stimulates competition, promotes higher levels of thinking
Puzzles and mental games	**Cognitive:** helps child to develop both inductive and deductive reasoning
Electronic games	**Cognitive:** stimulates curiosity and problem solving
Books and storytelling	**Cognitive:** develops vocabulary and logic
	Emotional: provides an outlet for emotional development
	Cognitive and social: fosters language skills, creativity and social relationships
Drama	**Cognitive and social:** encourages imagination and new experiences, stimulates social planning within a group
Art	**Emotional and social:** stimulates creativity and self-expression

Construction toys	**Physical:** teaches hand-eye coordination
	Cognitive and social: stimulates creativity, invention and use of tools, teaches role imitation
	Cognitive: problem solving
Skipping with rope	**Physical and social:** teaches timing, rhythm and social interactions
	Physical: stimulates motor skills and balance
Sports activities	**Cognitive, emotional, and social:** teaches ability to apply rules, provides outlet for energy, reduction of tension, encourages fair play, teaches importance of team effort
	Physical: stimulates large muscle development
	Social: teaches cooperation and pro-social skills
Parties	**Social:** provides interaction with others, including those of the opposite sex, develops notion of social position and roles
	Emotional: sometimes reduces tension but can be very difficult for shy children
Swimming	**Physical:** enhances large muscle development
Cooking	**Emotional and social:** teaches creativity and self-expression
Films	**Cognitive and social:** enhances ability to concentrate in peer activity
Construction sets	**Cognitive:** stimulates creativity and problem solving
Drama	**Cognitive and social:** encourages imagination and new experiences, stimulates social planning as a group, also provides outlet for energy and reduction of tension

- Shared hobbies
- Electronic computer games

An environment such as a day room or social space can be suitable for arm chair aerobics, knitting, crochet, card games, dominoes, or music: a television may be useful in other settings.

Other factors to consider

Patient safety

For safety in the ward area (see Chapter 3), the following should be available (this applies equally to any setting, for example, home, school, or respite care):

Selecting activities suitable for adolescents

Action	Rationale
Encourage the adolescent to wear his or her own clothes	Individuality is important, as are choices, even if you are ill
Encourage adolescent to bring favourite things for decoration of cubicle and around bed space	This is especially important for long-term patients: security, ownership, and choice are important
The adolescent should be involved in planning his or her own care, to accept any restrictions of health teaching by having a better understanding of the situation	Empowering, educating, enabling, and encouraging are essential skills when working with adolescents
The need for privacy and periods of isolation should be respected	Some adolescents have a strongly felt need for privacy and this should be respected unless there is a clinical danger of self-harm or suicide
Allow time for some degree of regression	Being more childish can relieve stress
Introduce young person to the hospital youth club, to encourage interaction with others	Potential stress reliever
Allow time for recreational pursuits, and accept the level of performance achieved	Potential stress reliever
Be a good listener	To establish good interpersonal relationships with adolescents

- Cots for infants and young children, keep children within a safe space
- Beds of the right height (height adjustable) help to prevent falls or accidents for all patients
- Tables and chairs of the correct height facilitate eating, drinking, and most playing activities
- Unbreakable crockery not only reduces accidental breakage but is often easier to clean
- Supervision at all times prevents accidents
- All medication in locked cupboards conforms to NMC guidelines
- All cleaning materials out of sight and reach, not only conforms to COSHH regulations but will also prevent accidental consumption
- No toys with sharp edges, to prevent accidents in children. Similarly, safety issues apply to other settings, for example, do not leave a self-harming patient with anything sharp
- Toys checked for British Standard mark, ensuring safety and suitability. Similarly, defective or sub-standard equipment should not be used in adult sectors
- Children must be strapped in to baby chairs and prams with reins, to prevent potential head injuries and limb fractures. All potentially vulnerable patients should be monitored regularly; some may require constant supervision, This applies in all settings
- Nontoxic materials for use in play, for example, paint, prevent accidental poisoning. In the adult sector never leave potentially toxic materials unsupervised

Selecting activities suitable for all adult patients

Action	Rationale
Offer choices and allow for preferences	Respects the individual's independence and autonomy
Try, as far as possible, to maintain access to requested activities	If equipment is not available on site, aim for the venue that is closest to you
Treat each person as an individual. Give choices	Maintain individuality
Do what the patient or client wants. Explore patients needs and wants	
Monitor activity or engagement, as it may indicate alterations in physical or mental state	Ensures safety and adequate supervision

Many of the Health and Safety and COSHH regulations are also directly applicable to learning disability, mental health and elderly settings.

Education

Especially when working with children, continuation of education should be encouraged. This often helps alleviate boredom and allows children and young people to keep up with their peer groups at school. Falling behind with school work, appearing silly, or even being held back can lead to friendships flagging. This often worries young people, as everyone wants to belong, especially adolescents.

It helps to assess a child's or adolescent's intellectual skills. This enables staff to provide the necessary information required to use problem solving for dealing with the child's or adolescent's illness and admission to hospital.

Remember that children and adolescents may also regress developmentally while in hospital. They get comfort from performing skills with mastery, which they achieved at a younger age. It helps them feel that they do still have some say and control over the situation in which they find themselves.

Education, continuous professional development, or even maintaining one's competency level (mastery) is equally important in learning disability, mental health, and adult elderly settings.

Education continues in the hospital setting, and in some cases in the home environment. Many major paediatric units now employ both primary and secondary teachers skilled in adapting education delivery in both the hospital and home settings.

In adult, learning disability, and mental health settings, educational and care management may be the responsibility of other members of the multidisciplinary team, such as occupational therapists, physiotherapists, speech and language therapists, or dieticians.

Disruptive behaviour

It could be argued that sociopathic tendencies, disruptive behaviour, and various forms of deviant behaviour may be, to some degree, learned behaviour. Equally, it must also be recognized that not all behavioural disorders manifest early in childhood and regular monitoring, especially in the first years of life, will highlight the majority of cases that require further monitoring.

Why does everyone know about the 'naughty step', 'chill out chair' or other child control mechanisms? It would seem that behaviour can be modified or ameliorated with appropriate inputs. There is a lot of information available concerning behaviour modification and microscopic detail is not essential at this early stage of nursing. Theoretically, by positive and negative reinforcement; behaviour that is rewarded will be repeated and behaviour that is not rewarded will be extinguished.

Behaviour-modification programmes and cognitive behaviour therapy are two of the many therapies available in the adult sector that fundamentally work on the above principle: further reading may be required when you enter your branch programme.

Scenarios

Consider what you should do in the following situations, then turn to the end of the section to check your answers.

Further scenarios are available at 🌐 **www.oxford-textbooks.co.uk/orc/docherty/**

Scenario 1

Eighteen-month-old Cameron is visually impaired and, whilst he is able to mobilize relatively independently, he is hesitant to move or interact without parental presence. How can Cameron be encouraged to mobilize, interact, and play?

Scenario 2

Twelve-year-old Ashleigh has experienced multifactorial abuse leading to low trust with all adults and, as a result, has low self-esteem and is self-abusive. How can therapeutic play contribute to Ashleigh's recovery?

Scenario 3

Angela has a multiple-diagnosis learning disability causing spastic paralysis of her limbs. She is 18 years old with a mental age of 8. She is unable to communicate verbally and as a result of her **spasticity** is unable to utilize sign language. Her **aural** and vision senses are intact and she reacts to vocal input. How can play be utilized to contribute to Angela's care plan?

Scenario 4

Mabel, aged 83 years, is active, articulate but unsteady on her feet. How could you help to maintain her activity, in a safe manner?

Website

🌐 **www.oxfordtextbooks.co.uk/orc/docherty/**

You may find it helpful to work through our short online quiz and interactive scenarios intended to help you to develop and apply the skills in this chapter.

References

Brooker C and Waugh A (2007). *Foundations of Nursing Practice: Fundamentals of Holistic Care*. Mosby Elsevier, London.
A useful generic source of information concerning fundamentals of holistic care, potentially applicable to all branches as detailed and broad examples are utilized in text.

Darbyshire P (1994). *Living With a Sick Child in Hospital*, pp. 89–93. Chapman and Hall, Glasgow.

Ginsburg KR, the Committee on Communications, and the Committee on Psychosocial Aspects of Child and Family Health (2007) The importance of play in promoting healthy child development and maintaining strong parent-child bonds. *Pediatrics*, **119**(1), 182–91.

Grandis S, Long G, Glasper EA, and Jackson P, eds (2003). *Foundation Studies for Nursing*. Palgrave MacMillan, London.

Heath H (2001). *Foundations in Nursing Theory and Practice*, 4th edn. Mosby, London.

Hubband S and Trigg E (2000). *Practices in Children's Nursing, Guidelines for Hospital and Community*. Churchill Livingstone, Edinburgh.

Price J and McNeilly J (2006). Developing an educational programme in paediatric care. *International Journal of Palliative Nursing*, **12**(11), 536–41.

Russell-Johnson H (2000). Adolescent survey. *Paediatric Nursing*, **12**(6), 15–19.

Taylor J, Muller DJ, Wattley L, and Harris P (1999). *Nursing Children, Psychology, Research and Practice*, 3rd edn. Stanley Thornes, Cheltenham.

Townley M (2002). Mental health needs of children and young people. *Nursing Standard*, **16**(30), 38–45.

Useful further reading and websites

Barker PJ (2004). *Assessment in Psychiatric and Mental Health Nursing: In Search of the Whole Person*, 2nd edn. Nelson Thornes Ltd, Cheltenham.
As assessment is the first stage encountered in making a **holistic** plan of care, this is a potentially relevant source. It also has potential transferability to other branches, although it is primarily written from a mental health perspective.

Cooper M, Hooper C, and Thompson M, eds (2005). *Child and Adolescent Mental Health*. Hodder Arnold, London.
Specifically relevant to the developing child and adolescent, with or without a mental health issue.

Department of Health (2001). Valuing People:
A New Strategy for Learning Disability for the 21st Century, white paper. Department of Health, London.
A primary source of information concerning learning disabilities developments.

Done A (2001). The theraputic use of story-telling. *Paediatric Nursing*, **13**(3), 17–20.

Kaminski M, Pellino T, and Wish J (2002). Play and pets: the physical and emotional impact of child-life and pet therapy on hospitalized children. *Children's Healthcare*, **31**(4), 321–35.
Though written from a child nursing perspective, potentially transferrable to other branches where pets may have a therapeutic role to play.

Reid D (2002). Benefits of a virtual play rehabilitation environment for children with cerebral palsy on perceptions of self efficiency: a pilot study. *Pediatric Rehabilitation*, **5**(3), 141–8.
This text describes the potential use of alternative stimulatory environments as a means of reaching maximum potential.

Schober J, Hinchliff S, and Norman S, eds (2003). *Nursing Practice and Health Care*, 4th edn. Arnold, London.
Age Concern. www.ageconcern.org.uk.
Older adult issues.
www.bbc.co.uk/cbbc.
A general source of current issues and news suitable for children.

Childline. www.childline.org.uk.
Support for children.

Department of Health. www.dh.gov.uk/en/index.htm.

Health and Safety Executive. www.hse.gov.uk.

Health and Safety at Work. www.healthandsafety.co.uk/hsw.htm.

www.opsi.gov.uk/acts/acts1999.
Legislation information.

Literacy Changes Lives. www.literacytrust.org.uk/Database/earlydebate.html.

RNIB. *RNIB See it Right Guidelines*. www.rnib.org.uk/seeitright.
Blindness.

RoSPA. www.rospa.co.uk.
Accident prevention.

Scotland's Commissioner for Children and Young People (SCCYP). www.sccyp.org.uk.
Children's and young people's rights.

Scottish Child Law Centre. www.sclc.org.uk.

UNICEF. www.unicef.org.uk.

World Health Organization. www.who.int/en/.

Check ☻ **www.oxfordtextbooks.co.uk/orc/docherty/** for changes and new developments. Updated research, guidelines, or equipment will be added every four months.

Answers to patient scenarios

Scenario 1

Select or suggest toys that would encourage movement, recognition of colour; develop awareness of texture, sound, numeracy, and the beginnings of sharing/considering others. Cameron requires supervision, especially if the cot sides are not fully up. No baby should ever be left with cot sides down, or half down. Consistency of play is essential. Also it can be useful to consult Cameron's parents or carers and ensure that team members follow his care plan.

Branch links

● Named nurses; inclusion of relatives or carer according to Cameron's wishes

- Encouragement of socialization skills
- Voluntary and Governmental support, for example, RNIB, local groups

 ## Scenario 2

- Consult mental health professionals to assist in allowing psychologically orientated constructive play (therapeutic play)
- Encourage trust development through play
- Play could assist Ashleigh with moral issues that may arise

Branch links:
- Socialization skills
- Skills required to enable trust development
- Links with other healthcare professionals, for example, mental health, social work
- Ethical and moral **consent** issues, for example, confidentiality—how this affects trust

 ## Scenario 3

- Play that would stimulate and improve movement and interaction within Angela's capabilities
- Play that encourages communication, expression of self

Branch links:
- Encourage movement and socialization

 ## Scenario 4

- Occupation, industry, and stimulation help to maintain functionality
- Offer a range of activities and choice: for mobility, try skittles and aerobics; for cognition, talking and reminiscing; for socializing, group games and outings

Branch links
- No matter who the client group may be, nurses and therapists aim to preserve skills that are present

12 Dying

LINDA LOFTUS

Introduction

This chapter introduces some fundamental skills related to caring for patients with advanced disease. These include communication, **oral** care, patient assessment on admission, pain assessment and management, and performing the last offices.

Human life is precious. An integral part of everyone's life is the dying process. Dying may be defined as the body's preparation for death. It is regarded as a natural process that is a profound and personal experience for the patient (Quaglietti *et al.* 2004). Dying may be sudden, as in a cardiac arrest or a road traffic accident, or it may last for weeks, months, or even years, for example, in patients with genetic disorders or cancer. Many patients will, therefore, enter a stage of their illness that is termed palliative. Palliative care is defined by the World Health Organization as: 'The active care of patients and their families by a multiprofessional team at a time when the patient's disease is no longer responsive to curative treatment and life expectancy is relatively short.' The life expectancy of palliative-care patients may range from a very short time in a clinical environment, to several years, much of which will be spent in the community. The end stage of the disease process requires particular skills and interventions and is often referred to as the terminal phase (WHO 2008).

The multiprofessional team may consist of palliative care specialist doctors and nurses, generic physicians and nurses, district nurses, pharmacists, occupational therapists, social workers, and volunteers. The multiprofessional team often work together in an integrated way to help coordinate the patients' care more effectively.

The approach to palliative care is **holistic** and focuses on the physical, psychological, social, and spiritual aspects of care for patients with advanced disease. The needs of the family are also considered when assessing, planning, implementing, and evaluating care for this group of patients. This may also include some anticipatory loss and bereavement support before and after the patient dies. Patients and their relatives experience a lot of psychosocial distress when they are dying. It is an important activity of living and sensitive intervention is crucial.

Learning outcomes

These outcomes relate to numbers 2, 3, and 5 of the NMC's Essential Skill Clusters and specifically to Care Domains 1, 2, and 3 of the NMC's Standards of Proficiency for Pre-registration Nursing (outcomes to be achieved for entry to branch).

On reading this chapter and interacting with the web pages and undertaking supervised activities the student will be able to:

- Understand the concept of a **generic palliative care** approach
- Apply palliative care concepts to nursing practice
- Demonstrate the use of effective verbal communication skills to contribute to the assessment of patients with advanced disease
- Develop a professional relationship with palliative-care patients and their families
- Assess the patient's mouth and provide oral care
- Use evidence-based practice in implementing oral care

- Assess the patient's pain holistically
- Identify the appropriate analgesia for managing pain in advanced disease
- Identify other factors relevant to managing pain in advanced disease
- Identify psychosocial or spiritual factors that may adversely affect the patient's experience of pain
- Prepare the deceased patient for the mortuary in accordance with legal requirements and the deceased patient's cultural and religious beliefs
- Respect the deceased patient's cultural and religious beliefs
- Comply with legislation associated with sudden deaths and fiscal cases
- Minimize any risk of cross-infection from the deceased patient to health professionals and relatives

Prior knowledge

You will need to use all the skills that you have developed so far, such as communication, administering medicines for pain management, caring for a patient's skin, and so on. It would be helpful to reread the book up to this point.

Background

You may nurse patients who are dying in different clinical placements in your first year, for example, acute care, community settings, and hospices. The approach to the patients and their relatives may be a little different in each of these placements because of the context in which it occurs. For example, care in an acute placement may be affected because of limited resources, such as time, whilst some staff in care homes may not have all the necessary skills. Patients, including patients with **dementia**, usually prefer to die at home or in a hospice (Davies *et al.* 2004), but the majority of patients continue to die in the acute care hospital settings, or in care homes if they have dementia (Harris 2007).

In the UK in 2000, 66.6% of patients died in hospital whilst 19% died at home (Ellershaw and Ward 2003). Palliative care needs to be improved for patients who die in acute areas, since this clinical setting is the one

context that has been most negatively assessed by patients, and particularly by their families (Rogers *et al.* 2000).

Acute hospitals will have a palliative care nurse and access to a palliative care team if patients present with problems that are difficult to resolve. You may see these health professionals while visiting your clinical placement.

Generic palliative care

Generic palliative care involves approaching patients holistically, considering the patient and family or partners as one unit and improving quality of life by good symptom control. Patients with more complex problems require specialist palliative care (NCPC 2007). The focus of this chapter is to develop skills related to generic palliative care.

The aim of palliative care for patients who have not moved into the terminal phase is to improve their quality of life so that they enjoy the time that they have remaining. It also enables some patients to attend to unfinished business and, if necessary, to put their affairs in order.

As a student nurse, you will be expected to attend to the patient's needs in relation to personal cleansing, continence, and mobility. Control of temperature can be problematic in patients who are dying and they may perspire a lot. This may be a side effect of morphine (Pittelkow and Loprinzi 2003). It is important to maintain patients' dignity in relation to personal hygiene by taking time to assist them into their own nightdress or pyjamas and taking time to look after, in particular, female patients' hair. If the patient scores high on a Waterlow Score then a specialized mattress, for example, Autoexcell, may be ordered. Assessment of pressure-ulcer risk should be carried out within four hours of the patient's admission. Thereafter, an individualized approach is recommended, since each patient's downward trajectory will vary.

A downward trajectory

Your patients may become semi-conscious or unconscious at the end stage of their illness. It is probable that they can still hear quite well. It is important to continue to treat them with respect, to introduce yourself, and to explain what you are about to do before carrying out a procedure. The way you lift and lay your patient should be done in a sensitive manner. It is important to concentrate on being gentle when touching patients. This is particularly important with children. Parents will be highly sensitive to the way in which their ill child is handled.

If a patient is at the end stage of the illness, relatives may need to stay overnight. They will be stressed and you may have to make tea for them and check to see if there is anything that they need. Your mentor will be communicating with the relatives about the patient's condition. This is an opportunity for you to observe the support that your mentor gives to relatives. Relatives of the dying child will need some quiet time with them to say their goodbyes. Any interventions with the child should be managed in an unintrusive, sensitive way.

Sometimes, patients die suddenly and the mentor will need to ask the relatives to come in. The severity of the situation must be made clear. Kent and McDowell (2004) suggest that phrases such as *critically ill* or *seriously injured* should be used. They also state that it is useful to give the relatives a specific named person to ask for when they arrive at the ward. This will decrease their stress. Having a relatives' room is also helpful, since it gives relatives a little privacy during a stressful period. Policies in different hospitals may vary but generally relatives and friends are not told that the patient has died until they arrive at the hospital.

Occasionally, the relatives are not there when the patient is dying and you may be asked to sit with the dying patient for a short period of time. If you have known the patient, it is a privilege to spend a little time with him or her near the end. Acute surgical and medical wards, however, are very busy clinical areas and sometimes the best that can be managed is that you check the patient frequently. Since the ethos of care is on recovery, and the ward is very busy, these patients may be referred to a hospice.

If the patient is dying and is being nursed in the community, the district nurse will usually visit more frequently when the patient's condition begins to deteriorate. The district nurse will have built up a good relationship with the family and you will be able to observe her communicating with them. Relatives often need to be involved in the decision-making process.

They also require information on who to approach for advice, insight into the specific processes of dying, advice on suitable adaptations to the home to facilitate mobility, a contact number for emergencies, and psychological support (including advice on how to help siblings, especially if it is a child who is dying) (Darnhill and Garnage 2006; Lynch and Dahlin 2007).

12.1 Communication with the patients and their relatives

Definition

Communication is an important, specific skill to develop when caring for palliative-care patients and their relatives. You should also refer to Chapters 2 and 4.

Sometimes, we think that we are good communicators because we relate well to people in a social context. However, effective communication is crucial to patients at the end stage of their lives when they may be faced with some complex care decisions and separation from loved ones, as well as their own mortality. Clear, accurate communication is important for giving information, psychological care to reduce anxiety, and for continuity of care through interdisciplinary teamwork. Misunderstandings must be avoided to ensure that patients don't become needlessly anxious or relatives become more stressed.

Background

Various factors are known to affect how well we communicate with our patients. If you have experienced a bereavement, in particular a recent bereavement, then this can affect your ability to communicate with a dying patient. This can have the effect of causing you to worry about getting upset about your own situation, with the effect that you cannot fully help the patient. It is important to let your lecturer and mentor know about this to enable them to be sensitive to your situation.

In your first year, it may be that you are worried about difficult questions that may arise, whether or not you will be able to answer them, and if you do, whether you might say the wrong thing and cause the patient additional **emotional distress**. For reasons such as this, nurses will sometimes block communication with dying patients. This can be exercised in various ways, for example, asking closed or leading questions, blocking, or distancing. This type of communication can result in your patients losing trust in you at a time when they may find it hard to speak to someone else, leaving them physically and psychologically isolated (Fallowfield *et al.* 2002 and De Araujo *et al.* 2004).

Example of blocking

> *Nurse: Hi, how are you today?*
>
> *Patient: Not so good. The pain seems to be getting worse.*
>
> *Nurse: Have your bowels moved?*

We need to give some thought as to how we communicate with dying patients. It is important to reflect on your experiences of loss and consider how these might affect your communication. It may help to write about your experiences to help make sense of them. Reflecting effectively on difficult situations enables you to raise your awareness of who you are. This self-awareness helps to improve your communication skills.

Developing good communication skills will facilitate the nurse–patient relationship. Getting to know the patient who is dying and gaining some insight into him or her can be comforting for relatives. It is important to relatives that there is a sense of the nurse 'knowing the patient' when you are communicating with them. This is especially important if the patient is a child (Lidstone *et al.* 2006). This can only be gained through achieving a meaningful nurse–patient relationship. For example, you may be present when the doctor or senior nurse breaks bad news to a patient or relatives. Sharing this experience can help to bring you closer to a patient (Dunniece and Slevin 2000).

Active listening

An *active* listener is someone who listens to what is being said, picks up cues, observes nonverbal reactions, and is willing to explore them, for example, by asking, 'You seem to be anxious?' This is what your patient often wants, someone to listen. Patients are not always looking for answers but trying

to work things out for themselves. However, **active listening** to a dying patient is not always easy, since they may want to talk about things which are painful to them and this could, therefore, be emotionally painful to the nurse who is listening to them (White *et al.* 2004). Nurses usually look for peer support in these situations: as a student nurse, this may be your mentor or university lecturer.

Difficult questions

If the patient does ask difficult questions, such as 'Am I dying?' it is important not to lie. Trust is crucial in maintaining a nurse patient relationship: once it is lost, it is almost impossible to regain. Most patients, including a high number of patients with cancer and Alzheimer's disease (Turnbull *et al.* 2003), wish to know the truth about their diagnosis and prognosis. However, as a student you will require some help in responding to this question. It is OK, therefore, to acknowledge with the patient that they are *quite ill* but state that you need to ask someone else to come and talk to them about it.

Developing your skills

Consider your own verbal and nonverbal communication skills when communicating with staff in your clinical placement. If you feel yourself tensing your muscles, ask yourself why you are getting anxious. Write these reasons down in a reflective diary. This will make you more aware of tension when you are communicating with patients and will allow you to relax purposefully when talking to a patient with advanced disease.

Other factors to consider

Communicating with patients with cognitive impairments

Communication with the cognitively impaired patient is particularly challenging for health professionals. The Mental Capacity Act (2005) allows people to express how they would like to be treated if they lose the capacity to communicate effectively. The median expected lifespan for a patient with Alzheimer's disease is about eight years. These patients experience similar symptoms to those with cancer but for a longer period of time. They may die from end-stage dementia, another illness, such

Communicating with a patient with advanced disease

Key point: The most important skill that you can use with your patient is that of active listening. You will not be able to listen effectively to your patient if you are worrying about how you will respond, or thinking about what you did yesterday. Most people are better at talking than listening.

Communication style   Rationale

Communication style	Rationale
Talk to your patient socially.	It is important to maintain some normality in your relationship with the dying patient. Patients may use humour to talk about the fact that they are dying.
Use open questions.	Gives control to the patient.
Be attentive to the patient or relative's cues and use reflective skills to echo these cues.	This lets the patient or relative know that you are actively attending to what is being said. It gives you the opportunity to ask if the patient or relative wants to talk more about a specific problem, but gives him or her control to choose to discuss it in more depth or decide that he or she is not ready to talk about it.
	For example, if a patient or relative mentions being worried about the pain getting worse, but then goes on to talk about something else, wait until that person has stopped talking, and prompt: 'You said that you are worried about the pain getting worse?'
Demonstrate sensitivity to the patient's situation.	Acknowledge that it must be difficult for them.
Take the patient's hand if they are upset, and if their nonverbal cues indicate that they would be receptive to this gesture.	This demonstrates that you care. However, not everybody is comfortable with this and it is important to assess the patient's nonverbal communication. You will also need to consider your patient's cultural values.
Actively listen.	To ensure that you capture and understand the messages the patient is communicating. These messages may be verbal or nonverbal (Egan 2007).

as cancer or a combination of mental and physical problems (www.Alzheimers.org.uk/; Harris 2007). It is important to tell the cognitively impaired patient what you are going to do before you commence doing it and to consider any **sensory** impairment, such as difficulty with hearing.

Communicating with patients with learning disabilities

The main causes of death in people with learning disability are respiratory and cardiac conditions (RCN 2006). Tuffrey-Wijne (2002) states that a conspiracy of silence may develop when a patient with a learning disability has advanced disease. The Adults with Incapacity Scotland Act (2000) and the England and Wales equivalent provide laws aimed at protecting the rights and interests of this vulnerable group.

Gaining **consent**, however, can be problematic with this group of patients. Resistance to intervention may occur and be demonstrated through **aggressive** behaviour. It is important to consider that any aggressive behaviour may be a result of a lack of understanding or poor pain control (MENCAP 2007). A relative or nurse, preferably someone who knows the patient, needs to act as an advocate for a patient with a learning disability.

It is particularly useful to have someone with experience in communicating with the patient present when the patient is initially assessed. In the MENCAP (2007) report it was found to be common for relatives to find that they were often not listened to, although they were the experts in caring for their relatives, whether adults or children, in their homes.

People with learning disabilities may find it easier if the communication is related specifically to their symptoms. This may be through explaining why they are feeling sick or why they are in pain as a better alternative to giving their illness a specific name, which may be difficult for them to comprehend. Consistently reflecting on any feedback that is given can also facilitate communication with these patients. You will need to accept that the process will be slower and that you will need more time. As with all

patients, questions should be answered honestly and pictures can be used to aid understanding. As well as nonverbal communication, for example, touch, facial expression, and tone of voice, communication aids such as **Makaton** (a unique language programme that teaches communication using signs and symbols, see www.makaton.org) may be used to facilitate understanding.

Communicating with children and their families

When a child is dying, the impact is profound on for all concerned. The needs of the whole family must be considered. Each child and family will have unique psychological, physical, social, and spiritual needs. Siblings may have special needs, since the parents often focus all their energy on the dying child. Children may be able to express themselves more easily through art therapy. Books about death and dying for children and their parents may also be helpful. Parents are usually told first that their child is dying. The physician will then speak with the parents and the child together.

Although young children may not understand what is wrong, they will sense their parents' and health professionals' anxiety in any response to them. The child may perceive that family and peers treat them differently, and this can lead to a sense of isolation (Stevens 2003).

Since children may know intuitively that they are dying, when they ask a difficult question they will probably already know the answer. The child is seeking confirmation. Paediatric nurses can help by including the child and the family in any plan of care, encouraging expression of their feelings and giving them some choices with any planned interventions. Teenagers, in particular, need to feel that they are well informed and included in the decision-making process. Parents also have specific needs, since they will experience many different emotions, for example, anxiety, anger, or feelings of guilt (Lidstone *et al.* 2006; McGrath and Brown 2003; Stevens 2003). Families who know what to expect and feel able to deal with symptoms may cope better after their child dies.

12.2 **Communication skills for assessing the patient with advanced disease**

Definition

These communication skills will help you to assess patients with advanced disease more effectively and sensitively.

Background

End-of-life care: the Liverpool care pathway

The patient with advanced disease needs to be consistently assessed, since the illness trajectory is often downhill. It can be difficult at times to determine when exactly patients move into the terminal phase of their illness. This can be because of the environment, the culture of curing, and a reluctance to remove hope of cure. It is also more difficult to diagnose dying, when the patient is suffering from nonmalignant disease such as cardiac conditions or dementia (Harris 2007).

The criteria that Ellershaw and Ward (2003) identify as indicating the dying phase in cancer patients are:

- The patient becomes bedbound
- The patient is semi-comatose
- The patient is able to take only sips of fluid
- The patient is no longer able to take oral drugs

When using the pathway if two of the criteria are present, the patient with advanced disease is assessed as being in the end stage of their illness, that is, the dying phase. When patients are placed on the **Liverpool care pathway**, it replaces all other methods of documentation, such as doctors' case notes and nursing care plans (Ellershaw and Wilkinson 2003; Kinder and Ellershaw 2003). You may see this pathway being used in clinical practice. An abbreviated example is shown in **Fig. 12.1**.

Patients have often worked out for themselves that things are not looking too good. The Buckman (1997) model of the process of dying states that your patient may experience many different emotions in the initial stage for

example: fear, anxiety, shock, disbelief, anger, denial, guilt, and humour. In the chronic stage, Buckman (1998) suggests that the intensity of these emotions is diminished but the patient may become depressed. In the final stage of this model (acceptance), the patient may communicate normally and make decisions normally.

When to perform an assessment

The following communication skills will be used when you are assessing a palliative care patient. Privacy is not always possible, especially in acute hospitals. However, it is important to choose a time when the ward isn't too busy and the screens should be drawn.

Procedure

Use the SOLER system to attend to your patient's needs. Attending refers to the ways in which helpers can be with clients, both physically and psychologically (Egan 2007).

- Face the client *squarely*
- Ensure that posture is *open*
- *Lean* slightly forwards
- Maintain *eye* contact
- *Relax*

Aftercare

At the end stage of any illness the patient may find it difficult to get comfortable when lying in bed. It is important to take time to ensure that your patient is supported well using pillows (see **Fig 12.2**). This will aid communication.

Other factors to consider

If the patient has a learning disability, consider asking the carer what situations and circumstances have been known to prompt challenging behaviour. This will help if interventions are required. Patients with learning disability may resist implementation of care and it is important to find out what may trigger challenging behaviour to facilitate any care intervention (MENCAP 2007).

INTEGRATED CARE PATHWAY FOR THE TERMINAL/DYING PHASE

NAME: .... UNIT NO: .... DATE: ....

SECTION 1	PATIENT ASSESSMENT				
DIAGNOSIS	PRIMARY Date of In-patient admission		SECONDARY Ethnicity		

PHYSICAL CONDITION	Unable to swallow	Yes ☐ No ☐	Aware	Yes ☐	No ☐
	Nausea	Yes ☐ No ☐	Conscious	Yes ☐	No ☐
	Vomiting	Yes ☐ No ☐	UTI Problems	Yes ☐	No ☐
	Constipated	Yes ☐ No ☐	Catheterised	Yes ☐	No ☐
	Confused	Yes ☐ No ☐	Respiratory Tract Secretions	Yes ☐	No ☐
	Agitation	Yes ☐ No ☐	Dyspnoea	Yes ☐	No ☐
	Restless	Yes ☐ No ☐	Pain	Yes ☐	No ☐
	Distressed	Yes ☐ No ☐	Other	Yes ☐	No ☐

COMFORT MEASURES

(If 'No' chart as variance on the back page)

Goal 1: Current medication assessed and non essentials discontinued Yes ☐ No ☐
  Appropriate oral drugs converted to subcutaneous route and syringe
  driver commenced if appropriate
  Inappropriate medication discontinued

Goal 2: PRN subcutaneous medication written up for list below as per Protocol Yes ☐ No ☐
  (see blue sheets at back of ICP for guidance)

  Pain   Analgesia
  Nausea & Vomiting   Anti-emetic
  Agitation   Sedative
  Respiratory Tract Secretions   Anticholinergic

Goal 3: Discontinue inappropriate interventions Yes ☐ No ☐
  Blood Test
  Antibiotics
  I.V.'s (fluids/medications)
  Not for Cardiopulmonary Resuscitation (Please record below)

  Doctor's signature .... Date ....

Goal 3a: Decisions to discontinue inappropriate nursing interventions taken Yes ☐ No ☐
  Routine Turning Regime (turn for comfort only)
  Taking Vital signs

Goal 3b: Syringe driver set up within 4 hours of Doctors order Yes ☐ No ☐ N/A ☐

Nurse signature .... Date .... Time ....

Figure 12.1 Abbreviated version of the Liverpool care pathway. By permission of Oxford University Press. Ellershaw J, Wilkinson S (2003). *Care of the Dying: A pathway to excellence.* Oxford University Press, Oxford.

INTEGRATED CARE PATHWAY FOR THE TERMINAL/DYING PHASE

NAME: .... UNIT NO: .... DATE: ....

Codes (Please enter in columns) A.. Achieved   V.. Variance

SECTION 2	PATIENT PROBLEM/FOCUS	08:00	12:00	16:00	20:00	24:00	04:00
ASSESSMENT PAIN/COMFORT MEASURES							
Pain **Goal: Patient is pain free** ● Verbalised by patient if conscious ● Pain free on movement ● Appears peaceful ● Move only for comfort							
Agitation **Goal: Patient is not agitated** ● Patient does not display signs of delirium, terminal anguish, restlessness (thrashing, plucking, twitching) ● Exclude retention of urine as cause							
Respiratory Tract Secretions **Goal: Patients breathing is not made difficult by excessive secretions**							
Nausea & Vomiting **Goal: Patient does not feel nauseous or vomits** ● Patient verbalises if conscious							
Other symptoms (e.g. dyspnoea) a)							
TREATMENT/PROCEDURES							
Mouth Care **Goal: Mouth is moist and clean.** ● See mouth care policy ● Mouth care to be given at least 4 hourly							
Micturition Difficulties **Goal: Patient is comfortable** ● Urinary catheter if in retention ● Urinary catheter or pads, if general weakness creates incontinence							
MEDICATION (If not appropriate record as N/A)							
Goal: All medication is given safely & accurately. ● If syringe driver in progress check at least 4 hourly ● If medication not required please record as N/A							
Nurse Signature **Repeat this page 24 hrly. Spare copies on Ward**		Early		Late		Night	

Figure 12.1 Continued

Communication skills for assessing the patient with advanced disease

Action	Rationale
Introduce yourself to the patient and relatives.	It is important that the patient knows who you are.
Check who the other people in the cubicle are and that the patient doesn't mind you talking in front of them.	To maintain patient confidentiality.
Establish what the patient knows and what he or she would like to know.	This helps you to assess the patient's present understanding of the situation.
Have the confidence to say, 'I don't know' – patients may have to deal with uncertainty or they might need to talk to someone else.	Patients appreciate honesty.
Use open questions, for example, 'What problems do you have at present? What effect has this had on you? How much can you do for yourself?'	Gives the patient control over the communication process.
Pick up on cues or reactions.	This shows that you have been actively listening and observing.
Reflect back to ensure that there are no misunderstandings.	Evidence that you have been actively listening and are interested.
Don't be afraid of silence.	Sometimes patients need a little thinking time.
Acknowledge emotions, for example, anxiety or anger: 'You sound anxious, worried?'	Gives the patient the opportunity to discuss any worries.
Actively attend to, and report, any signs of depression, for example, feelings of hopelessness, worthlessness, excessive feelings of guilt, expressing thoughts on suicide.	Some patients may be clinically depressed and require some antidepressant medication.
Don't give false hope.	You need to develop a trusting relationship with your patient.
Summarize and establish a positive direction in which to move to maintain hope, for example, plans to control nausea and vomiting or to control pain.	To maintain realistic hope.

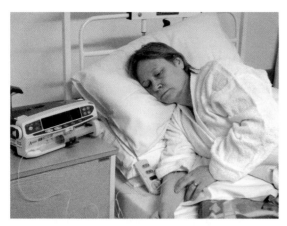

Figure 12.2 Patient propped up with pillows

12.3 **Oral care for the patient with advanced disease**

Definition

Oral care involves assessing the oral cavity and implementing care that is specific to the needs of the patient who is dying. Refer to Section 8.7 for general details.

Mouth care is extremely important in the dying patient. Effective mouth care will enhance the patient's ability to eat, drink, and communicate (Fitzpatrick 2000). It will also improve the quality of life for that patient (Lidstone *et al.* 2006).

When to provide oral care

The oral **mucosa** may need to be assessed daily using a pen torch and a gloved finger. Oral care will need to be provided about four to five times a day to keep the oral mucosa healthy.

Aftercare

Maintaining a positive fluid balance through the oral intake of fluids, and the act of chewing food (mastication), are important for a moist, healthy oral mucosa. Every effort should be made to maintain fluid balance in patients with advanced disease. However, near the end stage of illness, patients may be unable to swallow and may become dehydrated. Fluids may be given **subcutaneously** if patients are distressed; in particular, if they are agitated or are suffering from **hypercalcaemia** (Pitorak 2003; Zerwekh 2003).

Harris (2007) and the Alzheimer's Association both argue that quality of life in this area could be improved for patients with advanced dementia, since they are often fed and hydrated artificially when they develop problems with swallowing and that this extends a poor quality of life. Furthermore, there is some evidence that **dehydration** has benefits when patients are in the final stages of advanced disease. Dehydration decreases urine output and the patient will, therefore, remain drier and not have to extend limited energy on toileting; pulmonary secretions may be reduced, therefore reducing coughing and congestion, and there may be less need for oropharyngeal suction. If gastrointestinal secretions are decreased, the patient is less likely to vomit. Pain may also be reduced because of lack of pressure from oedema (Critchlow and Bauer-Wu 2002; Pitorak 2003; Zerwekh 2003). However, the unpleasant consequence of dehydration is that patients may complain of a dry mouth. Small amounts of iced water or an orange to suck can help alleviate the mouth dryness that many patients may experience.

Developing your skills

You will provide oral care to a range of patients either in acute care, care homes, or a hospice. Remember that this is an important skill and care should be taken with palliative-care patients since their mucosa may be more delicate than for other patients. Regardless of this, oral care is an important skill to practise and should be part of the basic comfort provided for patients.

Oral care for the patient with advanced disease

Key point: Care needs to be taken if cancer patients are on, or have recently had, active treatment, such as **chemotherapy** or **radiotherapy**. Such patients may have badly inflamed oral mucosa and will need more specialized care.

Action	Rationale
Introduce yourself to the patient.	It is important that the patient knows who you are.
Explain what you are about to do.	You need to gain consent.
Ask the patient about any problems he or she might have had with the mouth.	This will give you some insight into potential problems.
Cleanse hands prior to assisting.	To prevent cross-infection.
Dentures will need to be removed.	To give a clear view of the oral cavity.
Observe for any obvious problems with teeth, for example, dental caries, furred coated tongue, redness, bleeding, ulceration, white spots. White, cream, or yellow raised spots may indicate a fungal infection.	Any dental caries or broken areas on the mucosa may be a source of infection.
	If the patient has specific problems. like a **fungal infection**, such as thrush, drugs like Nystatin or **Fluconazole** may be prescribed.
Relatives are often anxious to help and it is worth asking them to bring in a soft toothbrush and fluoride toothpaste.	Relatives may be willing to be involved in this aspect of care.
Brush teeth with a soft toothbrush and a fluoride toothpaste and rinse with water afterwards.	Current evidence supports the use of regular brushing of teeth with a soft toothbrush and fluoride toothpaste and rinsing with water afterwards.
If the patient is unable or unwilling to use a toothbrush then normal saline may be used as a mouthwash.	This is in preference to more astringent substances such as chlorhexidine.
Advise the patient or relative that chewing sugar-free gum can help to stimulate the production of saliva and help to keep the mouth moist. Artificial saliva agents may also be used.	To prevent infection.
Use a mild lip balm for dry lips but not Vaseline (soft paraffin based). Relatives may bring this in for the patient.	Clinicians' experiences from hospice suggest that mild lip balms are useful but not Vaseline-type products like soft paraffin, since they are not easily absorbed and can solidify, causing the patient more discomfort.

If the patient has dentures these should be cleaned after each meal and soaked overnight in Milton (sodium hypochlorite).	To avoid infection.
	To help to stimulate appetite.
If the dentures have metal in them, they should be soaked in chlorhexidine to avoid staining (Bagg 2003; Miller and Kearney 2001; Milligan *et al.* 2001).	To improve patient comfort.
	To improve communication.
Cleanse hands after assisting.	To prevent cross-infection.

12.4 Assessment and management of pain for the patient with advanced disease

Definition

One of the main problems for patients who are dying is pain. Refer to Chapter 3. About 50–60% of patients in the UK who have advanced cancer and noncancer chronic conditions will suffer pain at the end stage of their illness. It is, therefore, important that pain is assessed using an appropriate pain assessment tool (Foley 2003).

Background

Patients with end-stage illness may present with pain, which can be physical, emotional, social, or spiritual. It is difficult to know and accept that you are going to die and that you will be leaving the people that you care about. Sometimes people have relationships that have been problematic, for example they may not have spoken to a brother or sister for many years. When faced with their own mortality, people try to make sense out of their lives and what has gone before, or they look to their religious beliefs to help them to cope. This means that managing pain for patients who are dying can be more complex than dealing with the physiological experience.

Pain is a very extensive and complicated subject and, as such, there are a large number of textbooks written on the theory of pain, as well as physiology books explaining the biological sensation of pain. It is worthwhile studying this subject.

Procedure: assessment of pain in adults

Pain assessment tools

To assess the level of a patient's pain, it is common to use a pain assessment tool. This can be used in acute and community settings. **Figure 12.3** shows an example. The ABBEY pain scale (**Fig. 12.4**) may be used to assess pain in patients with dementia and for some patients with learning disability (Cunningham 2006).

Procedure: assessment of pain in children

Pain control is also an important part of caring for the dying child. As with adults, children may experience pain from the disease process, interventions, and side effects, as well as psychosocial and spiritual distress. The child's age, cognitive ability, and **perception** of what is happening will affect the experience of pain. Reactions from parents, close relatives, and health professionals will also affect the child's experience of pain.

Date:_____

Patient's name:_____

DoB:_____

CHI number: _____

Use address label

NHS
Greater Glasgow
and Clyde
**Acute Services
Division**

Hospital: .... Ward: ....

Generic Pain Assessment Tool

- Ask the patient to **mark all his or her pains** on the body diagrams opposite.
- **Label each site of pain with a letter** (i.e. A, B, C etc).

1. Assess **the pain in each site. Score and record nature of pain.**

2. Ask the patient to rate his/her pain using the numerical rating scale. Enter the score in appropriate column overleaf.

3. Record pain score 4 hourly or more frequently if pain is uncontrolled.

   Record pain score approximately 45 minutes after analgesia is given orally; record pain score approximately 25 minutes after analgesia is given by subcutaneous injection.

4. If pain remains unimproved after two breakthrough doses, please ask for a medical review.

Using the numerical rating scale

Ask the patient to rate his/her pain by choosing a number between 0 and 10 - use the diagram on the right to assist the patient.

Note: 0 = No pain; 10 = Worst Possible Pain

VI MEDICAL ILLUSTRATION • PALLIATIVE • CARE 10520

```
0   1   2   3   4   5   6   7   8   9   10
|   |   |   |   |   |   |   |   |   |   |
No                                    Worst
Pain                                  Possible
                                      Pain
```

Likert Conversion Scale
0   = No pain
1–3   = Mild Pain
4–6   = Moderate Pain
7–10   = Severe Pain

Date	Time	Site	Score	Description of pain e.g. 'shooting' 'stabbing' 'burning' 'aching'	Action taken / analgesic given (Name, dose, route)	Comments from staff / patients / carer	Signature

Figure 12.3 Example of pain assessment scale. Courtesy of North Glasgow Hospitals Trust. Compiled by F Wylie, I Wotherspoon, J Wright, *et al.*

Talking to children about their pain, explaining what is being done to help it, encouraging them to remain engaged with their lives as fully as possible, teaching them strategies for coping with their pain, and ensuring adequate pain relief medication can improve management of the child's pain. Most toddlers above the age of two years can communicate their pain. The language that children use to describe their pain will develop from the language the family use to describe pain (Lidstone *et al.* 2006; McGrath and Brown 2003).

The Wong faces and colour scale (see **Fig. 12.5**) may be used for children and adults with a learning disability. Children aged about five may be able to use a visual analogue scale.

Procedure: management of pain

The principle of pharmacological management of pain in patients (including children) and administering analgesia to patients with advanced disease is that it is:

Abbey Pain Scale

For measurement of pain in people with dementia who cannot verbalise.

Q1. **Vocalisation**
eg whimpering, groaning, crying
Absent 0   Mild 1   Moderate 2   Severe 3

Q1 ☐

Q2. **Facial expression**
eg looking tense, frowning, grimacing, looking frightened
Absent 0   Mild 1   Moderate 2   Severe 3

Q2 ☐

Q3. **Change in body language**
eg fidgeting, rocking, guarding part of body, withdrawn
Absent 0   Mild 1   Moderate 2   Severe 3

Q3 ☐

Q4. **Behavioural Change**
eg increased confusion, refusing to eat, alteration in usual patterns
Absent 0   Mild 1   Moderate 2   Severe 3

Q4 ☐

Q5. **Physiological change**
eg temperature, pulse or blood pressure outside normal limits,
perspiring, flushing or pallor
Absent 0   Mild 1   Moderate 2   Severe 3

Q5 ☐

Q6. **Physical changes**
eg skin tears, pressure areas, arthritis, contractures,
previous injuries
Absent 0   Mild 1   Moderate 2   Severe 3

Q6 ☐

Add scores for 1–6 and record here ⟹ **Total Pain Score** ☐

Now tick the box that matches the
Total Pain Score

⟹

0–2 No Pain	3–7 Mild	8–13 Moderate	14 + Severe

Finally, tick the box which matches
the type of pain

⟹

Chronic	Acute	Acute on Chronic

Abbey, J; De Bellis, A: Piller, N: Esterman, A: Giles, L: Parker, D and Lowcay, B.
Funded by the JH & JD Gunn Medical Research Foundation 1998–2002
(This document may be reproduced with this acknowledgement retained)

Figure 12.4 The ABBEY pain scale. Reproduced with permission.

Assessing pain in the patient with advanced disease

Step	Rationale
1 Introduce yourself to the patient.	It is important that the patient knows who you are.
2 Ask the patient to describe the pain.	Patients with cancer may have many different types of pain, for example, visceral, which could be caused by infiltration of tumour into tissues and could result in a deep difficult-to-locate pain or squeezing sensation. Patients could also experience nerve or bone pain. Nerve pain, that is, neuropathic, can cause a constant dull ache, be vice-like, or create a burning sensation (Payne and Gonzales 2003). Pain may also be caused by interventions or treatment.
3 Using a pain scale, for example, a numerical scale, ask the patient to assess the intensity of the pain. For children or people with learning disabilities, consider a visual scale.	Evidence-based practice supports the importance of the patient knowing and assessing the pain (SIGN 2000).
4 Ask the patient if the pain is affecting daily activities, for example, mobility or sleep.	The patient may need more pain relief at certain times of the day.
5 Ask the patient how he or she is feeling.	If the patient is feeling low in mood, is very anxious, or very tired, this will increase the experience of pain.
6 Ask the patient if previous analgesia has been effective.	This is important since the medication may need to be increased.
7 Check, using the drug chart, that the patient has actually been getting analgesia. Look to see how much breakthrough medication they've required.	To ensure that the prescribed medication has been administered.
8 Consider the patient's situation as a whole.	Existential issues, for example, fear of dying, worry about family, could be causing distress.
9 In cognitively impaired patients who can communicate verbally, use words such as *sore* or *aching*.	To help the patient describe the pain.
10 Other visual cues, such as body scales and dolls can help with the cognitively impaired (Davies *et al.* 2004).	To aid understanding,

11	Use large print.	To aid understanding for the cognitively impaired.
12	Ensure adequate lighting.	To aid understanding for the cognitively impaired.
13	Consider sensory impairment, for example, difficulty with hearing.	You may need to talk more slowly and clearly if the patient is deaf.
14	Observe for signs of pain, for example, increased aggressiveness, restiveness, moaning, groans, and yelling. Patients with a learning disability may rock, pace, bite their hand, or become self-injurious (MENCAP 2007). If the pain is acute, the pulse may be raised (tachycardia) and the blood pressure may be lower (Partners in Change 2003).	Increased aggressiveness, restiveness, and vocalizations, such as moaning, are the three main manifestations of pain in the cognitively impaired (Miller *et al.* 2000).
15	Ask the patient with cognitive impairment if the pain is associated with eating, going to the toilet, moving, or vomiting (Partners in Change 2003).	It is important to use more specific criteria when assessing the patient with cognitive impairment.
16	Include the family and healthcare assistants in the assessment if the patient can't communicate verbally. It is important to know what is normal behaviour for the patient with a learning disability or dementia.	To aid understanding. Pain assessment and management needs to be improved for this group of patients (MENCAP 2007).

- By mouth
- By the clock, and
- By the 'ladder'

The 'ladder' refers to the World Health Organization's (WHO) pain ladder, shown in **Fig. 12.6**.

Analgesia in advanced disease should not be prescribed for administration when required unless for breakthrough pain, since inconsistency in administering such medication can result in the patient experiencing unrelieved pain. Giving **analgesics** by the clock ensures that the levels of analgesic within the bloodstream are kept fairly consistent and there are no peaks and troughs, which contribute to pain becoming more difficult to manage.

Steps 1 and 2 on the WHO pain ladder are used to control mild to moderate pain. Morphine, which is on step 3 of the WHO analgesic ladder, is often the drug of choice to relieve severe pain in patients with advanced disease, particularly cancer patients.

Morphine is produced naturally (endogenously) in small amounts in the body. When it is given as a medication it binds to naturally occurring opiate receptors. Morphine usually binds to the mu opiate receptor (Payne and Gonzales 2003). Drugs that bind to opiate receptors are termed opiates. Morphine is an agonist opiate drug. Agonist drugs will enhance the activity of receptor sites. Morphine, therefore, alters pain at the level of the spinal cord and in the central nervous system (CNS), were opiate receptors are located, as well as having some impact on the patient's emotional response to the pain and illness (British Medical Association and Royal Pharmaceutical Society of Great Britain 2006).

Opiates like morphine are **controlled drugs** by law because people can become addicted to them. They are

Wong-Baker FACES Pain Rating Scale

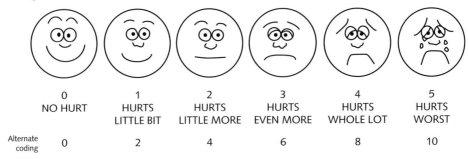

0 NO HURT	1 HURTS LITTLE BIT	2 HURTS LITTLE MORE	3 HURTS EVEN MORE	4 HURTS WHOLE LOT	5 HURTS WORST

Alternate coding	0	2	4	6	8	10

Brief word instructions: Point to each face using the words to describe the pain intensity. Ask the child to choose face that best describes own pain and record the appropriate number.

Original instructions: Explain to the person that each face is for a person who feels happy because he has no pain (hurt) or sad because he has some or a lot of pain. **Face 0** is very happy because he doesn't hurt at all. **Face 1** hurts just a little bit. **Face 2** hurts a little more. **Face 3** hurts even more. **Face 4** hurts a whole lot. **Face 5** hurts as much as you can imagine, although you don't have to be crying to feel this bad. Ask the person to choose the face that best describes how he is feeling.

Rating scale is recommended for persons age 3 years and older.

Figure 12.5 WONG faces scale from Hockenberry MS, wilson D, Winkelslein ML. *Wong's Essentials of Pediatric Nursing*, 7th edn, Lams, 2005, p. 1259. Used with permission. Copyright, Mosby.

WHO's Pain Relief Ladder

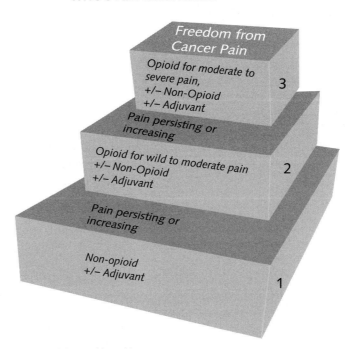

Figure 12.6 WHO pain ladder. Courtesy of the World Health Organization.

Assessment of pain in children

Step		Rationale
1	Introduce yourself to the child.	It is important that the child and parent know who you are.
2	Ask the child directly about their pain, for example, 'Where does it hurt? Does the pain or soreness move about?' Ask the child to tell you how it feels – young children may use babyish words. Ask the parent to describe the pain as well.	It is important to include the child in the pain assessment and accept their language to describe the pain.
3	Observe for signs of anxiety, frustration, or being withdrawn.	The child may be anxious or clinically depressed.
4	Observe for pain behaviours, for example, crying, grimacing, frowning, guarding, limb rigidity.	These are common behaviours exhibited by children in pain (Hall 2005).
5	Ask the parents and child to complete a pain scale, for example, a colour scale or faces scale.	To determine the intensity. Most children of five and above can differentiate a wider range of pain descriptions. Younger children may be limited to describing: *a little, some* and *a lot* (McGrath and Brown 2003)
6	Provide accurate age-appropriate information about interventions to relieve pain.	To relieve child's and parent's anxiety.

kept in a locked cupboard within a locked cupboard, with relevant documentation completed when they are administered. Two nurses, one of whom must be registered, need to administer controlled drugs. Psychological addiction, however, is not a problem when opiates are used correctly to relieve pain. Hartmann *et al.* (2000) states that the treatment of cancer pain leads to addiction in less than 1% of patients who have no drug addiction history.

Morphine can be given orally, subcutaneously, by the **buccal**, or **sublingual** routes, **nebulized**, **intramuscularly**, **intravenously**, and rectally (see Chapter 2). It can also be given by the **intrathecal** or epidural route. The two most common routes in palliative care are *orally*, and, when the patient has difficulty swallowing, *subcutaneously* via a syringe driver.

When drug abusers develop malignancies, a common-sense approach is to accept background drug maintenance therapy, for example, a methadone maintenance programme, and then to titrate the most appropriate opioid analgesic along with non-steroidal anti-inflammartory drugs (NSAIDs) and adjuvant analgesics, as appropriate (SIGN 2000). This is to ensure that patients with a drug abuse problem who develop pain have their pain managed well.

Some palliative-care patients, including children, who are being nursed in a medical or surgical ward, specialist centre, or in the community, may need to receive medication via the subcutaneous route (see **Fig. 12.7**). These drugs include opioids, anti-emetics, and anxiolytic sedatives. They will be administered using a syringe pump driver. Examples of syringe pump drivers that may be used are: the Alaris® syringe pump driver (often used in the acute sector) and the CME Mc Kinley T34 ambulatory pump, often used in community placements, specialist cancer centres, and hospices (see **Figs. 12.8** and **12.9**)

A significant advantage of this method of administration of medication is that plasma levels of the drug are

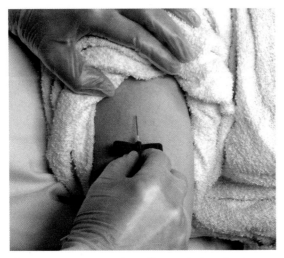

Figure 12.7 Inserting a butterfly cannula for subcutaneous infusions

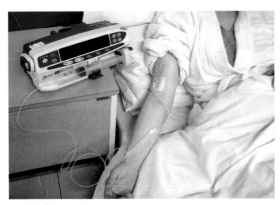

Figure 12.8 Using the Alaris® PK syringe pump driver. With permission of Cardinal Medical Alaris.

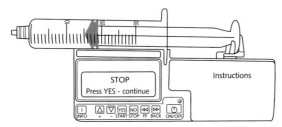

Figure 12.9 McKinley Syring Driver

more stable, and more than one drug may be administered, making it useful in controlling more than one symptom, for example, morphine for pain and midazolam for restlessness and agitation. It may be used for patients who have severe difficulty with swallowing (**dysphagia**), gastrointestinal obstruction (e.g. from tumour), frailty and weakness, poor absorption of oral drugs, unconscious patients, or those who have intractable symptoms:

Managing breakthrough pain

Breakthrough pain is unpredictable and can occur intermittently between regular doses of prescribed medication (Bennet 2005). You may find that your patient still complains of pain even when on oral medication or a morphine pump. Your patient will be prescribed further medication for breakthrough pain, for example, Sevredol or Oramorph, as required. These are oral forms of morphine.

If your patient is on the syringe-driver pump then it may mean that they will be given some additional subcutaneous injections. It is important to note how many times your patient needs medication for breakthrough pain since he or she may require an increase in the overall dose of morphine that is prescribed.

Each day, the dose of morphine administered over the previous 24 hours should be calculated. This would include any extra doses for breakthrough pain. Some patients are reluctant to take breakthrough analgesia. They may require an increase in their regular dose of morphine.

Aftercare

Hughes *et al.* (2005) argue that adequate analgesia for pain may help to combat some behavioural disturbances in patients with dementia. It may be necessary to contact a palliative-care specialist nurse or team for advice on pain control, since some mental health and learning disability nurses lack knowledge and expertise in this aspect of care (Ng and Li 2003).

Some side effects associated with the administration of morphine and diamorphine are:

● Constipation
● Drowsiness

- Sweating
- Dry mouth
- Urinary retention
- **Hallucinations**
- Respiratory depression (in larger doses that have not been titrated)

(Quigley 2005)

A high proportion of patients who take opiate-based drugs for pain will experience constipation. SIGN (2000) recommend the prophylactic use of aperients, such as movicol, senna, or lactulose. Small microlax **enemas** may be required for acute impaction.

Nausea and vomiting associated with the administration of morphine or diamorphine will normally settle in a few days. Drugs that may be used to alleviate nausea and vomiting are called **anti-emetics**. Examples of anti-emetics used in palliative care are ondansetron, cyclizine, and levomepromazine (British Medical Association and Royal Pharmaceutical Society of Great Britain 2007).

Developing your skills

When you are out on practice with your mentor you may observe her setting up a syringe pump driver and administering the medication to your patient. Syringe pumps drive the plunger of a syringe forwards at a controlled rate to deliver medication to the patient. Specific protocols are followed to ensure that these syringe pumps are running effectively and safely. For example, registered nurses follow guidelines to ensure the correct administration of medications and the correct use of the **diluent**. The registered nurse will also ensure that there is no air in the tubing, the syringe is correctly loaded onto the pump, and the pump is programmed and sited correctly, and take measures to prevent infection at the cannula site. The nurse will also ensure that there is no malfunction of the pump when it is running, for example, from inflammation at the cannula site, kinking or stretching of tubing, or insecure connections (Trundle *et al.* 2007). You may learn more about this method of administration of medications in your second or third year of practice.

Other factors to consider

Managing restlessness and delirium

Some opiate medications, such as methadone, increase agitation and delirium in cognitively impaired patients. Morphine may be used to relieve pain for this group of patients but is often commenced at a lower dose than the normal adult amount.

If patients are very restless or become delirious in the end stage of dying, midazolam may be given via a syringe driver to settle them (**Fig. 12.9**). Children may also be given midazolam if they have persistent seizures, although **noninvasive** routes, such as the buccal or intranasal route (Mahmoudian and Mohammadi 2004; Scott *et al.* 2002), may be preferred. Scott *et al.* (2002) state that buccal midazolam is as effective as rectal diazepam and the route is more socially acceptable. Phenobarbitone may also be given to children via a subcutaneous infusion pump.

Children may be give acetaminophen (paracetamol) for mild pain (step one of the analgesic ladder), codeine phosphate for moderate pain (step two) and an opiate for severe pain (step three) (Hall 2005). The dose of analgesics, including morphine, will vary widely with individual children. The age, weight, and frailty of the child, as well as the intensity of pain, need to be considered.

Morphine may also be given intranasally or via the buccal route for children. As with adults, the dose of morphine may need to be titrated to control the pain. Young children need you to be their advocate and to be sensitive to their potential needs for breakthrough analgesia. A child, as well as an adult on morphine, may still require night sedation to help sleep.

Antidepressants and anticonvulsants may be used to manage neuropathic (nerve pain) in adults and children. Gabapentin is a useful anticonvulsant medication for managing neuropathic pain in both elderly adults and children. However, relatives need to be educated about the use of morphine, antidepressants, and anticonvulsants for managing their children's pain. Morphine, in particular, can conjure up images of a drug addiction. Alternatively, parents may identify its use as meaning that their child is getting worse.

Nonsteroidal anti-inflammatory drugs, like ibuprofen, need to be used with caution in children with organ failure or a history of GI bleeding (Lidstone *et al.* 2006; McGrath and Brown 2003).

The route of medication is important for both adults and children since an injection is painful. Children may be given oral transmucosal fentanyl citrate (OFTC) (fentanyl lozenge). This provides rapid onset analgesia via a pleasant route. The fentanyl lozenge is suitable for children from 2 to 12 years. Fentanyl is a powerful opioid, which, like morphine, binds to mu receptors. It can also be given via a transdermal patch and has been effective in controlling pain for adults and children with cancer (Lidstone *et al.* 2006; McGrath and Brown 2003). A new sublingual form of fentanyl, currently under development, may be useful for breakthrough episodes of pain. Children may also receive pain medication via the subcutaneous route.

Neonates and infants also need pain control. They require special dosing regimens and careful monitoring. The starting dose of morphine for infants under 6 months is one-quarter to one-third of that for older children. Drug clearance of morphine in infants above the age of six months and for children is the same as that for the young adult (McGrath and Brown 2003).

Nondrug therapies

For adults, nondrug therapies to manage pain include:

- Relaxation exercises
- Music
- Distraction
- Aromatherapy
- Reflexology
- Hypnosis and guided imagery

Nondrug therapies for children include:

- Giving information to the parent and the child
- Teaching relaxation methods
- Music therapy
- Distraction

> *(http://www.health-first.org/health_*
> *info/your_health_first/kids/pain.cfm;*
> *McGrath and Brown 2003; Zeltzer 2005).*

Dyspnoea

When patients become distressed because of difficulty with breathing (dyspnoea) oxygen may have limited effectiveness. Patients may then be given a dose of morphine. This may also be given in a slow-release form (once daily). This helps to suppress the unpleasant feelings associated with dyspnoea and is unlikely to cause respiratory depression. If patients are also able to practice relaxation exercises, this may help to improve breathing. The physiotherapist may be able to teach patients to use other strategies (Abernethy *et al.* 2003; Andrewes 2002; Jennings and Davies 2002).

12.5 **The last offices**

Definition

The last offices are performed to prepare the body so that relatives can spend some time with the deceased and to transport the body to the mortuary.

When to perform the last offices

You may be required to carry out this procedure in your first placement. You will find that your mentor is supportive of you as a student when dealing with a death in the ward or community for the first time.

Special considerations

Religion

Last offices might need to be adapted to take account of the religious beliefs of the patient or the patient's family. Although people are of different faiths, some do not follow their faith strictly and so it is worth checking with the patient and family what their wishes are. The following, however, provides some important information about some religions. Remember that there are other religions not mentioned here. You may need to find information about what you can and cannot do.

You do not perform the last offices for patients of the Islamic faith. The family usually attend to them. Nurses should wear gloves and may be permitted to close the eyes, straighten the limbs, and turn the head towards the right shoulder (Mecca). Muslims are traditionally always buried, not cremated. They are buried quite quickly. Muslims are opposed to post-mortem examinations.

If a Muslim child is dying, it can be helpful to turn the foot of the cot in the direction of Mecca – south-easterly. If a baby dies shortly after birth, it is worth remembering that the Islamic faith forbids a woman from touching a dead body for 40 days after the delivery of her baby.

There is usually no objection to nurses preparing the patient of Hindu faith, although you may have to seek the family's permission to do this. Gloves should be worn when preparing the body. Sometimes a Hindu priest (Pandit) will attend. However, Hindus are very unwilling to consent to post-mortem examination. Both Sikhs and Hindus are cremated and Hindu funerals are held within 24 hours. Hindus and Sikhs prefer to prepare the body of a child themselves. Hindu children under five are buried.

The priest may need to be called if the patient is Catholic, or a rabbi may be called if the patient is Jewish. If there is no family member or rabbi in attendance for the Jewish patient, it is permissible for the nurse to close the eyes and mouth, keep limbs straight, remove any tubes, and wrap the body in a plain sheet. Parts of the body that have been removed by surgery may be retained and the Jewish burial society should be contacted. The bodies of Jewish people, however, are not normally left unattended and they are buried as soon as possible after death. Post-mortem examination is discouraged (McDonald 2002; NHS Greater Glasgow Last Offices Guidelines 2004).

Infection

If the patient has had an infection, extra precautions should be taken. This would mean protecting yourself with a plastic apron and disposable gloves prior to undertaking the last offices.

Drainage tube sites and open wounds should be sealed using waterproof dressings. If it is not possible to cover the body fluids with waterproof dressings, the body will be placed in a leakproof cadaver bag.

Where serious infection, for example, untreated tuberculosis, hepatitis B, C, or HIV, are present, the body must be placed in a leakproof cadaver bag labelled 'Danger of infection'. The label must be signed by the nurse and the doctor. 'Danger of infection' labels may be put on the wrists of the patient but are also affixed to the outside of the bag. Porters are advised of the risk. If any spillages occur from a patient with a suspected infection then decontamination should be undertaken by trained personnel. Individual trust policy will need to be consulted for this.

It is important to remember that relatives will be distressed and anxious if the infection risk is high. You may observe your mentor communicating with them sensitively.

Aftercare

After a child dies, the family will need some quiet time with the child. It is helpful if brothers and sisters can see the body, since this can help in the bereavement period. The family should not be rushed at this time and sensitivity to their child and their situation is crucial. Sometimes, if it is a small child or baby, the nurse will take the body to the mortuary. This can help a parent who finds it hard to let go.

Developing your skills

You may find it difficult to sever the relationship when a patient dies. Performing the last offices for a patient that you have known can help to bring closure. Discussing your feelings with other members of staff may also help.

The last offices are never easy, however, they can become less painful and emotional the more you perform them. If a **therapeutic** relationship has formed between the nurse, patient, and family, it will still be an emotional time for the nurse.

Other factors to consider

Sudden or unexpected death

A post-mortem examination will be carried out, usually as a legal requirement. This is known as a fiscal case. The funeral arrangements could be delayed for as much as one week. Cremation fees are paid to medical staff if patients are to be cremated. A cremation certificate is given to the family and the undertakers collect the fees.

Where a death is expected, some nurses can verify this death: for example some District Nurses have this authority and a specific protocol is followed.

The last offices

EQUIPMENT

- Last offices box,
- Shroud,
- Identification labels.

 ## Action   Rationale

Action	Rationale
The curtains around the bed are closed.	To ensure privacy.
The doctor is called.	The doctor will pronounce death and will issue a death certificate.
The doctor or nurse will inform the relatives.	The relatives may wish to attend the patient.
Note the time that the patient has died.	This is important, since there may be a further investigation into the death.
Collect items from the last offices box.	There is normally a special 'last offices' box in the ward.
Cleanse hands.	To prevent cross-infection.
Wear disposable gloves.	To prevent cross-infection.
The patient is washed. Nurses will often talk to the patient as they are doing this. The eyes are closed. The eyes may be gently taped (transpore).	To ensure that respect is ensured and the dignity of the individual maintained at this final stage.
A disposable hospital gown is put on, or if the family request it, the deceased patient's own clothes.	Relatives' wishes will be respected.
An incontinence pad is used and any wounds are padded. Any intravenous cannulae, catheters, or drains are removed unless the death requires legal investigation (you will be told of this by your mentor).	To protect from leakage of body fluids.
Rings, etc., may be removed or left on the body. If they are removed, this should be witnessed by two people and a signed account recorded. They are then stored safely until the relatives collect the patient's belongings. If rings remain on the body, by the relative's request, then the undertaker must be informed.	To ensure the safety of the patient's belongings.
Identity bands (containing the deceased patient's name, hospital number date of birth and ward) are put on the ankles and wrists of the patient (four in number).	For correct identification and security when transporting to the mortuary.
If the lower jaw of the deceased patient has dropped, consider using a chin support as shown in Fig. 12.10.	If advised in trust guidelines.

The body is wrapped in a blanket and tape is used to secure limbs.	To avoid any damage or harm to the corpse during transportation.
The bedlinen is changed.	The relatives may wish to spend some time with the deceased. It may help them a little to see that care has been taken in preparing the body.
Cleanse hands.	To prevent cross-infection.
A mortuary card is given to the porter and a card with the date and time of death is placed on the body.	This is to ensure accurate identification of the body and communication of the time of death to mortuary staff.
The relatives may want to sit with the patient. The room is tidied up and a vase of flowers may be put on the bed table. Religious beliefs should be considered if possible, for example, if the patient was a Christian then a bible may be placed on the locker.	This can help the relatives in the bereavement period.
The family may be escorted to the bedside and then left to sit with the patient alone. Alternatively, your presence might be appreciated. They may sit with the patient for some period of time.	This can help the relatives in the bereavement period.
The family may need support and help to get home safely, for example, a taxi may be ordered.	The family or friends could be in shock and their concentration may be poor.
The porters are informed, by phone, that the body is ready to be taken to the mortuary.	
The screens may be drawn around other patients before the porters come to take the body (corpse) to the mortuary.	To maintain privacy. To ensure that other patients don't become too distressed.
If a post-mortem examination is to be carried out, all the clinical records will be sent with the patient to the mortuary.	This is important because the circumstances of deaths that are referred for legal investigation need a full review.

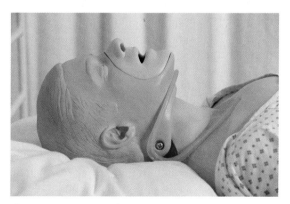

Figure 12.10 Using a chin support

There is no specific bereavement support for relatives and friends in acute hospitals but your mentor may recommend organizations such as Cruse. If your mentor has known the patient well, he or she may go to the funeral.

A bereavement pack may be given to the relative, for example, with instructions on how to register the death, or a leaflet may be given on bereavement support, particularly if the patient has died in the community or a hospice. Bereavement visits may then be made in the community after two weeks, three months, and six months. Hospices may have a 'drop in' bereavement group, a structured bereavement group, or one-to-one counselling services.

District nurses and paediatric nurses will often attend the funeral of patients they have cared for. This can mean a lot to the family.

 ## Scenarios

Consider what you should do in the following situations, then turn to the end of the section to check your answers.

Further scenarios are available at

🌐 **www.oxfordtextbooks.co.uk/orc/docherty/**

 ### Scenario 1

Sarah is a 37-year-old woman who is married and has two children, 14-year-old Abigail and 11-year-old Tom. She was admitted with a history of abdominal pain, severe nausea, and vomiting, and steady weight loss over a period of two months. After investigation, she was diagnosed as having an obstruction of her bile duct caused by a **cholangio carcinoma**. Sarah was restricted to oral fluids, a nasogastric tube was inserted, an intravenous infusion pump was set up and she was given ondansetron, an anti-emetic, to relieve her nausea and oramorph to relieve her pain. Sarah was informed that the tumour was not re-resectable and told that bypass surgery (gastrojejunostomy) could improve her symptoms.

Sarah felt quite positive about the bypass surgery and stated that it would be nice to enjoy her food without feeling constantly sick. She was also keen to get back to her family and spend some time with them. Her recovery from the bypass surgery was uneventful and she was discharged home.

One week after discharge, Sarah was readmitted to the surgical ward. She was in severe pain, felt nauseated, and was vomiting. Her urea, electrolyte, and liver function tests were deranged. She was restless, semi-comatose with some episodes of delirium. She was doubly incontinent. Her sisters accompanied her to the ward but her husband was not there.

1 Which communication skills would you use when talking to Sarah?
2 After readmission, which factors would you consider that might be exacerbating Sarah's pain?
3 What action could be taken to relieve Sarah's pain and distress?
4 Which medications would be suitable for controlling Sarah's nausea and vomiting?
5 Which criteria would indicate that Sarah is dying?

 ### Scenario 2

Jane was diagnosed with a neuroblastoma (brain tumour) when she was 4 years old. She had a history of headaches, which were worse when she lay down. She was also nauseated and vomited daily. She was admitted for surgery and had partial removal of a large tumour. She was readmitted to have the rest of the tumour removed but stopped breathing whilst under anaesthesia. She was ventilated for a lengthy period in the paediatric intensive care unit. As she could not support her breathing on her own, a **tracheostomy** tube was inserted.

Jane is now 6 years old. She still relies on a tracheostomy tube to maintain her own breathing. She attends a school for children with special needs. Tracheal suction is carried out at the school on a weekly basis when the tube is changed. This may be done more often when Jane is at home. She has a tendency to drool and she has been prescribed **hyoscine** patches for this. These are causing irritation of her skin. Jane is prone to chest infections and this debilitates her and affects her quality of life. The physiotherapist sees Jane each week.

Owing to damage to the nerves involved in swallowing, Jane has had a PEG tube inserted. Jane's parents feed her overnight so that she can be more mobile during the day. She has water inserted in the tube during the day. She requires regular mouth care.

Jane is confined to a wheelchair and needs support for her spine via a spinal jacket and splints to prevent her legs from contracting and in particular her feet turning in. She is doubly incontinent but she is not catheterized. She communicates using a **Dynavox system**.

Jane has remained debilitated since her surgery and her parents have been told that she will get steadily worse. She is on codeine phosphate for pain but this is not controlling her pain well. The physician is keen to commence her on morphine to manage her pain better but Jane's parents are unwilling to agree to this.

1 What would be the most effective way to keep Jane's mouth healthy?
2 Which step of the WHO ladder would codeine phosphate be on and why would the physician consider putting Jane onto morphine?
3 Why might Jane's parents be unwilling to agree to her commencing morphine?

 ## Scenario 3

Joseph developed normally until the age of 4 when he developed a degenerative disorder called adrenoleucodystrophy (ALD). This is a genetic disorder that causes progressive cerebral deterioration and dysfunction of the adrenal gland (Green 2004). He is now a frail 8-year-old who has learning disabilities. Joseph's limb movements are uncoordinated and he takes 5 mg baclofen twice daily to relieve muscle spasms. Joseph lives at home with his parents and older brother. He has been attending a school for children with special needs.

Joseph is supported in a wheelchair. He has difficulty with speech and swallowing. He is underweight for a child of his age and he can only communicate via head nods or blinking his eyes. He persistently takes seizures and has recently developed pneumonia. Joseph's mother has been told that he may only survive for a few months. Joseph has been moaning a lot recently and making facial grimaces.

1 What pain assessment tool could you use with Joseph?
2 Which drugs may be used to control his seizures?

 ## Scenario 4

Cameron is a 69-year-old man with a diagnosis of Alzheimer's disease. He also has advanced prostatic cancer with multiple bone **metastases**. Cameron and his wife Gloria have been told that he has only a few months to live.

He had been in a hospice for almost a year but was transferred to an organic admission ward in a local psychiatric hospital when his symptoms changed. Cameron had been a pleasant and amenable man during his time in the hospice but he had recently become violent, hitting out at staff and disrupting other patients, particularly during the night.

Initially, staff at the hospice thought that Cameron needed more pain relief and his analgesia was increased. This caused a temporary relief in his symptoms. However Cameron's aggressive behaviour returned and it was suggested that this was caused by a change in his mental state as a result of damage to his brain.

Cameron's behaviour was disruptive when he was admitted to the psychiatric assessment unit but since his medication was changed from haloperidol (an antipsychotic drug) to quetiapine, an antipsychotic drug that may be better tolerated than haloperidol (British Medical Association and Royal Pharmaceutical Society of Great Britain 2006), he has become more settled. Cameron's other symptoms included pain, reluctance to eat or drink, and double incontinence. His medication included oxycodone, an opioid analgesic (15 mg at 10 am and 10 pm), co-codamol (four hourly) and Oramorph for breakthrough pain. Oxycodone has a similar efficacy to morphine. The side effects are also similar to those experienced whilst on morphine. It is normally given by mouth every four to six hours (British Medical Association and Royal Pharmaceutical Society of Great Britain 2006) but may be given in a sustained release form twice daily.

Cameron's wife, Gloria, is angry because she thought that the hospice would take Cameron back once his behaviour improved. However, the hospice have informed her that they are unwilling to accept him and that his bed has already been filled by another patient. She feels that he is now in a ward that is unsuitable for a dying man. She points out that the quiet, calming atmosphere of the hospice was ideal for Cameron's last months and that the ward he is in now is far to noisy and that he has no one to speak to as all the patients there are too mentally impaired. She does, however, acknowledge that staff on the ward have managed Cameron's behavioural problems better than they did at the hospice but recognizes that it is an admission ward and not equipped for the care of a dying man.

1 What kind of pain assessment tool would be useful for assessing Cameron's pain?

2 Name three behaviours that are commonly demonstrated by cognitively impaired patients in pain.

3 Which intervention could help reassure Cameron's wife?

Website

◉ www.oxfordtextbooks.co.uk/orc/docherty/
You may find it helpful to work through our short online quiz and interactive scenarios intended to help you to develop and apply the skills in this chapter.

References

Abernethy A, Currow D, Frith P, Fazekas B, McHugh A, and Bui C (2003). Randomised, double blind, placebo controlled crossover trial of sustained release morphine for the management of refractory dyspnoea. *British Medical Journal,* **327**, 523–8.

Andrewes T (2002). The management of breathlessness in palliative care. *Nursing Standard,* **17**(5), 43–52, 54–55.

Bagg I (2003). Oral candidosis: how to treat a common problem. *European Journal of Palliative Care,* **10**(2), 54–6.

Bennet D (2005). Consensus panel recommendations for the assessment and management of breakthrough pain. Part 1: assessment. *Pharmacy and Therapeutics,* **30**, 296–301.

British Medical Association and Royal Pharmaceutical Society of Great Britain (2006). *British National Formulary.* British Medical Association and Royal Pharmaceutical Society of Great Britain, London.

British Medical Association and Royal Pharmaceutical Society of Great Britain (2007). *British National Formulary.* British Medical Association and Royal Pharmaceutical Society of Great Britain, London.

Buckman (1998). Communication. In Doyle D, Hanks G, MacDonald N, eds, *Oxford Textbook of Palliative Medicine,* 2nd edn, p.146. Oxford University Press, Oxford.

Critchlow J and Bauer-Wu S (2002). Dehydration in terminally ill patients: perceptions of long term care nurses. *Journal of Gerontological Nursing,* **28**(12), 31–9.

Cunningham C (2006). Managing pain in patients with dementia. *Nursing Standard,* **20**(46), 54–8.

Darnhill S and Garnage B (2006). The patient's journey: palliative care—a parent's view. *British Medical Journal,* **332**, 1494–5.

Davies E, Male M, Reimer V, and Turner M (2004). Pain assessment and cognitive impairment: part 2. *Nursing Standard,* **19**(13), 33–40.

De Araujo M, da Silva M, and Francisco M (2004). Nursing the dying: essential elements in the care of terminally ill patients. *International Council of Nurses,* **51**, 149–58.

Dunniece U, Slevin E (2000). Nurses' experiences of being present with a patient receiving a diagnosis of cancer. *Journal of Advanced Nursing,* **32**(3), 611–18.

Egar G (2007). *The Skilled Helper,* 8th edn, Thomson Brooks/Cole.

Ellershaw J and Ward C (2003). Care of the dying patient: the last hours or days of life. *British Medical Journal,* **326**, 30–4.

Ellershaw J and Wilkinson S (2003). *Care of the Dying: A Pathway to Excellence.* Oxford University Press, Oxford.

Fallowfield LJ, Jenkins VA, and Beveridge HA (2002). Truth may hurt but deceit hurts more: communication in palliative care. *Palliative Medicine,* **16**, 297–303.

Fitzpatrick J (2000). Oral health care needs of dependent older people: responsibilities of nurses and care assistants. *Journal of Advanced Nursing,* **32**(6), 1325–32.

Foley K (1998). Pain assessment and cancer pain syndromes. In Doyle D, Hanks G, and MacDonald N, eds, *Oxford Textbook of Palliative Medicine,* pp. 310–31. Oxford University Press, Oxford.

Green S (2004). Adrenoleukodystrophy: Where are we now? CLIMB update 215.

Hall J (2005). Validation of a paediatric pain assessment tool designed specifically for use in the A&E Department at The Royal London Hospital. *Progress in Practice,* **16**. www.rlhleagueofnurses.org.uk/ Education/Progress_Index/Progress_16/ PaediatricPain/paediatricpain.html.

Harris D (2007). Forget me not: palliative care for people with dementia. *Postgraduate Medical Journal,* **83**, 362–6.

Hartmann L, Zahasky K, and Grendahl D (2000). Management of cancer pain. *Postgraduate Medicine,* **107**(3), 267–76.

Hughes J, Robinson L, and Volicer L (2005). Specialist palliative care in dementia. *British Medical Journal,* **330**, 57–8.

Jennings A and Davies A (2002). A systematic review of the use of opioids in the management of dyspnoea. *Thorax,* **57**, 939–44.

Kent H and McDowell J (2004). Sudden bereavement in acute care. *Nursing Standard,* **19**(6), 38–42.

Kinder C and Ellershaw J (2003). How to use the Liverpool care pathway for the dying patient. In Ellershaw J and Wilkinson S, *Care of the Dying: A Pathway to Excellence,* pp. 11–15. Oxford University Press, Oxford.

Lidstone V, Delaney J, Hain R, and bir Singh-Jassal S (2006). *Paediatric Palliative Care Guidelines,* 2nd edn. South West London, The Surrey, West Essex and Hampshire, The Sussex Cancer Networks, and The Northern Ireland Palliative Medicine Group.

Lynch M and Dahlin C (2007). The National Consensus Project and National Quality Forum preferred practices in care of the imminently dying: implications for nursing. *Journal of Hospice and Palliative Nursing,* **9**(6), 316–22.

Mahmoudian T and Mohammadi Z (2004). Comparison of intranasal midazolam with intravenous diazepam for treating acute seizures in children. *Epilepsy and Behaviour,* **5**(2), 253–5.

MENCAP (2007). *Death by Indifference.* MENCAP, London.

McDonald P (2002). *Religions and Culture: North Glasgow University Hospitals Trust.* NHS Greater Glasgow, Glasgow.

McGrath A and Brown S (2003). Paediatric palliative medicine. In Doyle D, Hanks G, and MacDonald N, eds, *Oxford Textbook of Palliative Medicine,* 3rd edn, pp. 777–807. Oxford University Press, Oxford.

Miller M, Nelson L and Mezey M (2000). Comfort and pain relief in dementia: awakening a new beneficence. *Journal of Gerontological Nursing,* **26**(29), 33–40.

Miller M and Kearney N (2001). Oral care for patients with cancer: a review of the literature. *Cancer Nursing,* **24**(4), 241–54.

Milligan S, Mc Gill M, Sweeney M, and Malarkey C (2001). Oral care for people with advanced cancer: an evidence-based protocol. *International Journal of Palliative Nursing,* **7**(9), 418–26.

NCPC (The National Council for Palliative Care) (2007). *Palliative Care Explained.* www.ncpc.org.uk/palliative_care.html.

Ng J and Li S (2003). A survey exploring the educational needs of care practitioners in learning disability settings in relation to death, dying and people with learning disabilities. *European Journal of Cancer Care,* **12**, 12–19.

NHS Greater Glasgow (2004). *Last Offices Guidelines.* NHS Greater Glasgow, Glasgow. http://library.nhsggc.org.uk/mediaAssets/Nursing%20and%20Midwifery/1.9%20-%20Last%20Offices.pdf.

Partners in Change (2003). *Palliative Care and People with Learning Disabilities: A Report From a Conference Held in 2003.* Partners for Change, SHS Trust Edinburgh.

Payne R and Gonzales G (2003). Pathophysiology of pain in cancer and other terminal diseases. In Doyle D, Hanks G, and MacDonald N, eds, *Oxford Textbook of Palliative Medicine,* 3rd edn, pp. 288–98. Oxford University Press, Oxford.

Pittelkow M and Loprinzi C (2003). Pruritis and sweating in palliative medicine. In Doyle D, Hanks G, and MacDonald N, eds, *Oxford Textbook of Palliative Medicine,* 3rd edn, pp. 573–86. Oxford University Press, Oxford.

Pitorak E (2003). Care at the time of death: how nurses can make the last hours of life a richer, more comfortable experience. *American Journal of Nursing,* **103**(7), 42–52.

Quaglietti S, Blum L, and Ellis V (2004). The role of the adult nurse practitioner in palliative care. *Journal of Hospice and Palliative Nursing,* **6**(4), 209–14.

Quigley C (2005). The role of opioids in cancer pain. *British Medical Journal,* **331**, 825–9.

RCN (2006). *Meeting the Health Needs of People with Learning Disabilities.* Royal College of Nursing, London.

Rogers A, Karlsen S, and Addington-Hall J (2000). 'All the services were excellent. It is when the human element comes in that things go wrong': dissatisfaction with hospital care in the last year of life. *Journal of Advanced Nursing,* **31**(4), 768–74.

Scott R, Besag F, Nevelle B (2002). Buccal midazolam and rectal diazepam for treatment of prolonged seizures in childhood and adolescence: a randomised trial. *Lancet,* **353**, 62.

SIGN (2000). *Control of Pain in Patients with Cancer.* Publication 44. Scottish Intercollegiate Guidelines Network, Edinburgh. www.sign.ac.uk/guidelines/fulltext/44/index.html.

Stevens M (2003). Psychological adaptation of the dying child. In Doyle D, Hanks G, and MacDonald N, eds, *Oxford Textbook of Palliative Medicine,* 3rd edn, pp. 806–22. Oxford University Press, Oxford.

Trundle J, Lennon K, Walley J, Mauchline R, Bashford I, and Gravil J (2007). *Syringe Pump Guidelines: CME McKinley T34 (ml/hour). For use within Argyll and Bute CHP and Clyde.* NHS Greater Glasgow and Clyde, Howwood, Renfrewshire. www.palliativecareglasgow.info/pdf/ABC_syringe_pump2007_NT_FINAL.pdf.

Tuffrey-Wijne I (2002). *Cancer, Palliative Care and Intellectual Disabilities.* St. George's University of London, London. www.intellectualdisability.info/mental_phys_health/cancer_id.htm.

Turnbull Q, Wolf M, and Holroyd S (2003). Attitudes of elderly subjects toward 'truth telling' for the diagnosis of Alzheimer's disease. *Journal of Geriatric Psychiatry and Neurology,* **16**(2), 90–3.

WHO (2008). *Palliative Care.* www.who.int/cancer/palliative/en/.

White K, Wilkes L, Cooper K, and Barbato M (2004). The impact of unrelieved patient suffering on palliative care nurses. *International Journal of Palliative Nursing,* **10**(9), 439–43.

Zeltzer L (2005). Pain management. *Journal of Paediatric Psychology,* **30**(7), 623–8.

Zerwekh J (2003). Hospital nursing: end-of-life hydration—benefit or burden? *Nursing 2003,* **33**(2), 1–3.

Useful further reading and websites

Adults with Incapacity Scotland Act 2000. www.opsi.gov.uk/legislation/Scotland/acts2000/20000004.htm.

American Medical Association (2007). *Pediatric Pain Management.* www.ama-cmeonline.com/pain_mgmt/module06/index.htm.

King N, Bell D, and Thomas K (2004). Family carer's experiences of out-of-hours community palliative care: a qualitative study. *International Journal of Palliative Nursing,* **10**(2), 76–83.

This research study explores services supplied by GPs and district nurses to family carers outside of normal access hours in the community setting.

Kinghorn S and Gaines S (2007). *Palliative Nursing: Improving End of Life Care.* Bailliere Tindall, London.

The key themes in this book are pain control, symptom control, loss and grief, and handling loss.

Mental Capacity Act (2005). www.opsi.gov.uk/acts/acts2005/20050009.htm.

Nursing Midwifery Council (2004). *Standards of Proficiency for Pre-registration Nursing Education.* NMC, London. www.nmc-uk.org.

Perry J, Galloway S, Bototorff J, and Nixon S (2005). Nurse-patient communication in dementia: improving the odds. *Journal of Gerontological Nursing,* **31**(4), 43–52.

A study that investigates a range of conversational strategies in a nurse-led **socialization** group with long-term-care residents.

Scherder E and van Manen F (2005). Pain in Alzheimer's disease: nursing assistants' and patients' evaluations. *Journal of Advanced Nursing,* **52**(2), 151–8.

This research study examines the levels of agreement about pain experienced by patients when assessed by nursing assistants. The two groups of patients are elderly, some have Alzheimer's disease and others are more cognitively able.

www.childhospice.org.uk/.

www.first.org/health_info/your health_first?kids/pain.cfm.

www.nhslanarkshire.co.uk/Homepage.htm.

www.nice.org.uk.

www.palliativecareglasgow.info/index_pro.asp.

www.sign.ac.uk.

www.who.int/cancer/palliative/en/.

Check **www.oxfordtextbooks.co.uk/orc/docherty/** for changes and new developments. Updated research, guidelines, or equipment will be added every four months.

Answers to scenarios

Scenario 1

1 Which communication skills would you use when communicating with Sarah?

Open questions, honesty, active listening, reflecting, and summarizing.

2 After readmission, which factors would you consider that might be exacerbating Sarah's pain?

Worries, fears about dying, worries about her family, spread of the cancer.

3 What action could be taken to relieve Sarah's pain and distress?

Subcutaneous morphine pump, midazolam, communication skills.

4 Which medications would be suitable for controlling Sarah's nausea and vomiting?

Cyclizine, Ondansetron, Levomepromazine.

5 Which criteria would indicate that Sarah is dying?

Sarah becomes bedbound,

Sarah is semi-comatose,

Sarah is able to take only sips of fluid,

Sarah is no longer able to take oral drugs (Ellershaw and Ward 2003).

Scenario 2

1 What would be the most effective way to keep Jane's mouth healthy?

Assess daily, observe for any problems, such as infection, clean with a soft toothbrush and fluoride toothpaste, and rinse with water.

2 Which step of the WHO ladder would codeine phosphate be on and why would the physician consider putting her onto morphine?

Children may be give acetaminophen for mild pain (step 1 of the analgesic ladder), codeine for moderate pain, and an opiate for severe pain (McGrath and Brown 2003).

3 Why might Jane's parents be unwilling to agree to her commencing on morphine?

They associate it with drug addicts and addiction,

It is a sign that their daughter is getting worse,

They do not want to acknowledge that their daughter is dying.

Scenario 3

1 What pain assessment tool could be used with Joseph?

Abbey pain assessment scale or the faces scale.

2 Which drugs might be used to control his seizures and which methods of administration could be used?

Midazolam or phenobarbitone: buccal, intranasal, or subcutaneous route.

Scenario 4

1 What kind of pain assessment tool would be useful for assessing Cameron's pain?

The Abbey pain scale.

2 Name three behaviours that are commonly demonstrated by cognitively impaired patients in pain.

Increasing aggressiveness, restiveness, and vocalizations, such as moaning.

3 Which intervention could help to reassure Cameron's wife?

Asking the palliative care nurse or team to become involved in his care.

Glossary

Abduction   Movement away from the mid line (median) in the coronal plane

Acetone   A ketone, which is the by-product of fat metabolism that is excreted in sweat and urine and can be detected on the breath as a 'pear drop' type of smell

Acromegaly   Enlargement of the bones through over-secretion of growth hormone: most noticeable in the hands, feet, and face

Active listening   The ability to capture and understand the messages patients are communicating

Active movement   Movement initiated by voluntary muscle

Adduction   To move towards the mid line in the coronal plane

Adenocarcinoma   Malignant tumour of glandular epithelial origin

Adenoma   Benign tumour of glandular epithelial origin

Aggressive   Responding with anger and the potential for violence or disrespect

Agonal breathing   Infrequent, irregular gasping breath

Alimentary   Pertaining to food or the digestive or gastrointestinal tract

Alkaline   (see pH) a pH greater than 7 on a logarithmic scale from 1–14

Altered conscious level   A decreased level of alertness and awareness of the environment, and decreased ability to make deliberate and intentional decisions

Ampoule   A sterile glass or plastic container that contains a single dose of a solution to be administered parenterally

Anaemia   A state where there is insufficient iron in the blood

Anaesthetic   An agent that reduces or abolishes sensation; affecting the whole body (general) or a particular area (local)

Analgesics   Drugs that relieve pain

Anaphylaxis   A life-threatening reaction to a foreign protein or other substance

Anorexia   Decreased food intake

Anthopometric   Measurement of the human body (derived from the Greek words anthro—meaning 'man'—and metron—meaning 'measure')

Antibiotic   A substance that destroys or inhibits the growth of other microorganisms (usually bacteria or fungus) that are sensitive to it

Anticoagulant   A drug that dissolves and decreases blood clot formation

Anti-emetics   Drugs that relieve nausea and vomiting

Antimicrobial   Something that kills microbes

Antipyretics   Drugs that reduce fever by lowering the body temperature

Anuria   Absence of urine: usually less than 100 ml in 24 hours

Anxiety   A condition characterized by fear, trepidation, and worry resulting in physical, psychological, and behavioural reactions.

Apyrexia   The absence of fever, that is, normal body temperature

Arrhythmia   An unusual heart rhythm

Arthritis   Painful inflammation of a joint

Aspiration   The breathing in of liquid (can be from the stomach, that is, vomit) into the lower airways (lungs)

Assertiveness   Making your feelings and wishes known without anger and giving respect to the other person. For example, when told to do something by another when you do not have the time, saying, 'No, I can't do that now—perhaps if I have time later, I'll be able to help you.'

Assistive technology   Assistive, adaptive, and rehabilitation technological devices and the process used in selecting, locating, and using them with the aim of promoting greater independence

Attachment   Infant–parent bonding

Aural   Relating to the ear

Auscultation   Listening to the sounds in the thorax with a stethoscope

Autoimmune disorders   These occur when the body's normal immune response is exaggerated and reacts excessively to minor or even absent stimuli. Rheumatoid arthritis is one example

Biochemical   Chemical substances in the human body

Biomechanics   The study of how the body moves and the stresses placed on it

Blanching hyperaemia   The skin whitening that occurs when pressure is applied, indicating that microcirculation is intact

Blood clotting   The process by which factors in the blood combine with platelets to form a solid mass that, in the body, blocks any leaking vessel and allows it to be repaired

Body mass index   A calculation using height and weight to determine whether the patient is underweight, a healthy weight, or overweight

Bradycardia   A decrease in heart rate below normal

Bradypnoea   A decrease in respiratory rate below normal

Bradypnoeic   Slow rate of breathing

Braille   A tactile language used to communicate with the partially sighted or blind

Bronchodilator   Drug commonly used to dilate the bronchioles

Buccal   Between the gum and the cheek

Cachexia   Abnormally low weight, weakness, and decline of the patient; most often associated with cancer

Calibration   The process of determining and, if necessary, adjusting the measurement given by an instrument and the measurement standard, within a specified accuracy

Calpol   Paediatric oral suspension of paracetamol

Cannulation   The process of inserting a cannula into a vessel

Canthus   The angle formed by the junction of the eyelids: in each eye, there is an outer and inner canthus

Capsule   A soluble case in which certain drugs are administered

Cell metabolism   The sum of the biochemical changes undergone by a cell

Cerebral lesion   A structural change in the cerebrum, resulting from injury or disease

Chemotherapy   Pharmacological treatment designed to kill certain types of cell: often used in the treatment of cancer and autoimmune diseases

Cheyne–Stokes respiration   A striking form of breathing, in which there is a cyclical variation in rate, which becomes slower until breathing stops for several seconds before speeding up to a peak and then slowing again

Chlorhexidine   Effective antiseptic that will inhibit plaque formation on the teeth

Cholangio carcinoma   A malignant tumour of the bile ducts

Coagulability   Tendency for the blood to clot

Cognitive   Age-related changes that occur in mental activities, for example, it takes a certain intellect to realize that steam, water, and ice are one and the same thing

Colloquial   Informal language, used in ordinary or familiar conversation

Commensal   An organism that lives in association with another organism, without benefiting it or causing it harm

Commode   A chair (often on wheels) containing a bedpan

Compression bandaging   One treatment for a leg ulcer

Confrontation   A face-to-face meeting, usually associated with conflicting ideas or opinions

Conjunctiva   The membrane that covers the front of the eye and lines the inside of the eyelids

Consent   To accept or agree. Informed consent is a legal condition whereby a person gives consent based on a full appreciation and understanding of the facts and implications of any actions. The individual must be in possession of all of faculties (not mentally retarded or mentally ill), and his or her judgement should not be impaired at the time of consenting (by sleepiness, intoxication by alcohol or drugs, or other health problems)

Contract (pupils)   Pupils get smaller or reduce in size

Contraction   Pulling together, tightening, shortening

Contracture   Deformity caused by shortening of muscles, tendons, and ligaments

Contraindication   A factor in a patient's condition that makes it unwise to pursue a certain line of treatment

Controlled drugs   Drugs that are subject to strict regulatory control owing to their addictive nature

Core temperature   The temperature in the deep tissues and organs

Covert   Secret or hidden

Crown   That part of the tooth that is visible above the margin of the gums

Cumulative strain   This can affect bones, muscles, tendons, and nerves and develops when small injuries occur repeatedly from over or misappropriate use of a body part or an external force applied to the body

Cutaneous   On or in the skin

Cyanosis   A blue or purple tint to skin colour or mucous membranes caused by a lack of oxygen in the blood. It can be central (for example, involving mouth, nose, or face) or peripheral (for example, involving fingers)

Cytotoxic   Capable of destroying cells, for example, in chemotherapy

De-escalation   Taking steps to reduce the likelihood that violence will occur when there tensions and heightened emotions in a situation

Decerebrate   Without cerebral function

Decorticate   Patients with decorticate posturing present with the arms flexed, or bent inward on the chest, the hands are clenched into fists, and the legs extended. Decorticate posturing indicates that there may be damage to areas of the brain, including the cerebral hemispheres, the internal capsule, and the thalamus

Defecation   The process of passing faeces

Deficiency   Lack of something

Dehiscence   The separation of the edges of a wound

Dehydration   A clinical condition in which the body has failed to replace fluid loss adequately

Delusions   A false, unshakeable belief that cannot be changed by rational argument and that is not shared by peers

Dementia   A chronic, irreversible condition leading to deteriorating mental functioning, caused by organic brain disease

Dental caries   The damage to teeth caused by bacteria

Dependent   Requiring support or assistance

Depilatory cream   Cream used to remove hair

Dermatitis   An inflammation of the skin caused by an outside agent

Detrusor   The muscle of the bladder wall

Diabetic foot ulcer   A foot ulcer or sore associated with the vascular problems that arise as part of the disease process of diabetes: often difficult to heal

Dilate (pupils)   When the pupil size increases

Diluent   A liquid used to reconstitute a powder to make a solution or a liquid used to weaken the concentration of the original solution

Direct spread   Spread of infection via contaminated hands

Down's syndrome   A chromosomal abnormality that results in learning disability and is often characterized by physical changes to facial features and body shape

Drain   A tube or device to help the drainage of blood or fluid from, for example, a wound

Dynavox system   A speech device that enables people with learning difficulties to communicate

Dysphagia   Difficulty in swallowing

Dyspraxia   An inability to make skilled movements with accuracy (in an organized way)

Dysuria   Difficulty in passing urine

Elixir   A preparation containing alcohol or glycerine used as a vehicle for bitter or nauseous drugs

Embolus   An unwanted solid body in the circulation—often a clot

Emollient cleanser   A cleanser that softens, moisturizes, and soothes skin

Emoticons   Images, used in text and email messages and often formed by symbols on a keyboard, which are used to express a particular feeling or emotion

Emotional distress   Suffering psychologically

Emotions   A subjectively experienced feeling, such as happiness, anger, or sadness—often associated with events and thoughts

Empathic   Showing an understanding of what other people are experiencing by trying to imagine what an experience is like for them and from their point of view

Enema   Fluid passed into the rectum, to be retained or returned

Engaging   Attracting and promoting someone's interest or attention and participating in their life in a professional way

Enteral   Through the intestine

Enteral feeding   Feeding by tubes into the gastrointestinal tract

Enteric-coated   Tablets that are coated with a substance that enables them to pass through the stomach to the intestine unchanged: this is to prevent them from being destroyed by the acid in the stomach

Epithelialization   The migration of epithelial cells over a wound

Ergonomics   The study of the effective use of energy in relation to human movement

Erythema   Reddening of the skin, usually associated with dilation of the blood vessels in the dermis

Expectorate   To clear out the chest and lungs by coughing up and spitting out matter

Expiration   Breathing out

Extension   Straightening movements in a sagittal plane (increasing the angle at a joint)

Exudate   Discharge from a wound containing protein and blood cells

Fissure sealant   Treatment used in the young to prevent caries by sealing the surface of teeth

Flexion   Bending movements in a sagittal plane

Fluconazole   An antifungal drug

Fontanelle   A membranous space between the skull bones

Fornix   An arched structure

Frank haematuria   Blood visible in the urine

Friction   Force produced by rubbing one surface against another, producing heat and superficial damage

Fungal infection   Cancer patients may develop an infection in the mouth. The most common type is thrush, which is also referred to as cardidiasis

Gait   The way that someone walks or moves on foot

Generic palliative care   Approaching patients holistically, considering the patient and family or partners as one unit and improving quality of life by good symptom control

Gerontology   The study of ageing

Gestures   Actions or movements of part of the body that express ideas or meaning, or convey a person's feelings or intentions

Glaucoma   A serious condition in which the fluid pressure within the eye builds dangerously and threatens to damage the delicate retina and which can cause blindness if untreated: it may happen suddenly and be associated with acute pain in the eye or, more likely, it is a chronic condition that can lead to gradual loss of vision if undetected

Glycosuria   Presence of sugar in the urine

Haematoma   The build-up of clotted blood in a confined space, causing a mass

Haemodynamic monitoring   Monitoring blood circulation, for example, input and output of fluid and electrolytes, blood pressure, pulse

Hallucinations   Perceptual experiences that occur without an external stimulus and that are usually not experienced by others

Heart failure   A condition in which the heart is no longer capable of meeting the demands of the body: it may be acute or chronic and may affect one side of the heart more than another, as in left ventricular failure Where the lungs become involved, as they inevitably do, this is described as congestive cardiac failure

Hickman line   A line inserted into a large central vein, tunnelled under the skin to ensure that the point of entry into the vein is at a distance from the point of entry through the skin, minimizing the risk of skin flora entering the circulation

Holistic   The whole person, or individual, including the mind and body

Homeostasis   The process by which the internal systems of the body (for example, blood pressure, temperature) are maintained, despite changes in external conditions

Hyoscine   Hyoscine butylbromide—may dry up excessive respiratory secretions

Hypercarbia   High level of carbon dioxide in the blood

Hypercalcaemia   The presence in the blood of an abnormally high concentration of calcium

Hyperinflation   Excessive air put into the lungs

Hypertension   Raised blood pressure

Hyperthermia   Exceptionally high body temperature (about 41 °C or above)

Hypnotics   Drugs that induce sleep by depressing brain function

Hypostatic   Lack of movement

Hypothalamus   The region of the forebrain that contains, amongst other things, the centre that controls body temperature

Hypothermia   A fall in body temperature below the normal range, in the absence of protective reflex actions such as shivering

Hypoxia   Lack of oxygen in the tissues

Incubator   Transparent container for keeping premature babies in controlled conditions

Indirect spread   Spread of infection via contaminated equipment or environment

Infestation   Being overcome with parasites

Inhaler   A portable hand-held device that delivers medication in a form that the person breathes in directly to the lungs

Inspiration   Breathing in

Integrated care pathway   A predicted route of care for a patient, which involves the multidisciplinary team. The pathway lists steps in the patient's progress to a suitable outcome and is often specific to certain clinical problems

Internal rotation   Rolling inwards

Intra-arterial   Within an artery

Intra-articular   Within a joint

Intracranial pressure   Pressure within the skull

Intracutaneous   Within the skin tissues

Intradermal   Within the skin

Intramuscular   Within a muscle

Intrathecal   Within the meninges, in the subarachnoid space

Intravenous   Within a vein

Invasive   Invades, or enters, the body

Ketonuria   Presence of ketones in the urine

Leg ulcer   A sore often associated with circulatory problems in the legs: it may be categorized as either arterial, venous, or mixed, with different treatment regimes for each type

Libido   In its common usage, this means sexual drive

Ligament   Tissue that attaches bones to each other and protects joints

Linctus   A syrupy, sweet liquid medicine, often used to treat coughs

Linear   Extending along a straight line

Liverpool care pathway   An integrated care pathway for the dying patient

Makaton   A unique language programme using signs and symbols for communication

Malnutrition   Lack of essential food necessary for health: this can be because of too much food as well as too little food

Manipulative   In relation to play, this term refers to manual dexterity, that is, it relates to gross and fine motor development

Meatus   The external opening of the urethra

Meninges   The surrounding membrane of the brain and spinal cord

Meningitis   Inflammation of the meninges due to viral or bacterial infection

Metastases   The spread of cancer from its original site

Micturition   The process of passing urine

Morbidity   The incidence of a disease: the amount by which a disease occurs in the population

Morbidity rate   The number of cases of a disease found to occur in a stated population

Mortality   A measure of the number of deaths in a population

Motor   Related to movement

Motor neuron disease   Progressive degenerative disease of nervous system causing muscle wasting and weakness

Mucosa   Mucous membranes

Myocardial infarction   Heart attack caused by a blood clot in the coronary arteries

Naso-lachrymal duct   The duct between the eye and the nose that normally functions to drain excess tears

Nebulizer   A device used to apply a liquid in the form of a fine spray

Neuro-   Of the nerves and nervous system

Neurological disease   A disease of the nervous system

Neurology   The science and study of the nervous system

Nocturia   Getting up more than twice in the night to pass urine

Nonblanching hyperaemia   There is no skin colour change when light finger pressure is applied

Noninvasive   Does not invade (enter) the body

Nystatin   An antifungal drug used principally for *Candida albicans* infections

Objective   Expressing or dealing with facts or conditions as perceived without distortion by personal feelings, prejudices, or interpretations

Occlusive   Sealed

Occult haematuria   Blood in the urine that is not visible in the urine to the naked eye

Oedematous   The increased collection of interstitial fluid in the tissues causing swelling and loss of function: often in the ankles, but can be anywhere: lungs, head and neck, buttocks, depending on the cause

Oestrogen   Hormone

Oliguria   A very small production of urine (less than 30 ml/hr): an output less than 400 ml in 24 hours

Opportunistic   Microorganisms that inhabit and thrive in areas where they would not normally be found, causing disease

Opportunistically   Taking advantage of a situation

Oral   Through the mouth

Oral hygiene   Providing the patient with a clean moistered mouth

Ortho   Of bones

Orthopaedics   The study or specialty concerned with conditions of the skeletal system

Osmolarity   The concentration of a solution, expressed as the total number of solute particle per litre

Osteo   Of bones

Osteoporosis   Loss of bony tissue, resulting in brittle bones that are prone to fractures

Pain threshold   The point at which a stimulus is perceived as pain by an individual

Pain tolerance   The level to which an individual can tolerate painful stimuli

Palate   The roof of the mouth. This is bony towards the front of the mouth (the 'hard palate') and more cartilaginous towards the back of the mouth ('soft palate')

Pallor   A pale colour of the skin most evident on the hands and face

Palpation   A method of examination by feeling the part of the body to determine its size, shape, firmness, or location

Paralinguistics   Oral information expressed through means other than the words being used, for example, tone of voice, inflection, sighing

Paraphrasing   Accurately conveying the meaning of what has been said using your own words

Parenteral   Other than through the alimentary canal, for example, by injection

Paroxetine   A drug that is used for people with depression, obsessive compulsive disorder, or anxiety states. It selectively inhibits the re-uptake of serotonin in the central nervous system. One of a group of drugs known as SSRIs

Passive movement   Movement without voluntary effort

Pathogenic   Microorganisms that are capable of causing disease

Peak flow   A measure which records the rate at which a person can expel air from their lungs

Perceptions   Beliefs or opinions of something based on appearances gained through the senses

Percussion   An assessment technique that produces sounds by the examiner tapping on the patient's chest wall: this produces sounds based on the amount of air in the lungs

Peripheral   The areas away from the centre of the body, for example, the arms and legs

Peripheral vasoconstriction   Describes the closing of small vessels on the periphery of the circulatory system, such as those in the legs, feet, arms, hands, and skin

Pessary   A medicated suppository inserted into the vagina or a device used to prevent vaginal prolapse

pH   An indication of the acidity or alkalinity of a substance. Neutral is 7 on a logarithmic scale from 1–14: alkaline is greater than 7, acidity is less than 7

Pinna   The flap of skin and cartilage that projects from the head at the exterior opening of the ear

Plaque   The combination of sticky mucopolysaccharide and bacteria that collects on teeth and causes local accumulation of toxic products damaging to enamel

Polyuria   Excess urine production

Portacath   A type of cannula

Prepubescent   Before onset of puberty

Pressure ulcer A sore caused by damage to tissues through pressure, shearing, and friction forces

Prone Lying on the front (anterior surface) with the face turned to one side

Proprioception The sense of position of various parts of the body/balance, regulated by stimuli of movement receptors

Proteinuria Protein in the urine

Provoke To cause response—usually associated with anger but can also be associated with other feelings (violence, mirth)

Psoriasis A chronic inflammatory skin disease, in which erythematous areas become covered with white, raised plaques

Pulmonary embolism A foreign body—usually a blood clot—that lodges in the circulation of the lungs

Purpura Small red spots or large red plaques appearing on the skin

Pus The result of microorganisms and body defence mechanisms interacting: often creamy yellow or green in colour, a sure sign of an active infection

Pyrexia A higher than normal body temperature (fever)

Pyuria Pus in the urine

Radiotherapy Electromagnetic waves used therapeutically, often in the treatment of cancer

Reflex Involuntary action

Resident bacteria Organisms that are present on the deeper layers of the skin and that are more difficult to remove

Residual More than 150 ml urine left in the bladder after voiding

Resolution When a situation has come to an end: resolution often suggests that something has ended satisfactorily

Rigor An attack of uncontrollable shaking and a sensation of coldness, accompanied by a rapid rise in body temperature: often suggests the onset of fever

Rotation Rolling or revolving—may be internal or external in direction

Ruga A fold or crease

Saliva The substance produced by salivary glands, containing alpha amylase (ptyalin), an enzyme that begins the process of carbohydrate digestion: about 1.5 litres are produced per day

Salivary glands Exocrine glands that secrete saliva: parotid, sublingual, and submandibular

Sebaceous glands Exocrine glands that secrete sebum

Semi-recumbent Reclining but not flat

Sensory Referring to stimulation of the senses, for example, touch, vision or sight, talking or communicating, hearing, and smelling

Sharp Any piece of clinical equipment that has the potential to pierce the skin

Shearing forces Forces deeper in the tissues, caused by opposing forces: for example, the force of gravity pulling a patient down the bed opposes the adhesive forces of the patient's back and buttocks against pillows, keeping the patient upright. These forces meet in the deeper tissues of the back and buttocks, causing tissue damage

Skin flora Bacteria and other microorganisms that are normally present and live on the skin

Slough Tissue that becomes necrotic and separates from underlying healthy tissue

Sluice Room in a clinical environment where waste is disposed

Social stigma An adverse consequence of an individual's position or behaviour, perhaps associated with stereotyping but carries negative attitudes

Socialization The acquisition of social skills and moral values, that is, when and where it is acceptable, if at all, to display certain behaviours

Sociopathic Antisocial, offensive, or unacceptable

Spasticity An increase in muscular tension or tone

Stimulate Arouse, encourage, excite, induce, inflame, prompt, promote, or trigger a response

Stimulus Something that causes a particular response

Stridor A high-pitched sound resulting from turbulent gas flow in the upper airway: can be caused by an obstruction in the trachea or larynx

Stunting Reduced height for age: a basic indicator of malnutrition

Subcutaneous The fatty layer under the dermis of the skin

Subjective Pertaining to or perceived by the affected individual—personal to the individual

Sublingual Under the tongue

Supine Lying flat on back, facing upwards

Suppository A medicine in a solid form that is inserted in the rectum

Sustenance   That which supports life: food, victuals, provisions, means of living

Sympathetic   Showing understanding, sharing, or support of another person's feelings of sorrow or suffering

Systemic   Pertaining to the whole body

Tachycardia   An increase in heart rate above normal

Tachypnoea   An increase in respiratory rate above normal

Tendon   Tissue that attaches muscle to bone

Therapeutic   Having a helpful or beneficial effect on the mind or body

Thermoregulation   Regulation of body temperature

Thirty degree tilt   Lying on the back with the body tilted at 30° to relieve pressure on parts of the body, for example, the sacrum

Thrombosis   A blood clot

Thyroid   An endocrine gland located in front of the larynx, which secretes hormones important for regulating metabolic rate

Tonic phase   Phase of a seizure when there is continuous muscle contraction and the casualty becomes rigid

Top-heavy movement   A top-heavy movement that results in imbalance, often caused by bending from the waist with the legs straight

Topical   Applied to the surface, for local effect: for example, a drug applied to the skin

Tracheostomy   A surgical operation in which a hole is made into the trachea through the neck

Traction   The application of tension—sometimes used in orthopaedics to hold a bone or limb in position and at a degree of stretch

Tragus   The projection of cartilage in the pinna of the outer ear that extends back over the opening

Transient organisms   Organisms that are present on the surface layers of the skin and can usually be removed by routine hand hygiene

Trigone   Triangular region of the wall of the bladder that lies between the openings of the ureters and the urethra

Tympanic membrane   The ear drum

Unintubated   Without an artificial breathing tube in the windpipe

Universal precautions   The steps that should be taken by all healthcare staff to reduce the risk of transmission of both known and unknown infections

Urethral meatus   The external opening of the urethra

Urinary stasis   Stoppage of flow of urine: stagnation

Urticaria   An allergic skin eruption, where multiple raised, pink, itchy weals appear: these usually subside in a few days leaving no trace

Vasoconstrictor   Any substance that causes narrowing of the lumen of the blood vessels

Vasomotor   The capacity of blood vessels to dilate and constrict

Void   Empty

Waterlow scale   A tool used to measure the risk of developing pressure sores

Whipple's operation   Removal of the pancreas and part of the duodenum

Index

The index entries appear in letter-by-letter alphabetical order. Page references in italics indicate information in figures and tables.